S

Antibodies
Volume II

a practical approach

The Practical Approach Series

SERIES EDITORS

D. RICKWOOD

Department of Biology, University of Essex
Wivenhoe Park, Colchester, Essex CO4 3SQ, UK

B. D. HAMES

Department of Biochemistry and Molecular Biology, University of Leeds
Leeds LS2 9JT, UK

Affinity Chromatography
Animal Cell Culture
Animal Virus Pathogenesis
Antibodies I and II
Biochemical Toxicology
Biological Membranes
Biosensors
Carbohydrate Analysis
Cell Growth and Division
Centrifugation (2nd Edition)
Clinical Immunology
Computers in Microbiology
DNA Cloning I, II, and III
Drosophila
Electron Microscopy in
    Molecular Biology
Fermentation
Flow Cytometry
Gel Electrophoresis of Nucleic
    Acids (2nd Edition)
Gel Electrophoresis of Proteins
    (2nd Edition)
Genome Analysis
HPLC of Small Molecules
HPLC of Macromolecules
Human Cytogenetics
Human Genetic Diseases
Immobilised Cells and
    Enzymes
Iodinated Density Gradient
    Media
Light Microscopy in Biology
Liposomes
Lymphocytes
Lymphokines and Interferons
Mammalian Development
Medical Bacteriology
Medical Mycology
Microcomputers in Biology
Microcomputers in Physiology
Mitochondria
Mutagenicity Testing
Neurochemistry
Nucleic Acid and Protein
    Sequence Analysis
Nucleic Acids Hybridisation
Nucleic Acids Sequencing
Oligonucleotide Synthesis
Peptide Hormone Action

Antibodies
Volume II

a practical approach

Edited by
D Catty

Department of Immunology, University of Birmingham Medical School, Vincent Drive, Birmingham B15 2TJ, UK

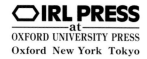
OXFORD UNIVERSITY PRESS
Oxford New York Tokyo

IRL Press
Eynsham
Oxford
England

First published 1989
Reprinted 1990

British Library Cataloguing in Publication Data

Antibodies.
  Vol. II/A practical approach
  1. Organisms. Antibodies
  I. Catty, D.   II. Series
  574.2'93

Library of Congress Cataloging-in-Publication Data

Antibodies: a practical approach
(Practical approach series)
Includes bibliographies and index.
1. Immunoglobulins—Laboratory manuals.
2. Serology—Laboratory manuals.
3. Immunoassay—Laboratory manuals.
I. Catty, David. II. Series. [DNLM: 1. Antibodies. QW 575 A6286]
QR186.7.A533 1988 616.07'93 88-26724
ISBN 0 947946 86 1 (v. 1 : hardbound)
ISBN 0 947946 85 3 (v. 1 : softbound)

ISBN 0 19 963018 6 (v. 2 : hardbound)
ISBN 0 19 963019 4 (v. 2 : softbound)

Previously announced as:

ISBN 0 947946 88 8 (v. 2 : hardbound)
ISBN 0 947946 87 X (v. 2 : softbound)

Printed by Information Press Ltd, Oxford, England.

Preface

This is the second volume of a book on antibodies which, like the first, is designed to serve primarily as a bench manual. In Volume I we described the principles and practice of antibody production (both polyclonal and monoclonal), immunoaffinity methods, and tests using unlabelled antibodies, including gel methods, agglutination and haemolytic assays. This second volume offers a further set of major antibody applications. These are of two categories. The first covers the use of antibodies in two highly significant clinical areas, red cell typing and HLA (tissue) typing. Methodology and specificities are under continuous review in these areas, and accounts of contemporary practice and nomenclature will clearly be of interest both to those wishing to update their own procedures and to those entering the field who need a practical guide. The second group of applications uses labels—radioisotopes, fluorochromes and enzymes—as a means to detect and/or measure antigens in solution, on tissues and cells, and to identify, quantify and quality-control antibodies. These are powerful techniques—some, such as the use of radiolabelled antibodies in tumour imaging (Chapter 8), are still very much in the development stage.

Fluorescence activated cell sorting is already a well developed method but one with growing applications as newer labels and increasingly sophisticated machines come into use: a good description of the principles, major operating parameters and versatility of the approach to cell separations and population studies (Chapter 7) should be considered in any book on antibody applications. Methods which are even better established but which are still nevertheless improving in sensitivity and specificity in the hands of experts are tissue immunofluorescence and immunoperoxidase staining; two recognized experts in these applications contribute Chapters 5 and 6 to this book. Finally, I have contributed Chapter 4 dealing with the principles, bench protocols and range of ELISA and related immunoassays, and (with my colleague, G.Murphy) an account (Chapter 3) of assays using radiolabels. These latter two labelled reagent approaches are the 'workhorse' systems of quantitative immunoassays.

We hope that these chapters provide useful guides to their performance and many applications.

D.Catty

Acknowledgements

In editing Volumes I and II of *Antibodies: A Practical Approach* I am particularly grateful for the help and patience of fellow authors without whose expertise these books would not have been possible. I owe a special debt of gratitude to the staff and students of my own laboratory who helped in many ways but especially with advice on protocols and illustrations. My special thanks go to Dr E.O.Bassey for his several contributions to the PAGE analysis of mycobacterial antigens and monoclonal antibodies, to Mrs C.Raykundalia for checking many chapters in which her expertise and practical knowledge were essential ingredients, to Mrs F.O'Reilly for preparing many of the manuscripts and to the World Health Organisation for allowing us freely to use data from bench protocols prepared for them.

Finally, I need to thank the staff of IRL Press and the Practical Approach Series editors for their patience and hard work in seeing these two volumes through to publication to such a high standard of presentation.

Contributors

B.A.Bradley
United Kingdom Transplant Service, Southmead Road, Bristol BS10 5ND, UK

A.R.Bradwell
Department of Immunology, University of Birmingham Medical School, Vincent Drive, Birmingham B15 2TJ, UK

D.Catty
Department of Immunology, University of Birmingham Medical School, Vincent Drive, Birmingham B15 2TJ, UK

P.W.Dykes
Department of Immunology, University of Birmingham Medical School, Vincent Drive, Birmingham B15 2TJ, UK

J.Gregory
Department of Pathology, University of Birmingham Medical School, Vincent Drive, Birmingham B15 2TJ, UK

D.G.Johnson
Department of Immunology, University of Birmingham Medical School, Vincent Drive, Birmingham B15 2TJ, UK

E.L.Jones
Department of Pathology, University of Birmingham Medical School, Vincent Drive, Birmingham B15 2TJ, UK

A.Milner
Department of Immunology, University of Birmingham Medical School, Vincent Drive, Birmingham B15 2TJ, UK

G.Murphy
Gastroenterology Unit, United Medical and Dental Schools of Guy's and St. Thomas's Hospitals, Guy's Tower, London SE1 9RT, UK

G.D.Poole
National Blood Transfusion Service, South Western Regional Transfusion Centre, Southmead Road, Bristol BS10 5ND, UK

T.C.Ray
United Kingdom Transplant Service, Southmead Road, Bristol BS10 5ND, UK

C.Raykundalia
Department of Immunology, University of Birmingham Medical School, Vincent Drive, Birmingham B15 2TJ, UK

G.D.Thomas
Department of Immunology, University of Birmingham Medical School, Vincent Drive, Birmingham B15 2TJ, UK

A.Vaughan
Department of Immunology, University of Birmingham Medical School, Vincent Drive, Birmingham B15 2TJ, UK

Contents

5. IMMUNOPEROXIDASE METHODS   155
E.L.Jones and J.Gregory

Abbreviations

ABCO	1,4-diazobicyclooctane
ABTS	2,3′-azino-di(3-ethyl)benzthiazoline sulphonic acid
ADCC	antibody-dependent cytotoxicity test
AEC	3-amino-4-ethyl carbazole
AFP	α-fetoprotein
AIHA	auto-immune haemolytic anaemia
AP	alkaline phosphate
APAAP	alkaline phosphate−anti-alkaline phosphatase
AS	ankylosing spondylitis
ASA	5-amino salicyclic acid
BCIP	5-bromo-4-chloro-3-idolylphosphate
β-Γ	β-galactosidase
bg	background
BP	Bromocresol purple
BSA	bovine serum albumin
CDC	complement-dependent cytotoxicity test
CEA	carcinoembryonic antigen
CFDA	carboxy-FDA
CFT	complement fixation test
CHO	Chinese hamster ovarian
CLL	chronic leukaemia
CNP	4-chloro-1-naphthol
CSF	cerebrospinal fluid
CREGS	cross-reactive groups
CV	coefficient of variation
DAB	diaminobenzidine
DASS	defined antigen substrate sphere
DGT	direct antiglobulin test
dithizone	diphenylthiocarbazine
DMF	dimethyl formamide
DMSO	dimethyl sulphoxide
DPH	1,6-diphenyl,-1,3,5-hexatriene
DTPA	diethylene-triamine-pentaacetic acid
DTT	dithiothreitol
EBV	Epstein−Barr virus
ELISA	enzyme-linked immunosorbent assay
EMIT	enzyme-modulated immunotest
FACS	fluorescence activated cell sorter
FBS	fetal bovine serum
FCS	fetal calf serum
FDA	fluorescein diacetate
FITC	fluorescein isothiocyanate
HIV	human immunodeficiency virus
HLA	human leukocyte series A
HRP	horseradish peroxidase
HSA	human serum albumin
HSP	highly sensitized patient

IAGT	indirect antiglobulin test
IF	immunofluorescence
Ig	immunoglobulin
IRMA	immunoradiometric assay
IS	iodine and starch
LISS	low ionic strength saline
Mab	monoclonal antibody
NAPFB	naphthol As-mx phosphate + Fast Blue BB salt
NAPR	naphthol As-mx phosphate + Red BB salt
NISS	normal ionic strength saline
NSS	non-specific staining
ONPG	O-nitrophenyl-β-D-galactoside
OPD	O-phenylenediamine dihydrochloride
PAP	peroxidase – anti-peroxidase
PBS	phosphate-buffered saline
PE	phyloerythrin
PFCDC	platelet fluorescence CDC
PG	penicillin G
PHA	phytohaemagglutinin
PLL	poly-L-lysine
PNPP	N-p-nitrophenylalkaline phosphate
PRA	panel reactive antibody
RAID	radioimmunodetection
Rh	rhesus
RIA	radioimmunoassay
SACT	serum antibody competitive test
SHPP	succinimidyl-3-(p-hydroxyphenyl)propionate
SPDP	N-succinimidyl-3-(2-pyridyldithio)propionate
SRBC	sheep red blood cells
TAA	tumour-associated antigens
T_c	cytotoxic T cells
TMB	tetramethyl benzidine
TRITC	tetramethyl rhodamine isothiocyanate

CHAPTER 1

Antibodies in blood group serology

GEOFFREY D.POOLE

1. INTRODUCTION TO BLOOD GROUP SEROLOGY

Karl Landsteiner described, in 1900, the clumping of one person's red cells by the serum of another person. One year later he suggested that these results could be explained by the existence of three phenotypes A, B and O and, in 1902, a fourth phenotype AB was added. More than 80 years later, further complexity at the ABO locus has been well documented, the mechanism of action of the A and B genes has been unravelled and the biochemical make-up of the A and B antigens determined. Nineteen blood group systems are now established (see Section 12). Some of these are highly polymorphic: the Rh (Rhesus) system comprises more than 40 antigens. Many blood group antigens, usually of very high or very low incidence in the general population, are not (yet) part of a blood group system, as antithetical antigens have not been described. In excess of 600 blood group antigens have been recognized.

Despite the complexity of blood groups, blood grouping is essentially very simple. Unless intact red cells are not available, such as when grouping stains in forensic work, haemagglutination is the standard technique used in blood grouping. The only modestly expensive item of equipment is a small centrifuge and perhaps a very simple microscope. Because of the clinical importance of blood groups in blood transfusion, reagents are available at a reasonable cost from several diagnostic companies. Commercially available antibodies are usually potent and carefully standardized and there is likely to be little difficulty in establishing the correct ABO and Rh group of red cells. A higher level of technical competence is needed in antibody identification work, and this can only be obtained by careful technique and experience.

The purpose of the following sections of this chapter is to introduce the reader to techniques used in blood group serology. There is little discussion on the relative merits of different techniques for various applications, and those involved in the specialized fields of blood transfusion, or forensic science, are advised to seek additional texts.

2. PRINCIPLES INVOLVED

A full discussion of the theoretical basis of antibody — antigen reactions with particular reference to blood group antibodies will be found elsewhere (1). However, a very brief summary of the main points involved may assist the reader in using the techniques described in this chapter.

Maximal binding of red cell antibodies usually occurs under conditions of neutral pH, of normal or low ionic strength (the reaction mixture must of course be isotonic

1

with red cells) and with antibody in high concentration. Using red cells with a high antigen site density will usually enhance agglutination, and this should be borne in mind in antibody screening or antibody identification, when selection of cells with a homozygous expression may be beneficial. The concentration of red cells should, however, be kept within certain limits according to the test system: for example concentrations of $2-5\%$ are usually used in tube techniques. Temperature is also important, as the equilibrium (binding) constant is for some blood group antibodies higher, and for some lower, at a higher temperature: hence the terms *warm (37°C) active* and *cold active* antibodies. Haemagglutination can only occur when close proximity of red cells can be effected. Some antibodies, usually IgM, can effect haemagglutination in a simple test using red cells suspended in isotonic saline and these are said to be saline-agglutinating or *complete*. Many IgG antibodies are not capable of directly effecting haemagglutination (i.e. are *incomplete*) since the forces involved in antibody binding are insufficient to overcome the net repulsive force between red cells at the small intercellular distance involved. Binding of IgG antibodies may be demonstrated by haemagglutination if an anti-IgG serum is used, as in the antiglobulin techniques, since this allows lattice formation at greater intercellular distances. Alternatively, haemagglutination with certain antibodies may be potentiated by modification of the red cell membrane using proteolytic enzymes, by addition of high molecular weight substances such as albumin, or by addition of a cationic polymer such as polybrene. Haemagglutination will also be affected by sedimentation conditions: the sensitivity of a tube test will be greater than a tile test and may sometimes be further enhanced by centrifugation.

3. APPLICATIONS OF BLOOD GROUP SEROLOGY

3.1 **Transfusion science**

(i)   Blood grouping of donors and patients.
(ii)   Provision of blood for patients: donor red cells are tested (cross-matched) against the patient's serum.
(iii) Identification of red cell antibodies in serum.
(iv)   Establishing whether red cells have been coated *in vivo* with antibody, as in auto-immune haemolytic anaemia (AIHA) and haemolytic disease of the newborn.

3.2 **Forensic science**

(i)   Exclusion of paternity.
(ii)   Criminal investigations: blood grouping of stains of blood and other body fluids can exclude a suspect.

3.3 **Anthropology**

Description and classification of populations.

3.4 **Cell biology**

Investigating the nature of membrane components.

3.5 **Hybridoma technology**

Screening culture supernatants for monoclonal antibodies (Mabs) of blood group specificity.

4. GENERAL PRACTICAL CONSIDERATIONS

Although the number of basic techniques available to the blood group serologist is not large, there are many variations and the worker may wish to adapt the technique according to his/her own requirements. The purpose of this section is to discuss the selection of equipment and materials with particular reference to differing circumstances.

4.1 **Blood samples**

Venous blood is used, taken into sterile containers. A blood sample which has been allowed to clot naturally is ideal for antibody investigations as the use of plasma sometimes leads to clot formation or rouleaux of red cells in the test. Red cells available from a clotted sample are usually suitable for blood grouping work provided the volume is sufficient. An EDTA anticoagulated sample can be taken if larger volumes are required or if the direct antiglobulin test is to be performed. For quantitative work on red cell antigens it is recommended that citrate−phosphate dextrose anticoagulant is used (collect 20 ml of venous blood into 2 ml of a sterile solution containing 89 mM trisodium citrate, 16 mM citric acid, 16 mM sodium dihydrogen phosphate and 128 mM dextrose).

4.2 **Pipettes**

Short form Pasteur pipettes which deliver drops of approximately 35 μl when fitted with a rubber teat are often used by the serologist. Their use has much to recommend them in terms of speed and flexibility but some practice is required. They must be clean and have a smooth delivery end. In use, the Pasteur pipette should be held vertically and sufficiently far away from the tube or microplate well for total release of the drop, otherwise a reduced volume will be delivered. After use it should be rinsed at least five times in physiological (isotonic) saline, but if a potent antibody-containing serum has been used the pipette should be discarded. Infectious material should be handled with plastic pipettes or pipette tips. In the following sections drop volumes, as delivered by a Pasteur pipette or a reagent dropper bottle, are used for brevity.

4.3 **Physiological (isotonic) saline**

A simple 0.15 M NaCl solution is often used for washing and suspending red cells but phosphate-buffered saline (PBS) is to be preferred: dissolve four PBS (Dulbecco 'A') tablets (Oxoid Ltd), 86 g of NaCl and 10 g of sodium azide in 10 litres of water. Check that the pH is between pH 7.2 and 7.4.

4.4 **Centrifuges**

A wide variety of bench centrifuges is available. An important factor when choosing is size as larger machines, although more versatile, have a longer acceleration and deceleration time and this may be a considerable nuisance when washing red cells. If antiglobulin testing is to be performed frequently the purchase of a cell washer should also be considered: this is discussed in Section 5.5.2. Infectious material should be centrifuged in sealed buckets.

4.5 **Tubes, microplates, tiles and capillaries**

Glass tubes are recommended for most applications. They are versatile, reasonably cheap and particularly suitable for the screening and identification of red cell antibodies. Tubes (12 × 75 mm or 10 × 75 mm) are usually used for macroscopically read techniques and for washing red cells (note that some cell washers accept only 12 × 75 mm tubes) while 7 × 50 mm ('precipitin') tubes are often used for microscopically read techniques. Plastic tubes may also be used instead of glass for reasons of economy or safety but the reader is advised to establish that the non-wettability and static of the plastic does not interfere with performing and interpreting the tests.

Microplates (96-well) are ideal for large-scale testing, particularly if potent antibodies are being used, as in red cell phenotyping. They are invaluable to workers engaged in the production of Mabs. V-well plates are used by a streaming technique which has good sensitivity. U-well plates are useful for washing red cells and serological tests may be performed by a streaming or resuspension technique. Polyclonal sera, unless diluted, may produce reaction patterns in microplates which are difficult to interpret. PVC plates should not be used for liquid-phase serology. Microplate techniques are more fully discussed elsewhere (2,3), in particular, ref. 2 contains several relevant contributions.

Some tests can be performed directly on a white tile or microscope slide. This has the advantage that no specialist equipment is needed and so tests may be performed in the field. However, sensitivity is inferior to that using tubes and microplates.

High sensitivity and good reagent economy are features of tests performed in glass capillary tubes. However, they are rather cumbersome in use and have not gained widespread popularity. Weiland (4) reviews the subject.

5. SEROLOGICAL TECHNIQUES

5.1 **Washing red cells**

Wash red cells from clotted and anticoagulated samples to remove plasma proteins as follows.
(i)   Remove approximately 200 μl of packed red cells from the sample into a 12 × 75 mm tube.
(ii)   Fill with approximately 4 ml of PBS and ensure that all red cells are resuspended.
(iii) Centrifuge at 500−1000 g for 1−2 min to pellet the cells.
(iv)   Aspirate the supernatant to waste and repeat the resuspension, centrifugation and aspiration twice more.
(v)   Resuspend the red cells to approximately 3% (v/v) in PBS or as directed in the technique protocol.

5.2 **Time and temperature**

Saline tests may be left to incubate and sediment naturally for 60−90 min or centrifuged following a shorter incubation time. Most commercial blood grouping antisera are standardized for use by a 'spin' technique and instructions for their use should be followed. Antiglobulin and potentiated techniques can often be performed following a short incubation time. In the technique protocols which follow, a sedimentation test and, where appropriate, an alternative spin test are described.

Tube tests can be conveniently performed at any temperature by incubating in a water bath, heating block or in a dry (preferably fan-assisted) incubator. Manufacturer's instructions should be followed regarding the optimal incubation temperature for blood grouping reagents. In blood transfusion work the temperature dependence of auto- and allo-antibodies in the patient will provide useful information regarding clinical significance of the antibody.

5.3 Reading and scoring tests

5.3.1 *Tube tests—macroscopic reading*

After incubation, hold the tube over a light box or white background and examine for haemolysis. Then use a combination of tipping, rolling and gentle shaking of the tube until the button of cells is completely resuspended. Examine the contents under a simple magnifying lens (or a low power microscope with a specially adapted stage) during this process for maximum sensitivity. Spin tests will need rather more agitation.

5.3.2 *Tube tests—macroscopic or microscopic reading*

Tests performed in tubes may also be read by transferring the reaction ingredients onto a slide. This is useful whenever careful examination of weak reactions is required, but is not generally necessary for blood grouping work using potent reagents.

After incubation, examine for haemolysis and then carefully draw up approximately 30 μl of the cell button into a Pasteur pipette and gently deposit as a streak or circle on a microscope slide. Examine macroscopically and, if desired, under a low power microscope ($\times 100$). Rock the slide gently if necessary to disperse any cohesion of unagglutinated cells.

5.3.3 *Tile tests*

Reading is described in the technique protocol (*Table 3*).

Table 1. Scoring results.

Numerical grade	Alternative	Appearance
6	C or $++++$	Complete agglutination. No free cells.
5	V or $+++$	Easily detectable visual agglutination (large clumps). Only very few free cells present.
4	$++$	Agglutination detectable with the naked eye. Some free cells detectable microscopically.
3	$+$	Agglutination just detectable with the naked eye.
2	$(+)$ or $\pm$	Agglutination only visible microscopically. Clumps consist of five to ten cells. Numerous free cells.
1	W	Microscopic agglutination, with clumps of two to five cells. Many free cells.
0	Neg or $-$	Negative reaction. All cells evenly distributed.

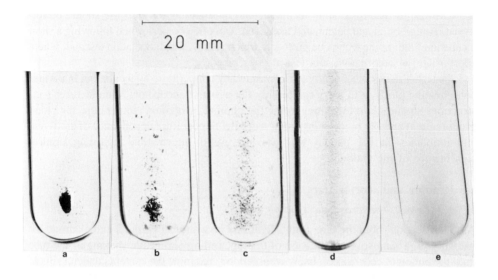

Figure 1. Macroscopic interpretation of haemagglutination tests in 75 × 12 mm tubes. The grades assigned were (**a**) 6 (**b**) 5 (**c**) 4 (**d**) 3 (**e**) 0.

5.3.4 *Scoring results*

A numerical scheme for scoring reaction strengths is given in *Table 1*, together with commonly used alternatives. Examples are shown in *Figures 1* and *2*.

If mixed red cell populations are present, as when grouping a post-transfusion blood sample or a sample from a chimaeric twin, a 'mixed field' reaction may be seen if the populations differ in their antigen content. Mixed field reactions can only be satisfactorily determined under the microscope. Note that some free cells are present in all weak reactions. An example of a mixed field reaction is shown in *Figure 3*.

5.4 **Saline techniques**

These will detect saline-agglutinating (complete) antibodies. Protocols for tube and tile techniques are given in *Tables 2* and *3*.

5.5 **Antiglobulin (Coombs) techniques**

5.5.1 *Direct and indirect tests*

Antiglobulin or Coombs techniques fall into two main categories: the direct antiglobulin test (DAGT) and the indirect antiglobulin test (IAGT). The DAGT is used to determine *in vivo* coating of red cells with globulins and therefore does not involve an incubation phase *in vitro*. Antibody identification and red cell phenotyping are sometimes performed by the IAGT, where antibody is incubated *in vitro* with red cells. In both direct and indirect tests, addition of an antiglobulin serum allows haemagglutination of globulin (antibody or complement components)-coated red cells which have been washed to remove free globulin.

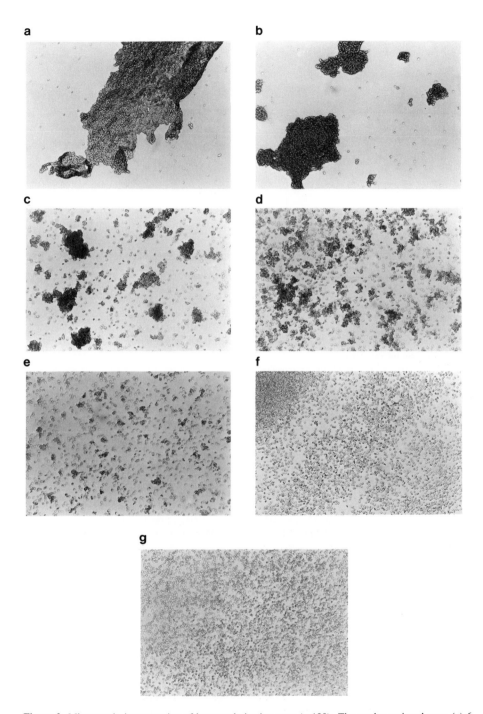

Figure 2. Microscopic interpretation of haemagglutination tests (×100). The grades assigned were (**a**) 6 (**b**) 5 (**c**) 4 (**d**) 3 (**e**) 2 (**f**) 1 (**g**) 0.

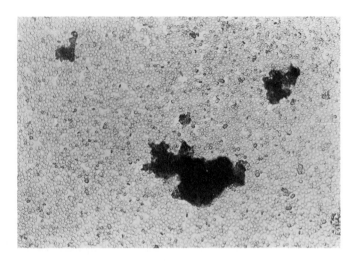

Figure 3. Mixed field agglutination (×100).

Table 2. The saline technique.

1.	Add two drops[a,b] of serum to a 75 × 12 mm or 75 × 10 mm tube.
2.	Add two drops[a,b] of a 2−3% suspension of washed red cells in PBS. Mix well.
3.	Incubate for 60−90 min.
4.	Read macroscopically or microscopically[c].

[a]Use a one drop vol. if 50 × 6 mm tubes are being used.
[b]A higher serum:cell volume ratio may be desirable for antibody identification work.
[c]See text for discussion of reading techniques.

Table 3. The saline technique for tiles.

1.	Add one drop of serum onto a white tile or microscope slide and spread this into a circle ∼20 mm in diameter using the bottom of a clean test tube.
2.	Add one drop of a 20−30% suspension of washed red cells in PBS.
3.	Rock the tile or slide gently such that the cells tend to move around the perimeter of the circle.
4.	Incubate for not more than 10 min, with occasional rocking of the tile or slide.
5.	Read tests on translucent tiles over a light box. Read slide tests macroscopically or microscopically.

5.5.2 *Washing red cells*

The protocol given in Section 5.1 is not suitable as contaminating globulins may not be completely removed. Three or four changes of PBS are only adequate if a very small volume (<3 μl) of packed red cells is used: this will be the case if the protocols in *Tables 4−6* are followed. Furthermore, great care must be taken when aspirating the supernatant not to cause re-introduction of globulin components. It is recommended that the supernatant is decanted by flicking the tube; with practice the button of cells will remain intact. Cell washers are available from several manufacturers and these should be considered if large numbers of tests are being performed. They may have 12-place or 24-place heads and some have a facility for automatic addition of antiglobulin serum (e.g. DiaCent 2000, G.S.Ross Ltd, and CW-2, Ortho Diagnostic Systems Ltd). Cell washers should not be used for washing larger volumes (>5 μl) of packed red cells.

Table 4. The direct antiglobulin test (DAGT).

1.	Prepare a 3−5% suspension in PBS of red cells from a freshly obtained blood sample[a]. Add one drop of this suspension to a 75 × 12 mm tube.
2.	Wash[b] the cells three or four times in PBS and decant the final supernatant.
3.	Add two drops[c] of antiglobulin serum. Mix well.
4.	Centrifuge at 500−1000 g for 20 sec or at 150−200 g for 60 sec.
5.	Read macroscopically or microscopically[c]. Confirm negative reactions (if using anti-IgG or polyspecific antiglobulin serum) as follows.
	(i) Add one drop of a 4−6% suspension of IgG-coated control cells. Mix well.
	(ii) Repeat step 4 and read macroscopically. The result must be moderately strong positive for validation of the test.

[a]Preferably an EDTA or citrated sample.
[b]See Section 5.5.2.
[c]Refer to antiglobulin reagent instructions.

Table 5. The normal ionic strength indirect antiglobulin test (NISS−IAGT).

1.	Add two drops[a] of serum to a 75 × 12 mm tube.
2.	Add one drop of a 3−5% suspension of washed red cells in PBS. Mix well.
3.	Incubate for 60−90 min.
4.	Proceed as in steps 2−5(ii) in *Table 4*.

[a]A higher serum:cell volume ratio will give greater sensitivity.

Table 6. The low ionic strength indirect antiglobulin test (LISS−IAGT).

1.	Add one drop of serum to a 75 × 12 mm tube.
2.	Add one drop of a 3−5% suspension of washed red cells in LISS. Mix well.
3.	Incubate for 20−60 min.
4.	Proceed as in steps 2−5(ii) in *Table 4*.

5.5.3 *Normal and low ionic strength saline tests*

In the standard IAGT, good uptake of antibody is obtained by using a 60−90 min incubation period and a serum:cell ratio of 2:1 or greater, with red cells suspended in PBS. However, a greater and quicker uptake of antibody can often be obtained using red cells suspended in an isotonic medium of low ionic strength. An incubation time of 20 min is usually quite sufficient for the low ionic strength saline (LISS) IAGT.

When using LISS, two important points should be noted. First, although LISS is sometimes used instead of PBS for all cell suspensions, red cells should be washed in PBS before resuspension in LISS, as non-specific uptake of globulin components may occur. Second, inadequate or non-specific uptake may occur if the serum:cell ratio in the LISS−IAGT is varied from 1:1.

LISS can be bought commercially or made up as follows.

(i)   Prepare a phosphate buffer by mixing 250 ml of 150 mM Na_2HPO_4 and 150 ml of 150 mM $NaH_2PO_4 \cdot 2H_2O$. Adjust to pH 6.7 by adding more NaH_2PO_4 solution.

(ii)   Prepare 500 ml of 480 mM glycine, adjust the pH to 6.7 with 1 M NaOH and add 20 ml of phosphate buffer, pH 6.7 and 100 ml of 306 mM NaCl; make up to 1 litre with water.

(iii)   Sterilize by passing through a 0.2 μ filter.

(iv)   The conductivity of the solution should be about 3.7 mS/cm at 25°C.

(v)   Keep sterile at 4°C.

5.5.4 *Choice of antiglobulin serum*

Anti-human IgA, IgM and IgG reagents are readily available commercially, standardized for use by the antiglobulin test. Reagents specific for IgG subclasses and for immunoglobulins (Igs) from other species are also available but these must first be standardized for antiglobulin testing. In blood transfusion work, polyspecific antigloblin serum is commonly used for the IAGT. This usually consists of rabbit anti-human IgG and rabbit (or mouse monoclonal) anti-complement. This is because some low affinity antibodies are strongly complement binding and are best detected by the use of anti-complement. Anti-IgM is not included as IgM antibodies can usually be detected by a direct agglutination (saline) technique. Human polyclonal red cell antibodies are rarely IgA only and so anti-IgA is also not included. The reader is referred elsewhere (1) for a discussion on the relative merits of various anti-complement components. In brief, polyspecific antiglobulin serum is recommended for antibody screening and identification and compatibility testing, and anti-IgG for red cell phenotyping using IgG antisera. The DAGT may be performed with polyspecific or monospecific antiglobulin sera, as desired.

5.5.5 *Controls*

It is useful to confirm that a negative reaction in the IAGT or DAGT has not occurred because of inadequate washing of red cells prior to addition of antiglobulin serum. This is particularly important using anti-IgG. Adequate washing can be confirmed by addition of red cells known to be coated with IgG. See *Table 7* for a simple method of preparation of IgG-coated cells.

5.5.6 *Methods*

Tables 4, 5 and *6* give protocols for the DAGT, the normal ionic strength (NISS)−IAGT and LISS−IAGT. Other strategies are outlined in ref. 1. One such alternative is the enzyme−IAGT. This is performed as in *Table 5* but using enzyme-modified red cells (see *Table 10*).

Table 7. Preparation of IgG-coated control cells for the antiglobulin test.

1.	Add 1 vol.[a] of suitably diluted[b] IgG anti-Rh(D)[c] to 1 vol. of washed, packed Rh(D) positive red cells. Mix well.
2.	Incubate at 37°C for 30 min.
3.	Wash the IgG-coated cells in several changes (at least five) of PBS.
4.	Prepare a 4−6% suspension of the cells in PBS. Test one drop of this suspension with antiglobulin serum as in steps 3−5 of *Table 4*. A suitable control will give a moderately strong positive result.

[a]Volume depends on the number of tests for which the control is required.
[b]Dilution must be determined by titration.
[c]'Coating' anti-Rh(D) may be available commercially. Alternatively, antiserum standardized for the detection of D^u is suitable.

5.6 **Potentiated techniques**

5.6.1 *Albumin techniques*

Albumin displacement techniques are used to detect some non-saline-agglutinating antibodies and to enhance the reactions of some agglutinating antibodies. Albumin solutions (20%) can be bought commercially for serological use or they may be made up much more cheaply from 30% bovine serum albumin (BSA); in the latter case a high polymer content albumin may give better results but the worker will have to determine that clear specific reactions are given.

Albumin tests are best read microscopically because of the cohesive quality of the medium. Cohesion of red cells that are not agglutinated can be recognized with practice and can be dispersed by gentle rocking of the slide. A method is given in *Table 8*.

5.6.2 *Enzyme techniques*

Enzyme techniques are highly sensitive for the detection of certain IgG antibodies, for example those directed against the human Rh blood group antigens. Various proteolytic enzymes may be used: papain, bromelain, ficin and trypsin are the most commonly used. Fully standardized enzyme solutions may be bought commercially. Alternatively, crude extracts may be made in the laboratory and found to be completely satisfactory, although efficacy may vary from batch to batch (a serological titration of known antibody with known enzyme-treated red cells will give some indication of how new and old batches of enzyme solution are performing). A suggested method for the preparation and use of a crude bromelain solution is given in *Table 9*. The use of enzymes other than bromelain is described elsewhere (1,6).

Enzyme tests are best performed by enzyme treatment and subsequent washing of

Table 8. The albumin displacement test.

1.	Add one drop of serum to a 50 × 6 mm tube.
2.	Add one drop of a 2−3% suspension of washed red cells in PBS. Mix well.
3.	Incubate for 60−90 min.
4.	Allow one drop of 20% BSA[a] to slide down the side of the tube such that it overlays the cell button. Do not mix.
5.	Incubate for 10−20 min.
6.	Read microscopically.

[a]Prepare by mixing 2 vols of 30% BSA with 1 vol. of PBS.

Table 9. Preparation of a bromelain solution.

1.	Add 30 g of dipotassium EDTA dihydrate, 15 g of bromelain powder (Hughes and Hughes Ltd) and 3 g of L-cysteine−HCl monohydrate to 100 ml of 150 mM saline.
2.	Mix continuously for 8 h and leave at 4°C overnight.
3.	Adjust to pH 6.8 with 5 M NaOH.
4.	Make up to 150 ml with 150 mM saline.
5.	Centrifuge to sediment undissolved material and reserve the supernatant.
6.	Dilute the supernatant 1:12[a] in 150 mM saline and store frozen.

[a]Or use an azo-albumin method to assay the bromelain (see ref. 5).

Table 10. Bromelain treatment of red cells.

1.	Add two drops of bromelain solution to one drop of washed, packed red cells. Mix well.
2.	Incubate at room temperature for 5 min.
3.	Wash the red cells twice in PBS and resuspend to 2−3%.

Table 11. The enzyme (bromelain) two-stage technique.

1.	Add two drops[a] of serum to a 75 × 12 mm or 75 × 10 mm tube.
2.	Add two drops[a] of a 2−3% suspension of washed, enzyme (bromelain)-treated red cells in PBS. Mix well.
3.	Incubate for 45−60 min.
4.	Read macroscopically.

[a]Use a one drop vol. for 50 × 6 mm tubes.

the red cells before incubation with serum. This is known as the *two-stage* test. This is much preferred to the *one-stage* test where serum, enzyme solution and red cells are incubated together.

Interpretation of enzyme tests is often more difficult than with other techniques. First, enzyme-treated red cells have a reduced surface charge and so, after sedimentation, they may require rather more agitation to disperse non-reacting cells. Second, serum from normal healthy persons often contains antibodies which are reactive only or preferentially in an enzyme technique. Temperature is important as these troublesome panagglutinins may have a low thermal optimum. The use of proper controls is essential and this is referred to again in later sections. Microscopic reading of enzyme tests is not recommended. *Tables 10* and *11* describe a method for the two-stage bromelain technique.

5.6.3 *Polybrene technique*

The manual polybrene technique can be used to enhance the reactions of a wide variety of IgM and IgG antibodies. It is very quick and easy to use. It is as sensitive as the IAGT for Rh antibodies but less sensitive for some other antibodies, unless it is carried through to an antiglobulin phase. A method is given in *Table 12*.

5.7 **Absorption techniques**

In contrast to haemagglutination techniques, the objective of an absorption test is to remove antibody activity, or to establish if it can be removed. The serum:cell volume ratio in absorption tests is therefore much lower than in haemagglutination tests, in order to allow maximal antibody removal. If desired, enzyme-treated red cells may be used for antibody absorption, such as when removing unwanted panagglutinins from serum (a haemagglutination technique may be used beforehand to establish that the antibody reacts preferentially with enzyme-treated red cells). Time and temperature conditions depend on quantity and type of antibody. As a general rule, longer incubation times should be used when absorbing antibodies with a low thermal optimum. Shorter incubation times may often be used when using enzyme-treated red cells. If the antibody is in high concentration, sequential absorptions using fresh red cells each time may

Table 12. The manual polybrene technique.

1.	Add two drops of serum to a 75 × 12 mm tube.
2.	Add one drop of a 3−5% suspension of washed red cells in PBS.
3.	Add 1 ml of low ionic medium[a]. Mix well.
4.	Incubate at room temperature for 1 min.
5.	Add two drops of working strength polybrene[b]. Mix well.
6.	Incubate for 15 sec.
7.	Centrifuge at 1000 g for 10 sec.
8.	Decant the supernatant to waste.
9.	Add two drops of resuspending solution[c].
10.	Mix gently.
11.	Read macroscopically or microscopically within 3 min of step 9. Non-specific aggregation induced by polybrene should be completely dispersed within 10 sec of step 9 but specific agglutination will also become weaker if the test is not read promptly.

[a]0.28 M dextrose, 0.005 M disodium EDTA.
[b]Stock solution: 100 g/l polybrene (Aldrich Chemical Co. Ltd) in 0.15 M NaCl. Working strength solution: dilute stock solution to 0.5 g/l in 0.15 M NaCl.
[c]Mix 60 ml 0.2 M trisodium citrate with 40 ml 0.28 M dextrose.

Table 13. Absorption of antibody.

1.	Wash[a] a sufficiently large volume of red cells in PBS.
2.	Centrifuge[a] to pack the cells well and remove all supernatant PBS.
3.	Add 1−2 vols of serum to 1 vol. of packed cells. Mix well.
4.	Incubate for 30−120 min[b].
5.	Centrifuge[a] to pack the cells well.
6.	Remove the absorbed serum for testing. Keep the red cells if an eluate is to be prepared from them.

[a]Wash volume and centrifugation conditions depend on red cell volume.
[b]See Section 5.7.

be performed to increase antibody removal. The absorption protocol given in *Table 13* can be used as a starting point.

5.8 Elution techniques

Elution is the removal of antibody bound to red cells. It has two main uses in blood group serology. First, elution can be performed following incubation of antibody with red cells in order to establish whether antibody has been adsorbed; this adsorption/ elution technique is a highly sensitive way of demonstrating that an antibody−antigen reaction has occurred. In practice, the same method for absorption (without elution: see Section 5.7) and adsorption (followed by elution) may be carried out. Second, elution can be used to establish the specificity of antibody (or antibodies) bound *in vivo*, such as in AIHA, or haemolytic disease of the newborn.

A wide variety of elution techniques are available: only three are described here and the reader is referred elsewhere (1) for a more comprehensive summary. The Landsteiner/Miller or heat elution technique is suitable for a wide range of IgM and IgG antibodies and is particularly easy to perform. The Rubin or ether elution technique gives excellent results with IgG antibodies although similar techniques using xylene or chloroform may be preferred on safety grounds (1). The acid elution technique is

Table 14. Heat elution technique.

1.	Wash a sufficiently large volume[a] of red cells in PBS.
2.	Centrifuge[a] to pack the cells well. Remove all of the final supernatant and retain it for testing.
3.	Add 1 vol. of PBS, preheated to 56°C, to 1 vol. of the washed, packed cells. Mix well.
4.	Agitate continuously for 5 min in a 56°C water bath.
5.	Centrifuge[a,b] to pack the cells; immediately remove the haemoglobin-stained eluate.
6.	If the eluate is to be stored, add 100 μl of 30% BSA to each ml of eluate. Mix well and store at -20°C.
7.	Test the eluate in parallel with the final wash.

[a]Wash volume and centrifugation conditions depend on red cell volume. See Section 5.8.
[b]Use a heated centrifuge if a long (>3 min) centrifugation time is used.

Table 15. Ether elution technique.

1.	Proceed as in steps 1 and 2 in *Table 14*.
2.	Add 1 vol. of PBS, followed by 2 vols of AR brand ether, to 1 vol. of the washed, packed cells.
3.	Stopper the tube and invert continuously for 1 min, carefully loosening the stopper two or three times during this procedure.
4.	Centrifuge[a] to obtain three layers: a supernatant ether layer, a layer of red cell stroma, and a haemoglobin-stained eluate.
5.	Carefully remove to waste the ether layer and as much of the stroma as possible.
6.	Remove the eluate to a fresh tube and incubate for 15 min in a 37°C water bath, unstoppered, to remove residual ether.
7.	Proceed as in steps 6 and 7 in *Table 14*.

[a]Conditions depend on red cell volume. Use 1000 g for 10 min for 0.5 ml of packed cells.

Table 16. Acid elution technique.

1.	Proceed as in steps 1 and 2 in *Table 14*.
2.	Add 1 vol. of PBS to 1 vol. of washed, packed cells. Mix well.
3.	Chill on ice for 10 min. At the same time, chill a tube of pH 3 glycine solution[a].
4.	Add 1 vol. of chilled pH 3 glycine solution to 1 vol. of washed, chilled, 50% cells.
5.	Mix continuously at 0°C for 60 sec.
6.	Centrifuge[b] to pack the cells and immediately remove the supernatant eluate. If required for further serological tests, the red cells can be washed in PBS.
7.	Add 20 μl of pH 10.5 Tris buffer[c] to each ml of eluate.
8.	Mix well for ~1 min (a light precipitate may form: centrifuge if necessary).
9.	Proceed as in steps 6 and 7 in *Table 14*.

[a]0.1 M glycine, 0.1 M NaCl, adjusted to pH 3 with 0.1 M HCl.
[b]Conditions depend on red cell volume. Use the minimum time necessary (e.g. 2 min at 1000 g for 1 ml of packed cells).
[c]0.5 M Tris.

less efficient than ether elution but the eluate is not haemoglobin-stained and the red cells remain intact which may be useful in certain circumstances.

Whatever technique is used, it is important to ensure that red cells are washed free of Ig before elution. Sufficiently large volumes of wash solution must be used (e.g. five 4 ml washes of PBS using 0.5 ml of packed red cells) and the last wash supernatant should be retained for testing in parallel with the eluate. This supernatant should not contain detectable antibody. Elution protocols are shown in *Tables 14, 15* and *16*.

6. RED CELL PHENOTYPING

6.1 **Selection of reagents**

Antisera of most commonly used blood specificities are available commercially (see Appendix of Suppliers). Monoclonal and polyclonal reagents are equally suitable for routine blood grouping. Mabs clearly have an advantage however, if the worker wishes to use the reagent other than as directed by the manufacturer, as panagglutinating and heterophile antibodies will not be present. Only some specificities are available as monoclonal reagents.

Commercial reagents are usually standardized for use by the saline tube (*Table 2*) or antiglobulin (*Tables 5* and *6*) techniques. Sometimes variations of these techniques are recommended and these should be followed unless the reagent can be properly re-standardized.

6.2 **Controls**

Two types of control are needed in red cell phenotyping: a reagent control, and a diluent control.

6.2.1 *Reagent controls*

The purpose of the reagent control is to establish under test conditions that the reagent (i) will react with a weak expression of the antigen and (ii) will not react with red cells not possessing the antigen (i.e. to ensure that the reagent is avid and specific). Red cells with a heterozygous expression of the antigen are usually used as the weak positive control. For example, $Jk(a+b+)$ and $Jk(a-b+)$ red cells would be suitable positive and negative controls for an anti-Jk^a serum. Such cells can be selected from an antibody identification panel. Commercially available ABO and Rh phenotyping reagents are however usually very avid, and provided manufacturer's recommendations are followed, the controls described in Sections 6.3 and 6.7 may safely be used; red cells of these phenotypes are available at a lower cost than cells from an identification panel.

6.2.2 *Diluent controls*

The purpose of the diluent control is to ensure that the red cells do not possess characteristics which make them, under test conditions, agglutinable or apparently agglutinable in the absence of typing reagent. This may occur when the red cells (i) have been coated, either *in vivo* or *in vitro*, with IgG, IgM or complement components or (ii) are agglutinable by all normal sera (i.e. are *polyagglutinable*), a situation which may be acquired *in vivo* or *in vitro* or inherited. Globulin-coated red cells will give misleading results using antiglobulin or potentiated techniques but can usually be phenotyped using saline-active antisera. Polyagglutinable red cells may give problems by all techniques but fortunately these are rarely encountered.

Diluent controls are therefore essential when phenotyping using antiglobulin or potentiated techniques but can be omitted when using a saline technique. However, most commercial reagents of Rh specificity are used by a 'saline' technique but are in fact potentiated with macromolecular substances (e.g. albumin, Ficoll, Dextran).

15

Antibodies in blood group serology

Table 17. Reaction patterns in ABO grouping.

Reagent	Phenotype of sample				
	A	B	O	AB	
anti-A	+	−	−	+	} Reagent antibody tested against sample cells (cell group)
anti-B	−	+	−	+	
A cells	−	+	+	−	} Sample serum tested against reagent cells (serum group)
B cells	+	−	+	−	
O cells	−	−	−	−	

Table 18. ABO grouping.

(a) *ABO cell (forward) grouping*
1. Add anti-A[a] to each of four tubes.
2. Add anti-B[a] to each of four tubes.
3. Add washed red cells[a] from the blood sample to the first tubes of anti-A and anti-B.
4. Add washed group A, B and O red cells[a] to the second, third and fourth tubes, respectively, of anti-A and anti-B. These are the reagent controls.
5. Mix all tests well.
6. Incubate[a,b] for 60 min at room temperature.
7. Read macroscopically or microscopically[a].

(b) *ABO serum (reverse) grouping*
1. Add serum or plasma[a] from the blood sample to each of three tubes.
2. Add washed group A, B or O red cells[a] to these tubes. Mix well.
3. Incubate[a,b] for 60 min at room temperature.
4. Read macroscopically or microscopically.

[a]Refer to reagent antibody instructions and *Table 2* for details of volume etc.
[b]Alternatively incubate for 5−15 min at room temperature and centrifuge at 800 g for 30 sec.

Diluent controls should also be used with these reagents and are available from the manufacturer. An AB (inert) serum control or an autologous (patient's serum) control may be used in place of a diluent control when using enzyme and antiglobulin techniques.

6.3 ABO grouping

Determination of the ABO group of a person's red cells is undertaken using anti-A and anti-B, and normally confirmed by testing for the presence or absence of 'naturally occurring' anti-A and anti-B in the serum. The red cell ABO group is sometimes known as the cell group or forward group and the interpretation of tests for serum allo-agglutinins constitute the serum group or reverse group. *Table 17* shows reaction patterns for the four ABO phenotypes A, B, O and AB. A suggested protocol for ABO grouping is shown in *Table 18a* and *b*.

6.4 ABO subgrouping

The A antigen is produced by either of two commonly occurring allelic genes, A_1 and A_2. The products of these genes can be distinguished by subgrouping with anti-A$_1$, as shown in *Table 19*. Anti-A$_1$ is used like anti-A (*Table 18a*) or by a tile technique (*Table 3*). Reagent anti-A$_1$ is in fact a lectin preparation from the seeds of *Dolichos biflorus*

Table 19. Reaction patterns in ABO subgrouping.

Reagent	Phenotype of sample							
	O	A_1	A_2	B	A_1B	A_2B	A_3	A_x
anti-A	−	+	+	−	+	+	+[a]	−
anti-A_1	−	+	−	−	+	−	−	−
anti-B	−	−	−	+	+	+	−	−
anti-A,B	−	+	+	+	+	+	+[a]	+
% Caucasians	44	35	10	8	3	0.8	0.1	0.003

[a]Weak, mixed field agglutination.

and a crude extract which is adequate for subgrouping is easily made (6) or can be obtained ready for use from a number of sources (see Appendix of Suppliers).

There are many other subgroups of A and B. The most common of these phenotypes, A_3, has a frequency of about 0.1% in Caucasians; red cells of persons having the genotype A_3O or A_3B will give a characteristic weak mixed field agglutination with anti-A (*Table 19*). Most of the other subgroups of A (or B) will not be detected using anti-A (or anti-B). Red cells having the A_x phenotype can be distinguished using anti-A,B (*Table 19*) although some monoclonal anti-A antibodies also react with A_x cells. Subgroups of A and B are sometimes the cause of discrepant reactions in cell grouping and reverse grouping.

6.5 Discrepant reactions in ABO grouping

Occasionally cell grouping and reverse grouping results do not match as expected. It should be noted here that the reactions of red cells with reagent anti-A or anti-B should be very avid (grade 5 or 6 in *Table 1*) if the cells have A or B antigen and so weak reactions in cell grouping constitute an anomalous result. Weaker reactions (grade 3 or 4) in reverse grouping are not uncommon.

Causes of discrepant reactions may be summarized as follows.

(i)   'Missing' or very weak anti-A or anti-B in the reverse group: red cells belong to subgroup of A or B; blood is from an old, very young or ill person; or blood is from a chimaeric twin (this latter situation is very rare).

(ii) 'Unexpected' reactions with A, B or O cells: anti-A_1 in persons of group A_2 or A_2B or of a rare A subgroup; or an antibody directed against antigens of another blood group system (see Section 7.3).

(iii) Red cells give weak or mixed field reactions with anti-A or anti-B: red cells belong to a subgroup of A; red cells are polyagglutinable; or blood is from a chimaeric twin or a patient who has received a recent blood transfusion.

6.6 Rh(D) grouping

The *Rh group* or *Rh type* is the name commonly given to the result of phenotyping with anti-Rh(D) (usually simply called anti-D) alone. Note that it is more correct to talk of 'Rh' than of 'Rhesus'.

Weak expressions of the D antigen are more common than those of A and B. About 0.5% of red cells from Caucasian donors have a weak D antigen (the D^u phenotype),

Table 20. Rh(D) grouping.

(a) *Rh(D) grouping by a saline technique[a]*

1. Add anti-D to each of three tubes[b].
2. Add diluent control to one tube[b,c].
3. Add washed red cells[b] from the blood sample to the first tube of anti-D and to the diluent control.
4. Add washed Rh(D) positive and Rh(D) negative red cells[b] to the second and third tubes, respectively, of anti-D. These are the reagent controls.
5. Mix all tests well.
6. Incubate[b,d] for 60 min at 37°C.
7. Read macroscopically or microscopically[b].

(b) *Rh(D) grouping by an indirect antiglobulin technique (IAGT)[e]*

1. Add anti-D to each of three tubes[f].
2. Add diluent control or AB serum to one tube[c,f].
3. Add washed red cells[f] from the blood sample to the first tube of anti-D and to the diluent (or AB serum).
4. Add washed Rh(D) positive and Rh(D) negative red cells[f] to the second and third tubes, respectively, of anti-D. These are the reagent controls.
5. Mix all tests well.
6. Incubate[f] for 60 min at 37°C if using the NISS−IAGT (*Table 5*) or for 20 min at 37°C if using the LISS−IAGT (*Table 6*).
7. Proceed as in steps 2−5(ii) of *Table 4*.

[a]Suitable for IgM reagents without additives (e.g. MAD-2 anti-D, BPL Diagnostics) or chemically modified IgG reagents or IgG reagents with additives (several commercial reagents—see Appendix of Suppliers).
[b]Refer to reagent antibody instructions and *Table 2* for details of volume etc.
[c]Available from the supplier of the anti-D reagent; may be omitted if using an IgM reagent.
[d]Alternatively incubate for 5−15 min at 37°C and centrifuge at 800 *g* for 30 sec.
[e]Suitable for IgG reagents selected for the detection of the D[u] phenotype.
[f]Refer to reagent antibody instructions and *Table 5* and *Table 6* for details of volume etc.

which has been somewhat arbitrarily divided into low grade and high grade types, depending on reactivity with certain types of anti-D. To summarize a rather confusing state of affairs:

(i) non-commercial IgM anti-D reagents which are used by a saline technique generally fail to react with high grade and low grade D[u];

(ii) non-commercial IgG anti-D reagents which are used by an albumin displacement technique generally react with high grade D[u] antigen but fail to react with low grade D[u];

(iii) non-commercial IgG anti-D reagents which are used by an antiglobulin technique react with high grade and low grade D[u];

(iv) commercial IgM or IgG anti-D reagents which are used by a saline technique generally react with high grade D[u] and often react with low grade D[u]. Note that these reagents usually contain additives of high molecular weight and should always be used with a diluent control.

Suggested layouts for Rh(D) grouping by saline and antiglobulin techniques are shown in *Table 20a* and *b*.

6.7 **Phenotyping with other Rh antibodies**

Although antibodies define more than 40 antigens associated with the Rh locus, the term Rh phenotyping is usually used to describe the results of tests with anti-D, anti-C,

Table 21. Reaction patterns in Rh phenotyping.

Reagent	Phenotype of sample								
	R_1r	R_1R_1	rr	R_2r	R_1R_2	R_0r	R_2R_2	$r'r$	$r''r$
anti-D	+	+	−	+	+	+	+	−	−
anti-C	+	+	−	−	+	−	−	+	−
anti-c	+	−	+	+	+	+	+	+	+
anti-E	−	−	−	+	+	−	+	−	+
anti-e	+	+	+	+	+	+	−	+	+
% Caucasians	32	17	15	11	11	2	2	0.8	0.9

Table 22. Designation of red cell phenotypes: some examples.

Blood group system	Antigens*	Example genotype	Phenotype
ABO	A_1, A, B	A_1B	A_1B
Rh	D, C, c, E, e	CDe/cde or R^1r	DCce or R_1r
MNS	M, N, S, s	MS/Ns	MNSs or M+N+S+s+
P	P_1	P^1/P^1	P_1 or $P_1{}^+$
Lewis	Le^a, Le^b	See footnote+	Le(a−b+)
Kell	K, k	$K\ k$	K+k+
Duffy	Fy^a, Fy^b	$Fy^a\ Fy^b$	Fy(a+b+)
Kidd	Jk^a, Jk^b	$Jk^a\ Jk^b$	Jk(a+b+)
Lutheran	Lu^a, Lu^b	$Lu^a\ Lu^b$	Lu(a+b+)

*Many other antigens in these systems have been described.
+The Lewis antigens are derived from the plasma and result from the interaction of genes from the *H, Se,* and *Le* loci.

anti-c, anti-E, anti-e and sometimes anti-C^w. These reagents are normally quite sufficient for phenotyping Caucasian samples, but the presence of other low frequency Rh antigens and differing haplotype frequencies may complicate the situation when phenotyping non-Caucasian samples: see ref. 1 for further details.

The method described in *Table 20a* will be suitable for Rh phenotyping with commercial anti-C, -c, -E and -e reagents. The following reagent controls should be substituted for those in step 4 of the table.

(i) R_1R_1: positive control for anti-C and anti-e and negative control for anti-c and anti-E.

(ii) R_2R_2: positive control for anti-c and anti-E and negative control for anti-C and anti-e.

An interpretation table of results is shown in *Table 21*.

6.8 Phenotyping with other blood grouping reagents

The general principles outlined above are applicable to the use of other blood grouping reagents. Red cells suitable for reagent controls will usually be found in an antibody identification panel (see Section 7.3). A sound knowledge of the blood group systems (see ref. 1) will be necessary for those who wish to undertake paternity testing or other family studies.

For historical reasons, the way of expressing red cell phenotypes varies between blood group systems. Some examples are shown in *Table 22*.

7. ANTIBODY SCREENING AND IDENTIFICATION

7.1 **Definition of terms**

The aim of screening is to establish the presence of a red cell antibody or antibodies as simply as possible, and is usually achieved by testing against two or three examples of red cells of known phenotype, selected to cover as wide a range of antigens as possible. Identification of the antibody is necessary to determine the exact specificity, and for this a panel of red cells from several individuals is required.

7.2 **Choice of technique and red cells**

The technique or techniques which are selected for antibody screening will depend upon the work that is being undertaken. For example, the serum of a hospital patient (who may require a blood transfusion) must be screened using techniques and red cells which will detect all clinically significant antibodies. It is generally considered that the antiglobulin technique (*Tables 5* and *6*) will detect most clinically significant antibodies. An enzyme (*Table 11*) or manual polybrene (*Table 12*) technique usually supplements an antiglobulin screen because of their values in detecting very weak Rh antibodies.

Great care must be taken in choosing the screening cells themselves. It is relatively easy to select three or four persons whose red cells possess, cumulatively, a wide range of antigens. The cells may be pooled into two sets for screening. However, a weak antibody directed against an antigen which is expressed on only 50% of the pool may pass undetected. It is far better to use two or three carefully selected *single donor* screening cells, such as are available commercially. For blood transfusion work the red cells should cover the following antigens: D, C, c, E, e, M, N, S, s, P_1, Le^a, Le^b, K, Fy^a, Fy^b, Jk^a, Jk^b. Ideally, homozygous expressions of the Rh and Jk^a antigens (i.e. the phenotypes R_1R_1, R_2R_2 and $Jk(a+b-)$ should be present.

On the other hand, if it is desired to screen culture supernatants for Mabs of reagent potential, there is little point in using highly sensitive techniques to detect antibodies with a wide range of specificities. For example, reagent quality anti-A might be screened for using only a saline technique (in microplates if desired) and using red cells with a weak (e.g. A_2B) or very weak (e.g. A_x) expression of the A antigen.

Table 23 lists the techniques by which some commonly encountered antibodies of blood group specificity usually react, although there are many exceptions. Note that saline-reactive antibodies vary greatly in their thermal optimum: anti-P_1, for example usually has optimal reactivity below 20°C while anti-D generally reacts well between 4°C and 37°C. With this in mind, a screen using the saline and antiglobulin techniques may be performed as a single test by reading for agglutination after incubation (step 3 in *Tables 5* and *6*) and before washing.

7.3 **Antibody identification**

This section is necessarily brief and can only present the salient points. The reader is referred elsewhere (1) for a fuller discussion.

Table 23. Modes of reactivity of blood group antibodies.

System	Antigen	Mode of reactivity of antibody			
		Saline 20°C	Saline 37°C	Enzyme 37°C	IAGT 37°C
ABO	A, B	Yes[1]	Yes[1]	Yes[1]	Yes[1]
Rh	D, c, e	Some	Some	Yes	Many
Rh	C^w, C, E	Many	Many	Yes	Some
Lewis	Le^a	Many	Some	Many[1]	Many
Lewis	Le^b	Many	Some	Some[1]	Some
Lutheran	Lu^a	Many	Some	No	Some
P	P$_1$	Yes	Some	Many	Some
MNS	M, N	Yes	Some	No	Some
MNS	S, s	Some	Some	No	Most
Kell	K, k	Some	Some	Many	Yes
Duffy	Fy^a, Fy^b	Rare	Rare	No	Yes
Kidd	Jk^a, Jk^b	Rare	Rare	Some	Yes
Ii	I, i	Yes[1]	No	Some[1]	Some[1]

[1]May be haemolytic.

7.3.1 Scope

Many of the blood group antibodies found in screening the sera of patients and healthy donors can be identified with the careful use of a single identification panel. Sections 7.3.5−7.3.7 allude to situations which are outside the capabilities of many laboratories because of the need for red cells of unusual or rare phenotypes (reference laboratories are listed in Appendix of Suppliers). Note that mouse hybridoma antibodies to human red cell antigens often have a specificity which may be difficult to interpret.

7.3.2 The identification panel

A blood group antibody identification panel should consist of red cells from between eight and 12 individual group O donors. For each of the more commonly encountered blood group antibodies there should be at least two phenotypes lacking and at least two phenotypes carrying expressions of the corresponding antigen. In addition, the panel should be able to resolve as many antibody mixtures as possible: for example, D−K+, D−Fy(a+) and c−K+ phenotypes should be represented. Red cells from the cord blood of a group O neonate will be useful for identifying anti-I and related antibodies.

Panel red cells from commercial sources are normally suspended in a preservative medium which gives them a 3 or 4 week shelf life at 4°C. Saline, NISS−IAG, albumin and polybrene tests (*Tables 2, 5, 8* and *12*) can be performed using these preservative-suspended cells but LISS−IAG and enzyme tests (*Tables 6* and *11*) can only be performed if the cells are centrifuged, packed and then washed and resuspended in LISS or enzyme-treated (*Table 10*).

7.3.3 Principles of antibody identification

For brevity it is assumed here that an antibody-containing serum from a patient (or donor) is being investigated. Clearly, if a culture supernatant is being investigated, any tests using the patient's own red cells would be omitted.

(i) The patient's serum should be tested by an appropriate technique against the identification panel of red cells and against the patient's own red cells. Correlation of positive and negative results with the presence and absence of an antigen (or antigens) on the red cells indicates an antibody (or antibodies) of corresponding specificity. *Table 23* lists the expected mode of reactivity for several blood group antibodies. Note that some antigens (e.g. P_1 and I) are expressed to a variable extent on different red cells, and that some antigens show dosage (i.e. are present in larger quantities on red cells when the person is homozygous for the appropriate gene).

(ii) The specificity of the antibody should only be assigned with confidence when it reacts with at least two examples of red cells possessing the antigen and fails to react with at least two examples of red cells lacking the antigen. Where the presence of more than one antibody is suspected, only results with red cells which possess one or none of the appropriate antigens will be informative unless the antibodies are working by different techniques or unless their strengths of reaction by a single technique are very different.

(iii) When one or more antibodies have been positively identified, the presence of other antibodies should be excluded by ensuring that the panel cells which fail to react cover as many antigens as possible, especially those corresponding to antibodies which are likely to be detected by that technique only. Different techniques may be used to exclude other antibodies.

(iv) The patient's red cells should be phenotyped using antiserum of appropriate specificity. If the cells do not possess the antigen and the patient's serum does not react with the patient's cells, then the antibody is an *allo-antibody*. If the cells do possess the antigen, and the patient's serum does react with the patient's cells, then the antibody is an *auto-antibody*, although this is not necessarily so if the patient has had a recent blood transfusion. If an auto-antibody is suspected, the use of a diluent control or AB serum control (see Section 6.2.2) is particularly important. Examples of interpretation of panel investigations are given in *Table 24*.

7.3.4 Anti-A₁

7.3.4 *Anti-A$_1$*

A small proportion of persons whose red cells are group A or AB have an antibody that reacts with group A red cells in the reverse ABO group. The antibody responsible is often found to be 'naturally occurring' anti-A_1; if so, the red cells will be found to lack the A_1 antigen (i.e. their phenotype will be A_2 or A_2B: see *Table 19*). Anti-A_1 is also often found in the serum of persons whose red cells possess a weakened expression of the A antigen, such as those of the phenotypes A_3 or A_x (see *Table 19*). To confirm the presence of a suspected anti-A_1 the following steps should be taken.

(i) Test the patient's serum against group A_1, A_2, B and O red cells by the saline technique as for standard reverse ABO grouping (*Table 18b*). Anti-A_1 will react with A_1 but not A_2 or O cells. Ideally, additional examples of A_1 and A_2 cells should be tested for further confirmation. If the serum reacts with A_2 or O cells

Table 24. Four sera tested using an antibody identification panel.

ABO	Rh						MNS				P_1	Lewis		Lu	Kell		Duffy		Kidd		Serum 1			Serum 2			Serum 3			Serum 4		
	D	C	C^w	c	E	e	M	N	S	s	P_1	Le^a	Le^b	Lu^a	K	Kp^a	Fy^a	Fy^b	Jk^a	Jk^b	S	E	I	S	E	I	S	E	I	S	E	I
$R_1^wR_1$ O	+	+	+	–	–	+	+	+	+	+	W	+	–	–	–	–	+	+	+	–	0 6 6			3 0 0			0 0 0			3 0 0		
R_1R_1 O	+	+	–	–	–	+	–	+	–	+	+	–	+	–	+	–	–	+	–	+	0 6 6			5 0 3			0 0 0			0 4 5		
R_2R_2 O	+	–	–	+	+	–	+	+	+	+	–	–	–	–	+	–	+	+	+	+	0 6 6			0 0 0			4 5 4			3 4 5		
R_0r O	+	–	–	+	–	+	+	–	–	+	W	+	–	+	–	–	–	–	+	+	0 6 6			2 0 0			0 0 0			3 0 0		
r'r O	–	+	–	+	–	+	+	+	+	–	W	+	–	–	–	–	+	–	+	–	0 0 0			5 0 3			0 0 0			5 0 0		
r"r O	–	–	–	+	+	+	+	+	+	+	+	–	–	–	+	+	–	+	+	+	0 0 0			5 0 3			4 5 3			0 0 0		
rr O	–	–	–	+	–	+	–	+	–	+	–	–	+	–	–	–	+	+	–	+	0 0 0			5 0 3			0 0 0			0 4 5		
rr O	–	–	–	+	–	+	+	+	+	+	W	–	–	–	+	–	+	+	–	+	0 0 0			0 0 0			0 0 5			3 0 0		
rr O	–	–	–	+	–	+	–	–	–	+	W	+	–	–	–	–	+	+	+	+	0 0 0			3 0 0			0 0 0			0 0 0		
rr O	–	–	–	+	–	+	+	+	–	–	–	–	+	–	+	–	+	–	–	+	0 0 0			0 0 0			0 0 0			5 4 5		

W = weak reaction; S = saline technique, room temperature; E = enzyme (bromelain) technique, 37°C; and I = LISS–IAGT, 37°C.
Interpretation: Serum 1 contains anti-D, Serum 2 contains anti-P_1, Serum 3 contains anti-E + anti-Kp^a and Serum 4 contains anti-M + anti-K.

then an antibody of different specificity is present and an antibody identification panel must be used.

(ii)   Subtype the patient's red cells (see Section 6.4).

7.3.5 *Antibodies to high frequency antigens*

A serum which is reactive against all the cells of an antibody identification panel may prove to be a difficult serological problem. It is quite possible that two or more blood group antibodies are present (see Section 7.3.3). It may be helpful to phenotype the patient's red cells for as many blood group antigens as possible prior to investigation, as this will indicate which allo-antibodies could have been made by the patient. Alternatively, a single antibody may be present, directed against an antigen which is present on the red cells of most individuals.

Many such antigens have been described (e.g. the H, Kp^b and Vel antigens). Although the pattern of reactivity with cells possessing the antigen may give a clue as to the identity of the antibody and in some cases (e.g. anti-Chido) inhibition tests may be useful, identification of antibody specificity will generally only be possible in those laboratories which have access to a comprehensive library of antisera and red cells.

7.3.6 *Auto-antibodies*

Sometimes a serum is found to react with the patient's own red cells by a particular technique. Identification of antibody specificity can be carried out as described in Sections 7.3.2−7.3.5. Occasionally however, no specificity can be determined. One such example is the presence of 'panagglutinins', reactive only by an enzyme technique, in the sera of many healthy individuals.

Anti-I is another commonly encountered auto-antibody. The I antigen is present on the red cells of most individuals, but is poorly expressed on the red cells of neonates. Antibody identification panels usually include red cells taken from the umbilical cord of a group O neonate so that anti-I antibodies can easily be recognized.

These auto-antibodies are generally benign and cause no clinical problems. In patients with AIHA, auto-antibodies directed against red cell antigens are responsible for shortening of red cell survival which may lead to severe anaemia. Two types of AIHA can be distinguished.

(i) *Cold-type AIHA or cold haemagglutinin disease.* The red cells from the patient will usually be DAGT strongly positive due to coating with complement (C3d) components (see Sections 5.5.1 and 4). The patient's serum is usually found to contain a saline-active antibody of wide thermal range (e.g. up to 31°C) and which may be of anti-I specificity. The antibody can also usually be detected by enzyme and IAGT at 37°C, unless careful pre-warming of cells and serum before incubation is carried out. Diluent controls (see Section 6.2.2) are particularly important when phenotyping the patient's red cells or performing the DAGT because of the possibility of auto-agglutination.

(ii) *Warm-type AIHA.* The red cells from the patient will usually be DAGT strongly positive due to coating with IgG and sometimes complement components. The patient's serum is often found to contain an auto- and panagglutinin reactive by enzyme and

IAGT, although sophisticated serology may reveal one or more antibodies of identifiable blood group specificity. Tests using an eluate (*Tables 14, 15* and *16*) prepared from the patient's red cells are more useful than those using serum when studying the auto-antibody because the latter may contain little free antibody. Phenotyping of the patient's red cells can only be performed using IgM or chemically modified IgG (complete) saline reactive antisera, unless IgG antibody is removed from the red cells by, for example, treatment with chloroquine diphosphate (1). Diluent controls are essential in either case.

7.3.7 *Antibodies to low frequency antigens*

It is estimated that about 1% of the population have anti-Wr^a in their serum. The Wr^a antigen is expressed on the red cells of about 0.1% of Caucasians and is just one of a large number of serologically distinct antigens of low incidence. Antibodies to these antigens are frequently found in the same serum; they rarely appear to have been stimulated by red cell transfusions or pregnancy. A serum which appears to react with red cells from one person, but does not react with cells from one or two identification panels, probably contains such an antibody. Another possibility is that the incompatible red cells are polyagglutinable (e.g. have become infected) or are DAGT-positive.

8. USES OF ABSORPTION AND ELUTION TECHNIQUES

Sections 6 and 7 have illustrated the principles involved in red cell phenotyping and antibody identification, where haemagglutination techniques are widely used. In some circumstances the absorption and elution techniques described in Sections 5.7 and 5.8 are useful. Some examples are given below.

8.1 **Mixtures of antibodies**

Identification of the individual components of a mixture of antibodies may be aided by one or more absorptions using red cells of known phenotype. For example, a serum which is suspected of containing allo-anti-D and allo-anti-Jk^a may be absorbed using cells which are D$^-$Jk(a+) or which are D$^+$Jk(a−). Absorbed serum is then tested against a red cell panel to identify the remaining activity (if any). If the specificity of one component is known with reasonable certainty, for example anti-D (perhaps because a panel of enzyme-treated red cells gives clear-cut anti-D specificity), it is better to absorb with red cells which are D+ but which lack as many as possible of the antigens which are not expressed on the patient's red cells. In this way all of the allo-antibodies except anti-D should be present in the absorbed serum.

This procedure can also be used to separate mixtures of auto-antibodies such as are often present in the sera (and eluates) of patients with warm AIHA. Absorptions with R$_1$R$_1$, R$_2$R$_2$ and rr cells may reveal 'simple' antibody specificities such as anti-e. Sera from these patients may also contain allo-antibodies. Repeated absorptions with patient's red cells can be used to remove all auto-antibody and reveal the specificity of any allo-antibody present (1).

The preparation of blood grouping reagents may require the absorption of unwanted antibodies. For example, the serum of a group A donor might contain anti-Fy^a but would have to be absorbed with group B or AB Fy(a−) red cells before it could be used to determine the Fy^a phenotype of the cells of persons of all ABO groups. Note that repeated absorptions may be necessary to remove all antibody activity: in the above example several examples of group B Fy(a−) red cells should be used to test for complete absorption of anti-B.

8.2 Confirmation of phenotype

In some circumstances it is better to use an adsorption and elution technique rather than a haemagglutination technique to phenotype red cells. Two examples illustrate this.

Red cells of the A_x phenotype (see Section 6.4) do not react with most anti-A grouping sera. Blood group A antigen can however be demonstrated on the cells by incubating them with an anti-A serum, washing away free antibody and eluting antibody from the cells. The antibody in the eluate will be found to have weak anti-A activity; enzyme-treated A (and control B and O) cells may be necessary to detect the antibody. The adsorption and elution should be performed also with group O cells in place of the suspected A_x cells to act as a negative control.

Anti-Wr^a and other antibodies to low frequency antigens are often found together in a serum (see Section 7.3.7). A positive reaction of red cells with an 'anti-Wr^a' grouping serum should therefore be interpreted with care as the serum may not have been tested against a comprehensive panel of cells possessing low frequency antigens. However, if anti-Wr^a can be adsorbed onto and eluted from the red cells (i.e. an eluate

Table 25. Determination of ABH secretor status.

Selection of antisera

1. Choose conventional monoclonal or polyclonal (IgM) anti-A and anti-B for the test. The lectin from *Ulex europaeus* is the best source of anti-H.
2. Titrate[a] the anti-A, anti-B and anti-H in PBS to a maximum dilution of 1:512.
3. Test using a saline technique[b] each dilution of anti-A with A_2 red cells, each dilution of anti-B with B cells and each dilution of anti-H with O cells.
4. Select the highest dilution of each antiserum at which good macroscopic agglutination (grade 4[c]) is obtained.

Preparation of saliva

1. Place a tube containing ~ 2 ml of saliva in a boiling water bath for 10 min (to destroy enzyme activity).
2. Centrifuge at 1000 *g* for 5 min.
3. Remove the supernatant and dilute 1:2 in PBS.

Secretor status

1. Add one drop of diluted saliva to each of three 75 × 12 mm tubes.
2. Add one drop of PBS to each of three 75 × 12 mm tubes. These are the controls.
3. Add one drop of diluted anti-A to a tube of saliva and a control tube. Repeat for diluted anti-B and anti-H.
4. Mix all tubes well.
5. Incubate for 10−20 min at room temperature.
6. Add one drop of a 3−5% suspension of washed A_2 red cells to the tubes containing anti-A, and similarly add B and O cells to the tubes containing anti-B and anti-H, respectively.
7. Mix all tubes well.
8. Incubate for 60−90 min at room temperature.
9. Read macroscopically. A negative result indicates inhibition by A, B or H blood group substance. The control tubes should all show positive reactions.

---

[a]See Chapter 7.
[b]See *Table 2*.
[c]See *Table 1*.

prepared after adsorption reacts with Wr(a+) but not Wr(a−) cells) then this is convincing evidence of the presence of Wr^a antigen. Alternatively, an 'anti-Wr^a' serum can be adsorbed onto and eluted from red cells which have been confirmed as Wr(a+); the eluate can then be used as a grouping reagent.

9. USES OF INHIBITION TECHNIQUES

Haemagglutination inhibition techniques for detecting and quantifying antigens are described in Volume 1, Chapter 7. Their main uses in blood group serology are:

(i)   to determine whether a person is a 'secretor' of ABH substances, that is whether his or her saliva contains soluble blood group ABH substances; and, in forensic work, to establish which ABH substances are secreted. Group A secretors secrete A and H substances, group B secrete B and H substances, group AB secrete A, B and H substances and group O secrete H substance (see *Table 25* for method of determination of secretor status);

(ii)   to aid the identification of an antibody because of its inhibitability by saliva, serum or other fluids which may contain antigen in a soluble form;

(iii) to aid the identification of mixtures of antibodies by inhibiting one or more components of the mixture with soluble antigen. Non-inhibited components can then be identified by haemagglutination techniques.

These uses are more fully discussed in ref. 1.

Table 26. Freezing red cells in liquid nitrogen and their reconstitution after storage.

(a) *Freezing red cells in liquid nitrogen*

1. Centrifuge^a an anticoagulated blood sample to pack the red cells well. Discard all of the supernatant plasma and buffy coat.
2. Add 1.5 vols of cryoprotective solution^b to 1 vol. of packed red cells.
3. Mix by continuous inversion on a rotary mixer (~18 r.p.m.) for 10 min.
4. Aliquot into labelled 2 ml or 5 ml cryotubes^c and stopper tightly.
5. Freeze the red cells by totally immersing the tubes in liquid nitrogen. This stage should be performed not later than 45 min after addition of cryoprotective solution.
6. When all bubbling has ceased, the tubes may be removed for storage in the liquid or vapour phase of liquid nitrogen.

(b) *Reconstitution of liquid-nitrogen-stored red cells*

1. Thaw the ampoule by gently agitating in a water bath at 37−42°C.
2. Transer the contents to a 75 × 12 mm test tube^d.
3. Wash out the cryotube with wash solution A^e to fill the test tube.
4. Mix and allow to equilibrate for 3−5 min at room temperature.
5. Centrifuge^d at 500 g for 90 sec. Discard the supernatant.
6. Gently resuspend the cell button in wash solution B^e.
7. Mix and allow to equilibrate for 3−5 min at room temperature.
8. Centrifuge^d at 500 g for 60 sec. Discard the supernatant.
9. Repeat steps 6−8 using wash solution C^e and then PBS^f. If necessary give the red cells further washes with PBS^f (without equilibration) until the supernatant is no longer haemoglobin-stained.

^{a}Centrifugation time depends on volume.
^{b}0.13 M NaCl, 0.14 M sorbitol, 2.77 M glycerol.
^{c}Sterilin Ltd, Hounslow, Middlesex, UK.
^{d}For a 2 ml cryotube.
^{e}Wash solution A is 0.14 M NaCl, 0.69 M sorbitol; wash solution B is one part wash solution A and one part PBS^f; wash solution C is one part wash solution A and three parts PBS^f.
^{f}Red cell preservative may be used in place of PBS (see text).

10. STORAGE OF RED CELLS AND SERUM

Whole blood taken into citrate (see Section 4.1) may be used for most blood grouping purposes up to 3 weeks after collection provided it is kept sterile at 4°C. Red cells from clotted and from EDTA anticoagulated specimens will only be usable up to 1 week after collection. Serum (or plasma) is best kept frozen at -20°C or below.

Suspensions of red cells in PBS may be used within 24 h of preparation provided they are kept at 4°C when not in use. Storage may be extended to several days or even weeks by suspending in a solution containing glucose and antibiotics. One such red cell preservative is an aqueous solution containing 0.11 M glucose, 20 mM trisodium citrate dihydrate, 20 mM $Na_2HPO_4.2H_2O$, 2.62 mM citric acid monohydrate, 0.27 mM $CaCl_2.6H_2O$, 34.2 mM NaCl, 0.59 mM adenine, 1.36 mM inosine, 0.99 mM chloramphenicol, 16 mg gentamycin sulphate (David Bull Laboratories). Dissolve 100 mg amphotericin B in 20 ml dimethyl sulphoxide and add 20 μl of this solution to 1 litre of the main solution. Check the pH is 7.0 ± 0.1. Sterilize by passing through a 0.2 μ filter. See Section 7.3.2 for the use of preservative suspended red cells in serological tests. Red cells may also be stored in the frozen state (see *Table 26*). Reconstituted frozen red cells will have a shelf life of about 8 h in PBS or 7 days in red cell preservative solution at 4°C.

11. REFERENCES

1. Issitt,P.D. (1985) *Applied Blood Group Serology*. Montgomery, Miami, USA, 3rd edition.
2. Knight,R. and Poole,G. (eds) (1987) *The Use of Microplates in Blood Group Serology*. British Blood Transfusion Society, Manchester, UK.
3. Dixon,M.R. (1984) In Myers,M. and Reynolds,A. (eds), *Micromethods in Blood Group Serology*. American Association of Blood Banks, Arlington, USA.
4. Weiland,D.L. (1984) In Myers,M. and Reynolds,A. (eds), *Micromethods in Blood Broup Serology*. American Association of Blood Banks, Arlington, USA.
5. Lambert,R., Edwards,J. and Anstee,D.J. (1978) *Med. Lab. Sci.*, **35**, 233.
6. Mollison,P.L. (1979) *Blood Transfusion in Clinical Medicine*. Blackwell, Oxford, 6th edition.
7. Race,R.R. and Sanger,R. (1975) *Blood Groups in Man*. Blackwell Scientific Publications, Oxford, 6th edition.
8. Sistonen,P., Hevanlinna,H.R., Virtaranta-Knowles,K., Pirkola,A., Leikola,J., Kekomäki,R., Gavin,J. and Tippett,P. (1981) *Vox Sang.*, **40**, 352.

12. APPENDIX: INHERITANCE OF HUMAN BLOOD GROUP ANTIGENS

Table 27 gives brief details of the inheritance of human blood group antigens. Many of the blood group systems are known to have multiple alleles, but for simplicity the

Table 27. Blood group genes and antigens.

Blood group system	Allelic gene or gene complex*	Antigen produced by allele	Gene frequency[+] in Caucasians	Notes
ABO	A_1	A_1, A	0.209	A_1, A_2, B (and H)
	A_2	A	0.070	genes are known to
	B	B	0.061	code for glycosyl
	O	None	0.660	transferases.
H	H	H	Very common	A and B red cell
	h	None	Very rare	antigens can only be synthesized in the presence of H gene.

Secretor	*Se*		0.523	A, B and H antigens in
	se		0.477	secretions can only be
				synthesized in the
				presence of *H* and *Se*
				genes.
Rh (Rhesus)	R^1 (*CDe*)	C, D, e	0.408	There is no d antigen.
	r (*cde*)	c, e	0.389	
	R^2 (*cDE*)	c, D, E	0.141	
	R^0 (*cDe*)	c, D, e	0.026	
	R^{1w} (*C^{w}De*)	C^w, D, e	0.013	
	r″ (*cdE*)	c, E	0.012	
	r′ (*Cde*)	C, e	0.010	
MNS	*MS*	M, S	0.237	The *MN* and *Ss* genes
	Ms	M, s	0.305	show very close
	NS	N, S	0.071	genetic linkage.
	Ns	N, s	0.387	
P	P^{1k}	P_1	0.540	The phenotype P_1- is
	P^k	None	0.460	also known as P_2.
Lewis	*Le*	Le^a, Le^b	0.816	Antigens are derived
	le	None	0.184	from the plasma by
Kell	*K*	K	0.046	interaction of genes at
	k	k	0.954	the *Le*, *Se* and *H* loci.
Duffy	*Fy^a*	Fy^a	0.425	
	Fy^b	Fy^b	0.557	
	Fy^x	Weak Fy^b	0.016	
Kidd	*Jk^a*	Jk^a	0.516	
	Jk^b	Jk^b	0.484	
Lutheran	*Lu^a*	Lu^a	0.039	
	Lu^b	Lu^b	0.961	
Xg^a	*Xg^a*	Xg^a	0.659	Xg genes are carried
	Xg	None	0.341	on the X-chromosome.
Diego	*Di^a*	Di^a	Very rare	Di^a antigen is more
	Di^b	Di^b	Very common	common in Mongolian
Cartwright	*Yt^a*	Yt^a	0.959	populations.
	Yt^b	Yt^b	0.041	
Scianna	*Sc^1*	Sc1	0.992	
	Sc^2	Sc2	0.009	
Dombrock	*Do^a*	Do^a	0.420	
	Do^b	Do^b	0.580	
Colton	*Co^a*	Co^a	0.956	
	Co^b	Co^b	0.044	
In	*In^a*	In^a	0	In^a antigen has only
	In^b	In^b	1.0	been found in Asian
LW	*LW^a*	LW^a	0.999	Indians.
	LW^b	LW^b	0.001	

*Alternative designation shown in brackets.

[+]Data taken from (7) except that for LW which is taken from (8).

table only shows alleles in these systems which have a frequency of greater than 0.01 or less than 0.97 in Caucasians. For example, there are many low frequency genes in the Rh system. Note also that alternative alleles may produce a common antigen (often therefore of high incidence); these antigens have not been included in the table with the exception of the CDE antigens of the Rh system. Some of the blood group systems have low frequency genes which, when inherited in a homozygous fashion, give rise to 'null' phenotypes, where the red cells show no expression of any antigens belonging to that system. In some systems, the blood group genes are known to be only expressed in the absence of unlinked rare inhibitor genes.

CHAPTER 2

Antibodies in HLA Serology

TERRY RAY

1. INTRODUCTION TO TISSUE TYPING

The HLA region is situated on the short arm of chromosome 6. The region consists of a series of linked genes which code for many of the proteins involved with the recognition and response to foreign antigens. The name HLA, which represents Human Leukocyte series A, is a permanent reminder of the origins of this branch of immunogenetics. The terms 'tissue typing' and 'HLA typing' are used interchangeably; it is too late for reform but it must be recognized that many tissue antigens are coded by genes not linked to the HLA region.

At the cell surface, two different polypeptides are always found in association to give the functional structure of class I and class II HLA molecules.

Class I molecules, which have a role in the presentation of antigen to the T cell receptor, consist of a glycopeptide of molecular weight 44 kd associated non-covalently at the cell surface with β_2-microglobulin, a 12 kd protein coded on chromosome 15. Substitution of just a few of the amino acids of the 44 kd heavy chain gives rise to the HLA-A, B and C series of polymorphic determinants (*Table 1*). Class I molecules, when associated with foreign antigen (e.g. of viral origin), seem to be favoured as targets by cytotoxic T (T_c) cells. When the molecule itself is presented as foreign allo-antigen on the fetus during pregnancy or on kidney transplants, for example, it is capable of initiating powerful humoral and cellular responses.

Class II molecules at the cell surface consist of a heavy (α) chain of 34 kd associated with a light (β) chain of 29 kd, they include HLA-DR, DQ and DP gene products (*Table 1*). In HLA-DR molecules the α chain is monomorphic and the amino acid sequence of the β chain alone is responsible for the polymorphism. In HLA-DQ both the α and the β chain contribute to the polymorphic determinants. Class II molecules have a more restricted distribution than class I antigens in normal healthy tissue, occurring mainly on B lymphocytes, macrophages, antigen presenting cells, activated T cells and vascular endothelial cells. The presentation of antigenic fragments to T and B lymphocytes in the initiation of an immune response seems to be the primary function of class II molecules.

1.1 The complement-dependent cytotoxicity (CDC) test

The most significant step in the technical development of HLA typing was the replacement of leuko-agglutination by the lymphocytotoxicity test using rabbit complement (1). The microlitre volumes of reagents required for the technique permit the testing of a wide range of sera from all parts of the world. The 1975 6th Interna-

Table 1. HLA specificities recognized by WHO Nomenclature Committee on Leukocyte Antigens 1988 (36).

Complete listing of recognized HLA specificities

A	B	C	D	DR	DQ	DP
A1	B5	Cw1	Dw1	DR1	DQw1	DPw1
A2	B7	Cw2	Dw2	DR2	DQw2	DPw2
A3	B8	Cw3	Dw3	DR3	DQw3	DPw3
A9	B12	Cw4	Dw4	DR4	DQw4	DPw4
A10	B13	Cw5	Dw5	DR5	DQw5(w1)	DPw5
A11	B14	Cw6	Dw6	DRw6	DQw6(w1)	DPw6
Aw19	B15	Cw7	Dw7	DR7	DQw7(w3)	
A23(9)	B16	Cw8	Dw8	DRw8	DQw8(w3)	
A24(9)	B17	Cw9(w3)	Dw9	DR9	DQw9(w3)	
A25(10)	B18	Cw10(w3)	Dw10	DRw10		
A26(10)	B21	Cw11	Dw11(w7)	DRw11(5)		
A28	Bw22		Dw12	DRw12(5)		
A29(w19)	B27		Dw13	DRw13(w6)		
A30(w19)	B35		Dw14	DRw14(w6)		
A31(w19)	B37		Dw15	DRw15(2)		
A32(w19)	B38(16)		Dw16	DRw16(2)		
Aw33(w19)	B39(16)		Dw17(w7)	DRw17(3)		
Aw34(10)	B40		Dw18(w6)	DRw18(3)		
Aw36	Bw41		Dw19(w6)			
Aw43	Bw42		Dw20	DRw52		
Aw66(10)	B44(12)		Dw21	DRw53		
Aw68(28)	B45(12)		Dw22			
Aw69(28)	Bw46		Dw23			
Aw74(w19)	Bw47		Dw24			
	Bw48		Dw25			
	B49(21)		Dw26			
	Bw50(21)					
	B51(5)					
	Bw52(5)					
	Bw53					
	Bw54(w22)					
	Bw55(w22)					
	Bw56(w22)					
	Bw57(17)					
	Bw58(17)					
	Bw59					
	Bw60(w40)					
	Bw61(w40)					
	Bw62(15)					
	Bw63(15)					
	Bw64(14)					
	Bw65(14)					
	Bw67					
	Bw70					
	Bw71(w70)					
	Bw72(w70)					
	Bw73					
	Bw75(15)					
	Bw76(15)					
	Bw77(15)					
	Bw4					
	Bw6					

tional Workshop in Aarhus adopted the microcytotoxicity method (2) developed by the staff of the National Institutes of Health (NIH), Bethesda, USA and this became the acknowledged international standard test procedure.

In the NIH microcytotoxicity test, 1 μl of antibody reacts with an equal volume of a preparation of separated lymphocytes in a polystyrene microwell tray. After 30 min incubation an excess of 5 μl of rabbit complement is added. The complement kills any cell sensitized with a complement-binding antibody—this is CDC. Dead cells are stained with eosin and the preparation is fixed with formalin. The proportion of viable and dead lymphocytes is assessed by eye using phase-contrast microscopy.

Fluorochromasia (3) is an alternative method of assessing cell death. The cells are pre-labelled with fluorescein diacetate (FDA) and tested in a CDC method. Viable cells retain the fluorescent dye, it is released from dead cells which are no longer visible under UV microscopy. A more stable label, carboxy-FDA (CFDA), has now been introduced; the signal is suitable for quantitation by the photomultiplier of automated reading systems (Section 5.2).

A range of antibody specificities is used in the different wells of the tray. The accurate assignment of an HLA antigen is based on the intimate knowledge of the characteristic, often idiosyncratic, reaction patterns of the sera used.

2. USES OF HLA TYPING

HLA typing has found widespread practical use in medicine, genetics and law. The major clinical application of HLA typing is the typing of potential transplant recipients' waiting lists and transplant donors, with the objective of matching the donor with the most suitable recipient. National and international kidney transplant databases show superior survival for well matched tissue.

Many blood transfusion centres throughout the world hold lists of HLA-typed blood donors. These lists are used to provide HLA-compatible platelets for thrombocytopenic patients sensitized to HLA antigens by previous transfusion. In many transfusion centres, donors have volunteered to donate bone marrow to matched unrelated recipients. Registries of these donors have been established and together they total in excess of 100 000 potential volunteers. The bone marrow registers are searched in an effort to find suitable donors for those patients with no HLA identical sibs.

Another application of HLA typing is in the study of the susceptibility to certain auto-immune diseases. The function of HLA antigens in initiating and regulating immune responses make it especially important in diseases caused, in part, by immune dysregulation. An extreme example of this phenomenon is the severe combined immune deficiency accompanying the 'bare lymphocyte syndrome', where there is a total absence of expression of HLA on tissue cells. If in auto-immune diseases an increased risk of disease is associated with one or more HLA phenotypes, for example HLA-DR4 and rheumatoid arthritis, then studies of the patterns of HLA and disease inheritance in affected families may provide information on susceptibility factors and eventually the pathogenesis of the disease process itself. Various publications (4,5) can be consulted as a first step in studying the association of HLA with a particular disease.

The association between HLA and disease can sometimes be spectacular: in narcolepsy almost all of the patients tested have inherited HLA-DR2 and over 90% of patients with ankylosing spondylitis (AS) possess the HLA-B27 antigen. This high incidence of B27 in patients with AS has led to a test for HLA-B27 antigen being used as a diagnostic indicator. The information gained by this test is of maximum value when the clinical evidence and radiography leave the rheumatologist in some doubt over the diagnosis.

The value of the HLA system in legal work arises from its extraordinary polymorphism. Over 100 antigens are recognized and the chance of two unrelated individuals sharing a phenotype is slim. In countries where the law encourages paternity and inheritance problems to be resolved by blood tests, HLA typing is used as the most discriminating of the serological methods. In many affiliation cases the HLA types can on the one hand exclude a falsely accused man or, on the other hand, may lead to a conclusion of a calculable high probability of paternity.

This chapter describes in detail some of the serological methods in use for the determination of the HLA types. The newer methods of biochemical analysis, gene probing and the techniques based on cell culture and cloning are outside the scope of this volume on antibodies. The reader is referred to ref. 6 and other texts for broader information on these other developments.

3. THE NIH MICROCYTOTOXICITY TEST

This section concentrates on the detailed procedure for performing an HLA type by the NIH method. This is followed (Section 4) by an alternative approach with a shorter incubation in which cells are separated and tested in the presence of monoclonal antibody (Mab) bound to magnetic beads. The bead technique offers substantial time savings. Procedures to identify, characterize and standardize the serological reagents for routine typing are described in Sections 5 and 6. A list of equipment, reagents and their suppliers is given in the Appendix of Suppliers. An outline of the major steps in HLA typing is shown in *Figure 1*.

Tissue typing involves many transfers of sample between containers. In order to avoid disaster, carefully label every container or tray, *before use*, and check the identity deliberately at each transfer. It is sound practice to transfer, layer or separate just one sample at a time into a single fresh bottle in a rack containing no other samples (*Figure 2*). In the interests of safety, wear surgical gloves if skin contamination with blood is likely, and take special care with the fine needles (although they should be 'squared-off' and thus blunted) on the microsyringes.

3.1 Preparation of HLA typing trays

It is conventional to use two, three or even four sera of each HLA specificity (if they are available) to give confidence in the assignment of an HLA phenotype. With such a polymorphic system most laboratories find it necessary to use two microwell trays of 60 wells (or 72 wells) to hold all the sera needed for an HLA-A and B type. HLA-C locus sera might use a third tray and HLA-DR and DQ sera, yet another. The trays of sera are prepared in batches at leisure and stored frozen. In order to prevent the evaporation of the antisera, in storage or in use, the trays are loaded with paraffin oil before the sera are dispensed. A minimum volume (3 μl) of a 'light' paraffin oil is

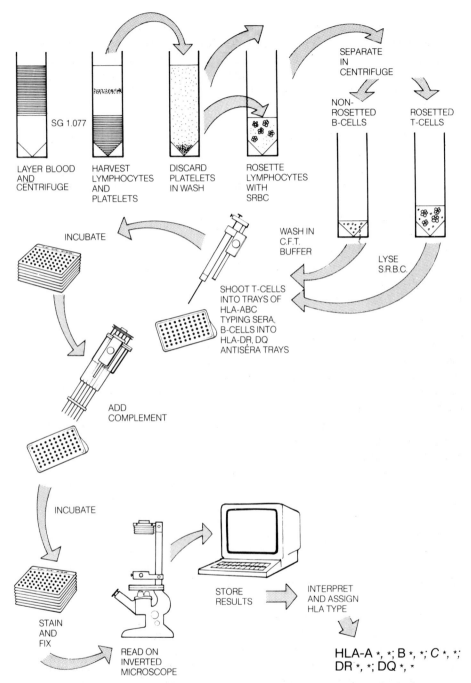

Figure 1. A summary of the procedures used in the determination of an HLA type by serology.

advisable when the 'shooting' technique is to be employed for dispensing the test lymphocytes (Section 3.6).

The contamination of one serum with another is the most frequent cause of poor

35

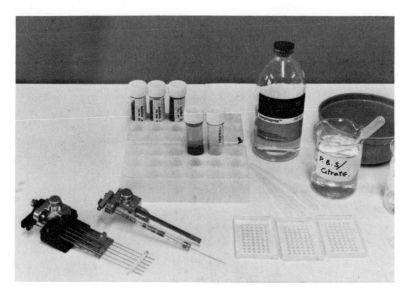

Figure 2. Lymphocyte separation and typing bench showing a syringe delivering 1 μl and a multiple unit delivering 6 × 5 μl operated by repeating dispensers.

Table 2. Preparation of HLA typing trays.

1.	Label microwell (Terasaki) trays with the serum batch number. Add 3 μl of light paraffin oil (sp. grav. 0.830−0.860) to each well using an automatic oiler or a six-way stream splitter fitted on a 1 ml disposable syringe operated with a 50-step repeating dispenser.
2.	Thaw a 200 μl reservoir tray (Greiner, Seromat) of serum rapidly at 37°C and check that the seal is intact, or thaw individual microfuge tubes of serum. Shake tray carefully to overcome any freezer concentration. Centrifuge the tray at 200 g for 2 min to deposit all the serum. Peel off the seal.
3.	Fill the syringes of an automatic dispenser with serum, discharge and refill, repeat until no more air bubbles are released.
4.	Discharge static electricity by pressing the microwell trays onto damp paper towels for a second or two. Add 1 μl of serum to all the wells of an entire tray by machine, or add one row of six sera manually to all the trays in turn using a repeating dispenser fitted with six 50-μl syringes. Place the needle tips below the oil surface before pressing the dispenser button; take care to avoid micro-droplet cross-contamination.
5.	Flush the syringes (or machine) thoroughly (10−12 times) in fresh CFT buffer[a] between serum sets.
6.	Inspect all the trays and mark the position of any missing antisera in felt tip pen on the underside of the tray.
7.	Fit lids, centrifuge the trays at 200 g for 2 min in a centrifuge with large buckets (Centra 7 or Beckman TJ6) or in microtitre plate carriers, to centre the sera in the bottom of the wells.
8.	Freeze and store the trays at −30°C or below.
9.	Make one copy of the tray map for each tray prepared.

[a]CFT or Veronal buffer, pH 7.2 (available as tablets from Oxoid): barbitone, 575 mg; barbitone soluble, 185 mg; $MgCl_2$, 168 mg; $CaCl_2$, 28 mg; NaCl, 8.5 g; water to 1 litre; sterilize in an autoclave.

reproducibility in HLA typing. Disposable pipettes or tips are advised for handling supplies of serum in bulk. When preparing trays or handling sera with permanent non-disposable equipment, a thorough washing of the syringe, pipette or machine between each serum is essential. When wiping or blotting dry the tips or the needles a fresh area of tissue should be used. The deliberate introduction of air bubbles will help to scour the walls of the syringes.

The following section gives guidelines on the handling of sera to prepare the batches of HLA typing reagents. *Table 2* gives details on the 'plating-out' of the sera into the individual typing trays.

The typing sera for a batch of typing trays are selected on the basis of their specificity, quality and volume, then listed in the specificity order desired on a paper chart or map of a microwell tray, or in a computer. The map order is arranged in a continuous serpentine fashion from the negative control to the last serum in the tray, to facilitate the rapid addition of cells. Well no. 1 is reserved for the negative control, the pre-tested serum of a non-transfused blood group AB male donor, and well no. 2 is reserved for a positive control of a cytotoxic monomorphic Mab or a mixture of multi-reactive cytotoxic allo-antisera.

The sera are thawed rapidly at 37°C and stored, when thawed, on melting ice. They are clarified and made lipid-free by centrifugation for 5 min at 13 000 g in a microcentrifuge to ensure good optical qualities on microscopy. The serum beneath the lipid layer is separated and stained with a 1% volume of a 1% (v/v) aqueous solution of phenol red to give a visual contrast in the tray. The food dyestuffs, certicol carmosine (red), certicol tartrazine (yellow) and brilliant blue (FCS 172291) can be added as an alternative, in concentrations of 1/2000−1/4000, as a colourful aid to inspection and identification. Sodium azide (10 μl, 10% w/v), is then added to each ml of serum to prevent bacterial contamination (Section 5.5). The sera are dispensed, with a calibrated pipette, in a standard volume into batches in a series of labelled polypropylene 400 μl microcentrifuge tubes or in the reservoir trays of an automatic dispenser.

The stock of 400 μl tubes are stored frozen at −30°C or below in racks which retain the preferred order of the typing batch. If a dispenser reservoir is used, non-toxic tray sealing tape is applied with firm pressure to obtain a perfect seal before the reservoirs of bulk serum are frozen. Do not remove or replace this seal until the batch is about to be dispensed—a replaced seal often fails.

3.2 The specimen for HLA typing

Ten ml of fresh anticoagulated blood is the minimum volume required although 20 ml is more usual. Store the sample at room temperature (not 4°C) for up to 24 h if necessary. Storage for more than 24 h gives increasingly unreliable results due to a rising background cell death. The more alkaline anticoagulants (*Table 3*), trisodium citrate and citrate phosphate−dextrose, are preferred to acid citrate−dextrose. Sequestrene (EDTA) is not usual in HLA typing. Defibrination is carried out immediately the blood is collected. It has an advantage in providing a platelet-free preparation but the lymphocyte yield is lower. Sterile preservative-free heparin is the anticoagulant of choice when lymphocyte culture methods are proposed.

3.3 Preservation of lymphocytes

Freshly collected blood must be HLA-typed within 36−48 h. Thereafter falling viability makes the cytotoxicity test impractical. For work of the very highest quality the typing should be completed within 24 h of sample collection.

Table 3. Anticoagulants for HLA typing.

Anticoagulant	Anticoagulant volume	Blood volume	Preparation
Trisodium citrate – dextrose	2 ml	20 ml	31.3 g Trisodium citrate (dihydrate) 10.0 g Dextrose 1.0 litres Distilled water Sterilize by filtration, pH 8.25
Liquid heparin	150 μl	20 ml	Liquid preservative-free heparin (1000 IU/ml)
Dried heparin	125 – 150 IU	10 ml	Dried preserved lithium heparin (collect 2 tubes)
Citrate phosphate – dextrose	3 ml	20 ml	26.3 g Trisodium citrate (dihydrate) 25.5 g Dextrose 3.27 g Citric acid (monohydrate) 2.22 g NaH_2PO_4 (monohydrate) 1.0 litres Distilled water Sterilize by filtration, pH 5.53
Defribination	Nil	20 ml	Gently swirl the blood, directly after collection, in a small sterile flask with 6 – 8 glass beads, 4 mm diameter, or 6 – 8 twisted paperclips or 4 – 5 applicator sticks for 8 – 10 min.

The life of the lymphocytes can be extended to about 2 – 3 weeks by sterile separation of the cells and storage in Park/Terasaki medium (7) which contains McCoy's 5A medium buffered with Hepes, 10% (v/v) fetal bovine serum (FBS) and antibiotics. Longer term storage involves freezing the cells using dimethyl sulphoxide (DMSO) as the cryoprotective agent. A final concentration of 10% (v/v) DMSO in the surrounding medium, followed by cooling at 1°C/min and storage in tubes or straws in liquid nitrogen is the conventional method. Thawing is rapid, with the temperature of the thawed material not being allowed to rise much above 0°C until the DMSO has been removed by washing (*Table 4*). Local variations on the basic method can be found in a booklet produced by the Council of Europe Committee of Experts in Histocompatibility (8).

Lymphocytes can also be frozen successfully in 7% (v/v) DMSO in microwell trays and stored in a deep freeze at −70°C (9). This approach allows a whole panel of cells to be stored on a single tray for the rapid identification of HLA antibodies.

3.4 Lymphocyte separation by density (isopyknic) centrifugation

The separation of lymphoid cells from whole blood by density (*Figure 3*) relies on a careful layering of diluted whole blood onto the surface of a medium which contains a red cell aggregating agent and which has a specific gravity of 1.077 (10). Suitable ready-made sterile lymphocyte separation media are available from most biological suppliers. Alternative approaches include: Sepracell® (Sepratech Corp.), a silica gel medium which requires mixing rather than layering, a shorter centrifugation time and an angle rotor (11); Lymphoquik® (One Lambda Corp.), a series of lymphocyte separation reagents based on lysing mixtures of Mabs; and Dynabeads® (Dynal UK),

Table 4. Freezing and recovery of lymphocytes in 10% dimethyl sulphoxide.

Freezing

1. Count lymphocytes and estimate the volume of diluent required to give a cell concentration of 1×10^7/ml. Take that volume of RPMI 1640 and mix with an equal volume of inert AB serum or autologous serum or plasma.
2. Add half the prepared diluent to the packed lymphocytes, resuspend gently and place in melting ice (concentration 1×10^7/ml).
3. Discard 20% of the volume of the diluent remaining, add DMSO to the diluent to restore the original volume. Place in melting ice for 10 min.
4. Gently stir the lymphocytes, add all the DMSO mixture a drop at a time to give 5×10^6/ml lymphocytes in 10% (v/v) DMSO.
5. Dispense the lymphocytes rapidly in small volumes into leak-proof tubes or straws.
6. Freeze in a controlled rate freezer with lymphocyte program (cool at $1-1.5°$C/min until $-30°$C, thereafter at $7°$C/min, with N_2 boost at critical eutectic point). Store in liquid N_2 vapour, **or** place cool tubes or straws in a cool polystyrene box, place in $-80°$C freezer overnight, store in liquid N_2 vapour thereafter, **or** place tubes or straws in freezing plug suspended in the neck of a liquid N_2 storage container, store in liquid N_2 vapour thereafter.

Recovery

1. Rapidly thaw cells by immersing in $37°$C water bath, swirl continuously until all the ice has nearly melted.
2. Gently add 10 vols of 50% (v/v) inert AB serum/RPMI 1640 medium, centrifuge at 400 g for 5 min.
3. Remove supernatant, wash cells at least twice (300 g, 4 min) in large volumes of CFT buffer to remove all traces of inhibiting soluble HLA material. Resuspend the cells in CFT buffer to $2-3$ times the volume originally frozen.
4. Add 1 μl 1% w/v trypan blue in phosphate-buffered serum (PBS)[a] to 1 μl lymphocytes in microwell tray, centrifuge at 100 g for 2 min, examine for viability—dead cells are large and pale blue, living cells are small and refractile. Adjust cell count if necessary.
5. If the material is irreplaceable and there are a large number of dead cells then the method below may allow an HLA type to be salvaged.

Removal of dead cells

1. Mix 4.5 ml of Percoll® (Pharmacia) with 0.5 ml 9% (w/v) NaCl to give an isotonic solution, add 6.25 ml PBS to give 40% isotonic Percoll.
2. Suspend the cell pellet in $3-4$ ml 40% Percoll, centrifuge at 800 g for 5 min.
3. Remove and discard the supernatant containing the dead cells and debris, wash the button of viable lymphocytes twice in CFT buffer, examine for viability and count as above.

[a]Available in tablet form from Oxoid; 200 mg KCl, 200 mg KH_2PO_4, 1.15 g Na_2HPO_4, 8.0 g NaCl, water to 1 litre, pH 7.3.

a Mab lymphocyte separation method using magnetized beads (12) described in detail in Section 4. A protocol for the density centrifugation method is described in detail in *Table 5*. Dilution of blood improves the lymphocyte yield.

The dilution fluid and first wash solution contain anticoagulant to avoid clotting and clumping of the platelet-rich suspensions. All the solutions are clarified by membrane filtration (0.45 μ) or centrifugation in order to remove small particles which interfere with microscopy. The final lymphocyte suspension fluid supports complement lysis. Hanks' buffered salt solution, or various tissue culture media with adequate calcium and magnesium ions, are as satisfactory as complement fixation test (CFT) buffer. The addition of a 2% volume of FBS to the wash fluids prevents the loss of B lymphocytes by adherence to plastic surfaces. Any glassware should be pre-siliconized.

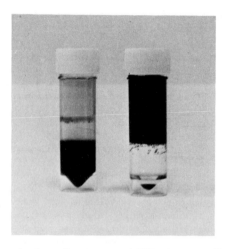

Figure 3. Blood layered onto density medium (sp. grav. 1.077) prior to centrifugation (right), small clumps of red cells can be seen settling in rouleaux. After centrifugation (left), showing diffuse layer of lymphocytes and platelets at the interface between the medium and the plasma.

Table 5. Density separation of lymphocytes from whole blood.

1.	Add 20 ml diluent to 20 ml whole blood, use PBS alone, PBS/citrate[a] or PBS/heparin[b] for diluting defibrinated, citrated or heparinized blood, respectively.
2.	Add 7−8 ml lymphocyte separation medium[c] (sp. grav. 1.077) to two 30 ml, 25 mm diameter sterile containers[c].
3.	Draw the diluted blood into a disposable polythene bulb pipette, rest the tip on the inside surface of the container for support just above the liquid—layer all the blood onto the surface by squeezing the bulb gently. Do not break the surface of the medium by over vigorous pipetting, move the pipette to the top of the tube as the level of blood increases.
4.	Centrifuge at 400 *g* for 20 min in swing-out buckets.
5.	Remove the entire cloudy layers of lymphocytes and platelets with a bulb pipette, combine into one bottle and wash at 300 *g* for 5 min in 25 ml PBS/citrate.
6.	Discard the supernatant platelets, resuspend the lymphoid cells initially in 1−2 ml PBS, then add 25 ml PBS and wash at 300 *g* for 4 min.
7.	Discard supernatant, wash the cells twice with 25 ml CFT buffer at 300 *g* for 4 min.
8.	Resuspend the cells in 6 ml of CFT buffer, place a drop in an Improved Neubauer counting chamber and count the cells in a defined area. Adjust the bulk with CFT buffer to achieve 200 cells in 1 mm^2: equivalent to 2×10^6/ml.
9.	Take 5 ml of standardized suspension for B lymphocyte enrichment and use the remainder for HLA-ABC type.

[a]PBS/citrate: 100 ml PBS, trisodium citrate·$2H_2O$.
[b]PBS/heparin: 100 ml PBS, 750 µl preservation free heparin (100 IU/ml).
[c]Sterilin.

3.5 B and T lymphocyte preparation

All peripheral blood lymphocytes may be typed for the HLA-ABC antigens (class I). The HLA-DR and DQ antigens (class II) are present only on the B lymphocytes and monocytes in normal peripheral blood. These cells constitute about 10−15% of the population harvested by density centrifugation. The B lymphocyte proportion is raised by enrichment of the B cells or depletion of the T cells, prior to class II typing.

Table 6. Separation of T and B lymphocytes by rosetting with sheep cells.

Reagents

Neuraminidase Type V (Sigma) Prepare 1 unit/ml stock solution, store frozen.

GET buffer Dissolve 1 g gelatine (Sigma), 3.72 g disodium EDTA·2H$_2$O, 2 g NaCl in 1 litre distilled water, adjust to pH 7.2 with 0.1 M Tris buffer. Sterilize by autoclaving. Add 1 g glucose to 100 ml buffer before use.

Polybrene (Sigma) 0.5 g Polybrene in 10 ml water, store stock solution at 4°C, dilute 5 μl in 150 μl PBS for use.

Neuraminidase-treated SRBC (N'ase/SRBC) Prepare weekly. Layer 10 ml of citrated SRBC onto 7 ml (sp. grav. 1.077) lymphocyte medium, centrifuge at 400 *g* for 20 min, discard all top layers to remove dead sheep lymphocytes and leave packed SRBC. Wash SRBC twice in PBS. Add 1 unit of neuraminidase to 1 ml of packed SRBC in 25 ml of PBS, incubate in a 37°C water bath for 30 min. Wash N'ase/SRBC three times in PBS, resuspend in 100 ml of GET buffer, store at 4°C.

Albuminized Ficoll/Isopaque Dissolve 26 g Ficoll 400 in 200 ml of distilled water, add 100 ml of 20% (v/v) bovine albumin solution. Adjust sp. grav. to 1.077 with Isopaque checking with hydrometer. Store frozen in 20 ml aliquots.

Method

1. Add 5 ml of peripheral lymphocytes at 2.0 × 10^6/ml in PBS/FBS to 5 ml of N'ase/SRBC and 100 μl of polybrene in a 8 mm diameter plastic centrifuge tube. Incubate at room temperature for 5 min with gentle mixing. Centrifuge at 200 *g* for 3 min to form firm rosettes, remove 5 ml of supernatant.

2. Resuspend cells by very gentle mixing or careful pipetting with a wide bore disposable Pasteur pipette. Add 5 ml of albuminized Ficoll/Isopaque by placing the tip of the plastic pipette at the bottom of the tube and under-layering with separation medium. Centrifuge at 400 *g* for 8 min.

3. Harvest non-rosetted cells (B lymphocyte enriched) from interface. Wash three times in CFT buffer/FBS, standardize after third wash at 2 × 10^6/ml in CFT buffer/FBS.

T cell recovery

1. Remove all fluid remaining above rosetted red cell button. Add 2.5 ml of 0.2% (w/v) NaCl, mix thoroughly to lyse all SRBC.

2. Quench lysing solution after 10 sec with 7.5 ml of 1.0% (w/v) NaCl. Centrifuge at 800 *g* for 3 min, discard supernatant, wash twice in CFT buffer, standardize in CFT buffer at 2 × 10^6/ml.

The protocol described in detail in *Table 6* is based on a T-rosetting method (13). Sheep red blood cells (SRBC) adhere to T lymphocytes—these 'rosettes' are particularly robust when the SRBC are first de-sialiated with neuraminidase and are enhanced by the presence of polybrene (14). 2-Aminoethylisothiouronium bromide (Sigma) treatment of SRBC has similar rosette-enhancing effects (15). The B lymphocytes are recovered by flotation on a density medium, T cell rosettes aggregate in rouleaux with the SRBC and sediment to the bottom of the tube.

Table 7. The NIH microcytotoxicity test (standard incubation).

1.	Thaw the selected typing trays at room temperature.
2.	Fill a 80 μl syringe fitted on a 80-step repeating dispenser (Robbins) with the lymphocyte suspension at 2.0×10^6/ml. Ensure the syringe is completely free of air and check the shooting efficiency before starting.
3.	For accuracy, hold the needle and position the tip about 4–5 mm from the surface of the oil. Shoot 1 μl of cells into each well by a firm press on the dispenser button and follow the serpentine order used in the serum distribution until all the appropriate trays have been seeded with the lymphocyte suspension.
4.	Inspect each well and check that the cells and serum have mixed together.
5.	Note the starting time and incubate at 22°C for 30 min.
6.	Completely fill and flush the syringe four or five times with clean CFT buffer before dispensing the next sample.
7.	Thaw frozen rabbit complement, or reconstitute lyophilized complement, 5 min before it is needed and store on melting ice.
8.	Rinse the syringes of a Robbins 250 μl multiple repeating dispenser with CFT buffer 4–5 times, then fill with complement and expel all air.
9.	When the 30 min initial incubation is completed, hold the mutiple syringe unit upright and carefully shoot 5 μl of complement into each row of the tray.
10.	Re-incubate the trays at 22°C for 1 h.
11.	Centrifuge 20 ml of formalin[a] and 20 ml of eosin[b] solution for 5 min at 400 g.
12.	Using dispensers fitted with stream splitters, add 2.5 μl of eosin to each well. When the 1 h second incubation is completed, 2–3 min later, add 8 μl of formalin to each well in a fume cupboard or exhaust filtered cabinet (*Figure 4*).
13.	Flatten the meniscus with a 75 mm $\times$ 50 mm glass slide or use a polystyrene coverslip with an adhesive seal (One Lambda).
14.	Replace tray lids, store the trays in an exhaust filtered cabinet or in storage boxes in a 4°C refrigerator.

[a]Formalin solution (37–41% w/v). Add one drop 1% (w/v) nitrazine yellow indicator to 100 ml formalin, add 10% (w/v) KOH until pale blue (pH ~7.2). The response of delicate pH electrodes is dulled by formalin. CAUTION. Never add HCl to re-acidify formalin—bis-chloromethyl ether can be formed: it is extremely carcinogenic.
[b]Eosin solution: 25 g eosin yellowish, 500 ml H_2O.

Another method in widespread use separates the B cells by adherence to a short column of scrubbed nylon wool (Fenwal 3-denier, 3.81 cm, type 200) contained in a wide plastic drinking straw (16). After a short incubation the non-adherent T cells are washed off and collected, the B cells are then released by vigorous squeezing of the flexible straw and recovered by washing.

The use of a fluorescent anti-immunoglobulin (anti-Ig) to tag the surface Ig of B lymphocytes is an alternative approach which allows class II typing of unseparated lymphocytes (17). The CDC test trays are examined with an inverted fluorescence microscope; the lymphocytes are classified as B cells or T cells by the presence or absence of fluorescent caps and the viability of each cell population visualized independently by ethidium bromide staining.

The rosetting method yields a higher proportion of class-II-bearing cells than the nylon wool adherence method, but non-viable cells are also enriched in the B cell fraction. T and B cell separation with Mab kits save time by replacing the lymphocyte preparation phase of conventional methods. The two-colour immunofluorescence method need glass bottomed trays and fluorescence microscopy. The magnetic bead separation method not only produces isolated cells more quickly, but also enables the CDC test incubation

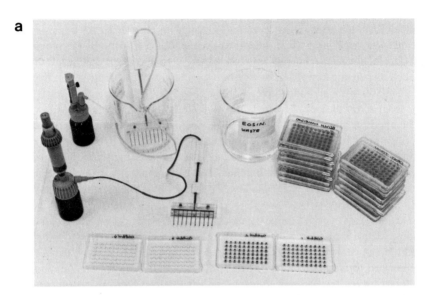

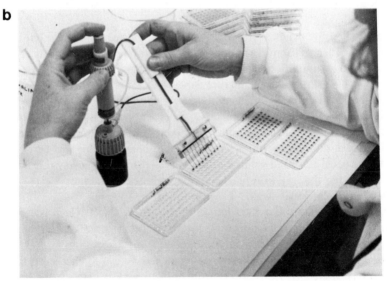

Figure 4. (**a**) Microdispensers and 10-way stream splitters in use for eosin staining and formalin fixation. (**b**) Microdispenser (25 μl) and 10-way stream splitter in use for eosin staining.

time to be shortened, giving a considerable overall saving in time. The trays must be examined, however, on an inverted fluorescence microscope.

3.6 The microcytotoxicity method

This section describes in detail (*Table 7*) an example of the type of procedures which have evolved to produce high quality, reproducible HLA typing results. The correct handling and use of the repeating 1 μl dispenser is a crucial factor in the quest for good

43

reproducibility, the contamination of one serum with another (carry-over) is a major cause of error especially when potent sera are under test—it must be avoided at all costs. Careful syringe technique can reduce these errors to a very low level, the needle of the cell dispensing syringe must never come into contact with the serum in the well. With a suitable syringe and needle, 1 μl of cells may be accurately ejected into the serum from a distance of 4—5 mm, the so-called 'shooting technique'.

To be good for shooting, a repeating dispenser must have a light, snappy action and the syringe must be mounted rigidly so none of the energy of the advancing piston is dissipated. The syringe must have a fine needle with a square-cut end and in use it must be rigorously checked for air bubbles. Two or three cycles of a vigorous discharge of the entire contents of the syringe followed by slow filling will usually clear any trapped air.

A study on carry-over in European laboratories (18), using potent Mabs, demonstrated that some methods of adding the cells were most unsatisfactory whilst 'shooting' and a careful 'no touch' technique (the needle never touching the serum, only the oil) reduced contamination to a bare minimum. For really accurate work it is recommended that up to three successive wells of diluent should be placed between potent monoclonal reagents to collect the traces of contamination and protect the monoclonals from each other.

Before use ensure that the syringe delivers the cell suspension in discrete 1 μl drops, which detach cleanly from the needle with no spray or micro-droplets, by shooting a few μl onto a tray lid and checking the droplet pattern. A fine cleaning wire and detergent can be used to clear internal debris and a fine-toothed file can be used by trial and error to modify the shape of the needle until intact 1 μl droplets of liquid are ejected cleanly from the needle tip.

Adding the cells to the tray in a consistent serpentine pattern ensures that any carry-over that does occur will always be in the same direction and may possibly be identified as such. If a 50 μl syringe is used for cell dispensing, always break off exactly halfway through the tray to refill the syringe with cells and thus locate consistently the position of the restart well.

Automatic dispensers (Lambda Jet, Bio-Tec) are available which add lymphocyte suspensions to the prepared typing trays by the 'shooting' technique, eliminating many of the problems of manual syringe handling and cell dispensing.

After cell dispensing, all the wells are examined by eye to check that the droplets have become mixed—a viewing box with suitable backlighting can be helpful. Any unmixed drops of cells and sera can be made to coalesce by use of a high frequency spark generator, or by careful prodding with a spare metal syringe piston which is rinsed and dried in absorbent tissue between wells.

The incubation times in *Table 7* are standard for typing unseparated cells and T cells. Class II antigens are tested in extended incubation. One hour is allowed for the first incubation period, followed by 2 h after the addition of complement.

3.7 **Reading eosin/formalin trays**

Formalin-fixed trays are readable for 2—3 days if they are stored in a box which prevents evaporation. Handle the trays gently so that air bubbles (which interfere with the phased light beam) are not introduced into the wells beneath the coverslide. Check the alignment

Table 8. Scoring of cytotoxicity by phase-contrast microscopy using eosin staining and formalin fixation.

Living lymphocytes

Intact cells are spherical and strongly refract the phased light, thus appearing as small yellowy discs shining with a bright halo, against a red background of eosin.

Dead lymphocytes

Dead lymphocytes are flattened and appear to be much larger than the bright viable cells, they are a dull grey-black, no brighter than the surrounding medium. Fragments of darkly stained material traces out the cell outline and gives a speckled appearance to the cell surface.

Scoring convention

Score	Microscopy	Interpretation
0[a]	Not readable	Void
1[a]	0−10% dead cells	Negative
2	11−20% dead cells	Doubtful negative
4	21−40% dead cells	Doubtful weak positive
6	41−80% dead cells	Positive
8	81−100% dead cells	Strong positive

[a]Some computer systems use the convention X = void, 0 or − = negative.
[b]The convention recommended by the American Society for Histocompatibility and Immunogenetics (ASHI) places the boundary between a score of 4 and a score of 6 at 50%.

of the phase annulus on an inverted microscope fitted with phase-contrast optics, a ×10 objective, ×10 or ×15 eyepieces and a 81 mm × 56 mm tray holder on a mechanical stage. All manufacturers have suitable models; check particularly the comfort of the working position and the operation of the stage controls.

(i)   Locate the microwell tray on the stage and check the orientation. Move well no. 1 into the light-path and assess the percentage of dead lymphocytes seen in the field of view of the negative control (*Table 8*). Examine this well thoroughly, it is the normal background cell death for this particular preparation. It is usual to estimate the percentage of cell death in each well over and above the background level seen in the negative control. If the absolute level of cell death in the negative control is around 50%, then grading of the results is abandoned and only strong positive reactions are recorded.

(ii)   Check that the positive control gives 100% cell death.

(iii)   Examine well no. 3 for a few seconds and assess the percentage cell death. Record the score on a copy of the appropriate tray map using the convention in *Table 8*.

(iv)   Examine the rest of the wells in sequence taking care to record the results in the correct map location.

B cell enrichment by rosetting and depletion of viable T cells concentrates any dead cells in the B cell fraction. This enrichment with non-viable cells, taken together with the toxic effects of the extended incubation, slows the reading process. Every well has to be thoroughly and skilfully surveyed to assess accurately the killing mediated by HLA antibody.

The discrimination becomes unreliable if the background rises over 40% no matter what the cell source. If the background is over 70% and a lymphocyte suspension is

Table 9. Interpretation of HLA typing results.

1.	Discard results if positive control well shows weak cytotoxicity only, or cell death of over 70% is seen in the negative control well.
2.	Interpret with caution any type with over 40% spontaneous cell death.
3.	Always consider alternative explanations to the obvious assignment, look for contradictory evidence in unusual or unexpected positive or negative serum reactions.
4.	Assign a 'broad' antigen to a cell when the pattern of reactions matches the documented antigen pattern established by previous experience with cells of known phenotype. Re-examine any well which is inconsistent with this assignment.
5.	Assign an antigen 'split' if the parent 'broad' antigen is present and the appropriate 'split' sera give a recognizable and unambiguous reaction pattern.
6.	Reconsider B locus interpretation in the light of the supertypic specificities Bw4 and Bw6.
7.	Reconsider the DR1-w18 assignment proposed in the light of the DRw52 and DRw53 supertypic specificities and the DQw1 − DQw9 types found.
8.	Compare mentally the known linkage disequilibrium in the population with the most likely haplotypes possible from the antigens assigned.
9.	Confirm that the type is consistent with any previous results on the individual or a family member.
10.	Make the interpretation and store with all the typing serum results on a computer or on a manual chart for later analysis, investigation and statistics.

Report the results, drawing attention to any weak, curious or otherwise doubtful findings and recommend further work, for example:

1.	Repeat typing on a fresh specimen and test on more comprehensive trays.
2.	Confirm that a blank antigen at any locus is due to homozygosity by a family study.
3.	Re-bleed and, with the agreement of an experienced or more specialized laboratory, send for investigation any HLA blanks which are unlikely to be due to homozygosity, cases of triple antigens as the products of a single locus and other cases of interest or uncertainty.
4.	Establish a lymphoblastoid cell line where weak reactions have been obtained, for repeat of the serology and possible analysis by molecular genetics or biochemistry.

still available, a type might be salvaged by re-testing after Percoll® separation (*Table 4*). If this is unsuccessful a repeat type is required on a fresh specimen.

3.8 **Interpretation of HLA typing results**

The assignment of an HLA type to a cell is dependent on the quality and the specificity of the antisera in the typing batch, the experience of the typer and the quality of the technical performance of the CDC test. An experienced typer knows the reaction patterns expected of the antigens of the local population and is also aware of the likely contaminants of the typing sera, of supertypic specificities, of antigen 'splits', of antigen frequencies and of the linkage disequilibrium (HLA haplotypes occurring more frequently than expected) demonstrated in the population being typed.

A routine typing batch contains reagents reacting with the antigens found in the local community. If a selection of sera is available, two or three (or more) examples of each specificity are used. Monospecific sera are capable of giving unambiguous results but sera containing multiple specificities are equally useful, providing the reactivity of the components is precisely defined.

A second batch of discriminating sera may be used to retype a cell where the interpretation is not clear or when the original type suggests homozygosity (i.e. when

Table 10. The splits of original broad HLA specificities.

Original broad specificities	Splits[a]
A9	A23,A24
A10	A25,A26,Aw34,Aw66
Aw19	A29,A30,A31,A32,Aw33,Aw74
A28	Aw68,Aw69
B5	B51,Bw52
B12	B44,B45
B14	Bw64,Bw65
B15	Bw62,Bw63,Bw75,Bw76,Bw77
B16	B38,B39
B17	Bw57,Bw58
B21	B49,Bw50
Bw22	Bw54,Bw55,Bw56
B40	Bw60,Bw61
Bw70	Bw71,Bw72
Cw3	Cw9,Cw10
DR2	DRw15,DRw16
DR3	DRw17,DRw18
DR5	DRw11,DRw12
DRw6	DRw13,DRw14
DQw1	DQw5,DQw6
DQw3	DQw7,DQw8,DQw9
Dw6	Dw18,Dw19
Dw7	Dw11,Dw17

[b]Bw4: B5,B13,B17,B27,B37,B38(16),B44(12),Bw47,B49(21),B51(5),Bw52(5),Bw53,
Bw57(17),Bw58(17),Bw59,Bw63(15),Bw77(15).
[b]Bw6: B7,B8,B14,B18,Bw22,B35,B39(16),B40,Bw41,Bw42,B45(12),Bw46,Bw48,Bw50(21),
Bw54(w22),Bw55(w22),Bw56(w22),Bw60(40),Bw61(40),Bw62(15),Bw64(14),Bw65(14),
Bw67,Bw70,Bw71(w70),Bw72(w70),Bw73,Bw75(15),Bw76(15).

[c]DRw52: DR3,DR5,DRw6,DRw8,DRw11(5),DRw12(5),DRw13(w6),DRw14(w6),DRw17(3),
DRw18(3).
[c]DRw53: DR4,DR7,DR9.

[a]The listing of a broad specificity in parentheses after a narrow specificity, e.g. HLA-A23(9) is optional.
[b]These specificities are generally agreed inclusions of HLA-B specificities Bw4 and Bw6.
[c]These specificities are generally agreed to be associated with DRw52 and DRw53.

a single antigen is detected as the product of a locus). Interpretation of the type from the serum reactions follows the guidelines of *Table 9*.

A new laboratory with only a little experience of the local antigen patterns must assess the reliability of the individual antisera by reference to the package inserts which accompany mailed antisera. The antigens are assigned initially by taking account of the most reliable antisera according to the paperwork—the information should include a 2 × 2 table for each specificity and the correlation coefficient (*r*), an indication of the serum strength (%8) and a quality indication (Q value).

The most frequent antigens in the population will be quickly recognized and the antigen patterns established, leading to a local assessment of the supplied sera and a critical

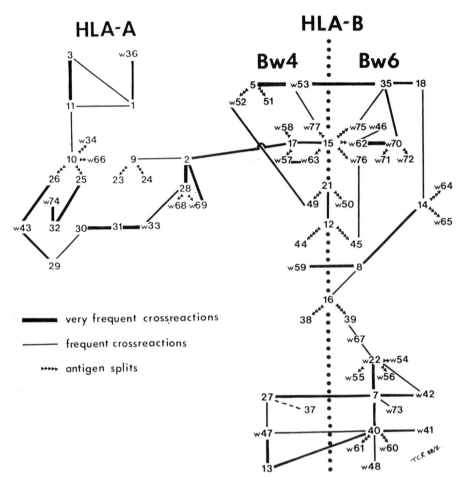

Figure 5. Frequent cross-reactions found in HLA-A and HLA-B antisera.

review of the HLA types assigned during the learning process. An arrangement should be made with an experienced laboratory to act in a reference capacity with all problem cells in order to ensure accuracy in all phenotyping and to secure entry into a regional quality assessment scheme.

3.9 The serology of the HLA system

This section charts the serology of the HLA system in terms of antigen splits, supertypic and cross-reactive groups and includes the WHO nomenclature (36) for the HLA system revised in November 1987 (*Table 1*).

A number of HLA antigens have distinct small variations named 'antigen splits' which are sub-divisions of the same broad antigen. The splits are assigned by the use of (usually) rarer sera which react with a single narrow specificity (*Table 10*).

In the HLA-B locus, the splits of the broad antigens are often associated with a particular Bw4 or Bw6 antigen. Determination of the Bw4/w6 status is extremely useful

	DQw Splits		DRw 52	DRw53
DQw 1	DQw 5	DR1,w10,w16(2)	DRw14(w6)	
	DQw 6	DRw15(2)	DRw13(w6)	
DQw 2			DRw17(3)	DR 7
DQw 3	DQw 7		DRw11(5),w12(5),w8 DRw13(w6),w14(w6)	DR 4
	DQw 8			DR 4
	DQw 9			DR 7,9
DQw 4			DRw18(3),w8	DR 4

Figure 6. The usual associations between HLA-DRw52-w53, HLA-DQw1-w4 and HLA-DR1-w18.

in its own right to help confirm a broad antigen assignment: it has the added value of lending confidence to the typing of many antigen splits.

An individual immunized with a single HLA antigen often produces antibodies which react with cells bearing different private HLA specificities but perhaps sharing a common epitope (19). This phenomenon defines a number of cross-reactive groups (CREGS). The unexpected extra reactions seen in HLA typing can usually be explained by weak and unreliable antibodies directed against CREGS. If the CREG antibody is strong then the serum would appear to have two, three, or more, private specificities.

Figure 5 represents the relationship of the antigen splits and the CREGS in a diagrammatic form. In the HLA-B locus diagram, the Bw4-associated antigens are shown on the left and the Bw6-associated antigens on the right. The lines are drawn to represent cross-reactivity; the heavier the line, the more frequent the presence of antibody directed against the shared epitopes.

Figure 6 shows the strong association which exists between the DR and DQ loci. Immunization by a single haplotype will often produce a mixture of antibodies; antibodies to a HLA-DQ product, for example, are frequently contaminated with antibodies directed against HLA-DR.

3.10 HLA typing of cell lines

Epstein−Barr virus (EBV)-transformed cells express more HLA antigen than normal cells. This phenomenon can be helpful in phenotyping patients with renal failure and other difficult cases possessing unreactive lymphocytes which defy typing and

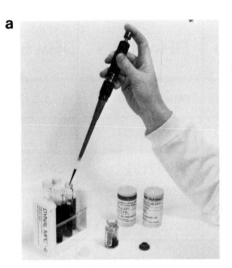

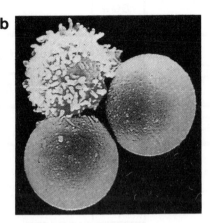

Figure 7. (a) Addition of Dynabeads® to blood samples held in magnetic separator. **(b)** Two beads adhering to a single cell. [Photomicrograph by courtesy of Dynal (UK) Ltd.]

interpretation. It is vital that the complement batch is screened before use, to demonstrate that it is not toxic in the CDC test to a selection of EBV-transformed cell lines (Section 6.1).

B lymphocytes are transformed by culture in the presence of EBV. A cell line is established in the presence of cyclosporin A (Sandoz) or phytohaemagglutinin (PHA; Wellcome) which are added to the culture to prevent T_c cells from killing the virus-infected cells.

The cell line should be recovered from liquid nitrogen and cultured for 2−3 days before attempting typing. Layering the cells onto 11% (v/v) Isopaque (Nycomed) and centrifuging at 400 g for 15 min, before routine washing and resuspension, removes cellular debris resulting in a clean preparation of viable cells (20).

The incubation times are shortened in the CDC test when typing cell lines: 30 min before complement and 60 min after for class II work, and 15 min plus 40 min for class I typing. With these incubation times the specificities of the class II typing sera will be a little broader than those assigned using full incubation with normal B cells—extra unexplained reactions will occur and careful records need to be maintained to help identify this reactivity. The same problem will occur with the HLA-ABC typing set, with an additional complication that contaminating class II antibodies, which do not interfere when peripheral lymphocytes are being typed for HLA-ABC, must be identified and the specific reactivity discounted, in order to avoid misinterpreting the results.

4. HLA TYPING WITH IMMUNOMAGNETIC BEADS

An alternative approach to the separation of lymphoid cells by flotation has recently been developed in Norway (12). T or B lymphocytes are selected and removed from whole blood by binding to magnetic beads of 4.5 μm diameter (*Figure 7*). The HLA typing beads have a magnetic core and a polystyrene surface which is coated with Mab

Table 11. HLA typing with magnetic beads.

Separation method

1. Centrifuge 20 ml of citrated blood for 5 min at 800 *g*. Aspirate the buffy coat in a maximum of 2.5 ml of plasma and make up to 10 ml with PBS/citrate (*Table 5*) pre-cooled to 4°C.
2. Divide the sample equally into two straight sided (non-conical) 10 ml tubes of 8 mm diameter, cool on melting ice to 4°C and add 100 μl of class I beads to the first tube and 100 μl of class II beads to the second. Incubate at 4°C for 5 min with very gentle mixing.
3. Apply a powerful magnet to the side of each tube for 3 min to attract all the beads and the attached lymphocytes. Decant or pipette off the free blood cells while keeping the magnet hard up against the side of the tubes.
4. From now on treat the bead−lymphocyte complexes with great care, they are fragile. Over-vigorous mixing, or resuspension, or squirting in the repeating syringe can disrupt some rosettes and produce a lower cell yield.
5. Remove the magnet, gently add 10 ml of PBS/citrate and carefully resuspend the beads. Reapply the magnet to the tubes; after 45 sec decant the wash fluid with the magnet in place as before.
6. Wash magnetically twice more in 10 ml CFT buffer containing 2% (v/v) FBS (CFT/FBS).
7. If CFDA pre-labelling is preferred, decant all the fluid after the last wash with the magnet in place. Remove magnet, add 0.5 ml CFDA labelling solution (*Table 19*), incubate at 37°C for 15 min, mixing occasionally. Wash twice magnetically in CFT/FBS.
8. After the last wash resuspend the beads in 500 μl of CFT/FBS. Count the lymphocytes contained in the bead clusters using a counting chamber and standardize the suspensions at 1.5×10^6 lymphocytes/ ml. Use the magnet if it is necessary to concentrate the cells further.

Typing method for class I HLA antigens

1. Thaw the typing trays, centre the serum by centrifugation at 100 *g* for 30 sec.
2. Ensure the class I bead/lymphocyte rosettes are thoroughly yet gently resuspended, fill a repeating syringe and add 1 μl of suspension without delay to all the wells using the shooting method (Section 3.6) to avoid carry-over.
3. After 30 min incubation at room temperature (22°C) add 5 μl of complement to each well using a careful 'no touch' method.
4. After incubation for 30 min at 22°C add 5 μl of stop/stain/quench (SSQ; see below) solution to each well using the 'no touch' method.
5. Centrifuge the trays at 100 *g* for 30 sec, or leave to settle for 15 min.
6. Arrange excitation/emission filter sets in the fluorescence microscope to permit simultaneous assessment of living and dead cell populations. Dead cells are red, viable cells are green with CFDA or yellowy with acridine orange.
7. Record the percentage cell death in each well using the convention in *Table 8*.

Typing method for class II HLA antigens
Follow method above except:

1. Use class II bead/lymphocyte rosettes.
2. Incubate for 40 min at 22°C after the addition of complement.

Fluorescent stain/quench reagent

Stock fluorescent dye mixture: dissolve 15 mg of acridine orange[a], 50 mg of ethidium bromide in 1 ml of ethanol, add 50 ml PBS. Store frozen in 1 ml aliquots.

Stop/stain/quench solution (SSQ) for daily use: dissolve 50 mg disodium EDTA·2H₂O in 9 ml PBS, add 0.5 ml 30% bovine serum albumin, 0.5 ml stock fluorescent dye mixture, 0.3 ml Higgins calligraphy ink (Faber−Castell)[b]. Store in the dark at 4°C. Make up daily.

---

[a]Some workers prefer to pre-label the lymphocytes with CFDA, in which case the acridine orange may be omitted from the stock dye mixture and the SSQ solution made up as described in *Table 19*.
[b]Higgins ink is purchased from a local stationery shop or an artists' supplier.

active against HLA class I or class II determinants. These are available from Dynal UK.

The beads are added directly to a sample of cooled citrated whole blood, or a buffy coat preparation (this generally gives a higher cell yield). *Table 11* outlines an HLA typing procedure with an initial separation of buffy coat by centrifugation. The low temperature prevents phagocytic cell attack on the rosettes.

After a few minutes incubation at 4°C, the beads and the affinity coupled lymphocytes are separated from the unbound cells with a magnet. After washing and standardization the lymphocytes are tested in a CDC assay whilst still bound in rosettes or clusters of beads. The incubation period is substantially reduced in this technique probably because there is some synergy between the Mab and the anti-HLA typing serum, in addition to the ability of ethidium bromide to enter a cell and combine with the DNA at an early stage of membrane damage. The initial separation is also quicker than the traditional flotation methods resulting in a total time saving of some 3.5 h in the determination of a single HLA-DR type.

It is prudent to check the typing serum set with cells of known phenotype before introducing the bead method into routine work as the shorter incubation and the different staining methods may change the operational specificities of some of the reagents.

A disadvantage of the technique is that an inverted fluorescence microscope must be used to examine the trays as the spherical beads outnumber and obscure the lymphocytes in routine phase-contrast microscopy. However, special glass bottomed typing trays are not necessary when detecting gross cellular fluorescence and routine polystyrene microwell trays are perfectly satisfactory.

The eosin/formalin staining procedure is replaced with an acridine orange/ethidium bromide combination, or the cells are pre-labelled with CFDA and counterstained with ethidium bromide. Under high intensity illumination, viable lymphocytes show a bright green fluorescence while dead cells appear red. The scoring of the cell death in the wells is not affected by the large drifts of beads surrounding and overlaying the lymphocytes.

The 'no touch' method is employed to deliver reagents used in 5 μl quantities. Although more likely to produce carry-over it is preferred because vigorous 'shooting' can wash the beads to the periphery of the wells and up the sloping walls, creating difficulties in microscopy.

A polythene separation device is available fitted with powerful cobalt–samarium permanent magnets in which six separations can be handled simultaneously (*Figure 7*). The device holds the tubes and magnets firmly together during the separation phase, yet allows the magnets to be slipped out when the beads need resuspending.

The major benefit of HLA immunobeads is the substantial time saving that can be achieved in the determination of an HLA-DR type. The saving when dealing with class I typing is proportionately smaller—it may therefore be convenient to combine HLA-DR typing by the bead method with a simultaneous conventional HLA-ABC method when urgency is not the primary consideration. The decanted blood from a class II magnetic separation will provide ample lymphocytes for a conventional class I method resulting in a complete HLA-ABC and DR type some 2.5 h after the receipt of the specimen, thus halving the time taken with conventional methods. If the typing is done exclusively with the bead method, then the total time taken for a single HLA-ABC and DR type can be as little as 1.5 h.

5. PROVISION OF HLA TYPING SERA

Many laboratories actively screen suitable donors for reagent-quality antisera. If screening is not possible, HLA typing reagents may be purchased (see Appendix of Suppliers).

HLA antibodies are produced in response to immunization by transfusion, transplantation or pregnancy. A successful HLA antibody screening programme is usually the reason for the high quality typing trays in use in today's leading laboratories. By investing time and effort in testing sera from potentially immunized individuals, a laboratory can provide the core of its own needs and use surplus material for exchange. With a source of local reagents to share with collaborators, specificities which are in short supply can rapidly be acquired. This collaboration can range from the exchange of a single serum to the supply of comprehensive typing sets within a sharing scheme (e.g. Eurotransplant, UK; Transplant and the Heidelberg Collaborative Transplant Study). The Council of Europe serum bank in Strasbourg is even able to supply a set of accredited reagents to laboratories within the European Community for use in establishing a reference cell panel. Access to regional and international workshop serum sets is gained by a deep interest and enthusiasm for HLA work, membership of the appropriate research group and an ability to contribute time, reagents and resources to the workshop programme.

The following section outlines one approach to the screening of sera for HLA antibodies.

5.1 Antibody screening with separated T and B lymphocytes

The serum of multigravida women is selected for HLA antibody screening after the completion of routine blood group tests. Screening of women in their first pregnancy is not cost effective because the yield in terms of useful antibodies is generally low. Transfused patients are not a good source, their antibodies are likely to be polyspecific. Transplant patients are screened regularly for HLA antibody as part of their clinical follow-up, they do not need screening as a special task.

The timing of the sample can have a dramatic effect on the antibody content as the titre and specificity often change substantially in the course of a pregnancy and post-delivery antibodies often rapidly weaken. A good source of large volumes of reagent is the placenta; it can express up to 200 ml of liquid if squeezed hard in a press. Some women become long-term producers; stable antibody of useful specificity can be found 20 years or more after antigenic challenge.

The selected sera are tested for HLA-ABC antibodies (*Table 12*) with a small panel of cells, each member of which expresses at least one rare antigen. A panel of some 15 – 18 cells can cover all the relevant class I specificities. It is constructed to ensure that rare antibodies are detected leaving the detection of common antibodies to fortune.

With appropriate insulated storage containers and a secure supply of liquid nitrogen, the screening panel can be frozen for regular use. *Table 4* outlines a method for freezing the lymphocytes in 10% (v/v) DMSO with storage in tubes or straws. The lymphocytes may be separated into the T and B cell fractions before preservation or frozen unseparated and processed after recovery.

An alternative approach (9) is to freeze an entire panel of cells directly in wells of

Table 12. Screening for HLA typing sera.

1.	Select and separate potential sera on a regular basis and store 1−5 ml volumes at −30°C until a suitable number have accumulated (several hundred sera are usual in a screening run).
2.	Batch the sera into tray loads of 60 or 72 in number, including positive and negative controls. Prepare 25−30 replicate microwell trays from each batch using 1 μl vol. of each serum (*Table 2*).
3.	Take one tray of each batch and test against a selected cell of the screening panel, using extended incubation for B cells and CLL cells, until the complete screening panel is tested.
4.	Record the results on a matrix, list the panel cell phenotypes and examine the serum reactions for specific HLA antibody patterns.
5.	Retain all sera with antibodies of interest or unidentified patterns, for titration and a comprehensive analysis with a large panel of well characterized cells.
6.	If the donor of an antiserum of high quality is pregnant, seek her consent for a donation of 100−200 ml after delivery and subsequent enrolment onto the regular donor panel.
7.	Treat any re-bleed as an unknown antibody and submit it to a full analysis with a comprehensive panel using several serum dilutions.
8.	Whenever possible, HLA type the antibody donor and the partner to be aware of the antigenic stimulus and the possible contaminating antibodies. Compare the serum for several months with standard typing antisera in routine conditions. Send aliquots to a collaborating laboratory for confirmation of specificity.
9.	If the serum is reliable and robust then bring into daily use, circulate its availability on the serum exchange list if there is sufficient quantity.

a Terasaki tray; this is especially useful when relatively small numbers of sera are to be screened. A fluorescent staining technique enables the background cell death to be discounted when reading tests with cells cryopreserved in-the-tray. The use of random fresh cells for screening, in parallel with the determination of the HLA type, is recommended for new laboratories seeking antibodies of relatively common specificity.

B cell reagents are screened with extended incubation against a 12−15 cell panel of splenic or peripheral B cells or with chronic lymphatic leukaemia (CLL) cells, or with the use of selected complement lymphoblastoid B cell lines and a short incubation (Section 3.10). Sera containing HLA-ABC antibodies must be absorbed with concentrated platelets prior to B cell screening (Section 5.3).

Two hundred and eighty pregnancy sera will make four batches of 70 sera (excluding positive and negative controls) distributed on 72-well microtest trays. Six cells per day can be comfortably tested by one worker against all four batches of sera giving 24 trays tested daily. A 30-cell screen can be completed in five working days using panel cells recovered from frozen storage.

The maternity services are requested to inform the laboratory when a women with a strong specific antibody is admitted. When the role of tissue typing in transplantation is explained, most potential serum donors in the UK give their consent when asked for a small donation of blood after the delivery of their baby.

HLA typing sera which are going to be distributed and used as a laboratory reagent must be tested and found negative for the antibody to human immunodeficiency virus (HIV) and hepatitis B surface antigen (HBsAg) [HM Govt Health Department's HN (86) 25]. The potential serum donor must be made aware of the implications of the virology screening and agree that the tests may be done.

Monoclonal antibodies produced against HLA antigens by methods outlined in Chapter 3 are screened against a more restricted panel than allo-antisera because the immunogen

Table 13. Absorption of unwanted HLA-ABC antibodies with platelets.

Platelet preparation

1. Collect 'outdated' platelet concentrates from the local transfusion department, or bleed volunteers on cell separators.
2. Pool concentrates together, add 1% vol. of 10% (w/v) NaN_3 (Section 5.5). Store at 4°C until 5 litres (~ 100 single units) have accumulated.
3. Centrifuge at 4°C for 30 min at 1750 g (Sorvall RC-5B), discard supernatant plasma, pool the deposited cells using an equal volume of PBS/azide[a].
4. Centrifuge at 300 g for 5 min, harvest platelet-rich supernatant.
5. Resuspend deposit in PBS/azide, repeat centrifugation, collect second harvest of platelet-rich supernatant and pool with first batch. Repeat if necessary. Discard the pellet of leukocytes and red cells.
6. Wash purified platelets twice in PBS/azide for 10 min at 800 g, resuspend in PBS/azide to a 50% packed cell volume, pool with similar preparations to a volume of 500 ml, representing the platelets of 300−400 donors.
7. Store at 4°C. Use within 6 months.

Absorption procedure

1. Remove supernatant from settled packed-down stock of purified platelets, replace with fresh PBS/azide, resuspend platelets.
2. Add 5 ml of 50% platelet suspension to each of two 30 ml tubes, wash once in 25 ml of PBS/azide at 800 g for 15 min. Resuspend platelets in each tube to 5 ml in PBS/azide, transfer to 5 ml polycarbonate tubes and centrifuge at 10 000 g for 30 min (Sorvall RC-5B).
3. Remove completely all supernatant after the second wash, add 2 ml of the anti-HLA-DR serum requiring absorption to first tube of packed platelets.
4. Incubate at 4°C for 2 h, centrifuge at 10 000 g for 30 min.
5. Recover serum, add to second tube of packed platelets, incubate at 4°C for 2 h.
6. Centrifuge at 10 000 g for 30 min, recover absorbed serum, take sample for test, freeze at below −30°C.
7. Screen absorbed serum thoroughly for HLA-ABC antibodies in CDC tests with 3 h incubation. Repeat absorption if contaminants are still active.
8. Check HLA-DR or DQ activity before allocating the serum to a typing tray.

is known more precisely. Enzyme-linked immunosorbent assay (ELISA) techniques are employed in addition to cytotoxicity in order to detect non-complement-fixing antibodies. Similar procedures are applied to human Mabs produced by EBV transformation. The screening of monoclonal reagents provides logistical problems of its own; the number of culture supernatants can escalate rapidly if limiting dilution is chosen as the cloning strategy.

With tissue cultured reagents the complement batch must be carefully pre-screened to ensure it gives no toxicity when tested against the target cells suspended in culture medium enhanced with 10% FBS (Section 6.1). Particular attention must also be given to the thorough washing of syringes and equipment and to other liquid handling techniques if the carry-over problems, common with these potent antibodies, are to be avoided. Laboratories experienced in the use of Mabs find that a useful ploy is to place one or two wells of fresh medium between wells of potent antibodies until the correct working dilution has been determined (18).

5.2 Screening with two-colour simultaneous fluorescence

With the use of two-colour simultaneous immunofluorescence it is possible to screen antisera against unseparated lymphocyte preparations and discriminate between class

I and class II antibodies (17). The surface Ig (sIg) of the B cells is pre-labelled with fluorescein isothiocyanate-conjugated anti-IgG (Chapter 7). On completion of the CDC test the dead cells are stained with ethidium bromide and the preparation examined on an inverted fluorescence microscope. The surface fluorescence is not so intense as that seen when the whole of the cell interior is labelled with a fluorochrome, so glass bottomed trays are used to transmit all the energy of the exciting radiation. The sIg aggregates in the membrane into green fluorescent patches or caps. Dead T cells appear as bright red discs while dead B cells are red with bright green caps. Full details of the technique are found in ref. 8.

5.3 **Removal of unwanted antibodies by platelet absorption**

If the NIH test is used for antibody screening with conventional staining and microscopy, then T and B cell populations must be tested in parallel on separate trays. If a serum is found to contain a class I antibody of broad reactivity then useful class II antibody may be obscured; alternatively a valuable class II antibody may be contaminated by a specific, though mundane, class I specificity. In these circumstances the class I component may be removed by absorption with a preparation of pure pooled platelets collected from a large number of random donors (*Table 13*).

If the HLA class I antibody is clearly defined, then a preparation of platelets containing that specific antigen may be used at the rate of 1×10^{10} platelets per ml of serum and two absorptions should suffice. If the specificity of the undesired antibody is uncertain, or if only untyped platelets are available, then 10 times that number should be used and the serum absorbed with an equal amount of packed platelets. *Table 13* gives details of platelet preparation and absorption.

5.4 **Conversion of plasma to serum**

The CFT buffer or cell culture medium used as the diluent for the final cell suspension in the microcytotoxicity test has an optimum level of calcium and magnesium ions to support complement-dependent lysis. These ions are consumed by chelating anti-coagulants; consequently HLA antibodies collected into blood bags cannot be used until the plasma has been recalcified and converted into serum. *Table 14* gives a method of dealing with plasma from a unit of blood. The volumes are scaled down for samples collected into a smaller volume of anticoagulant, but the plasma from a whole blood unit should always be treated as stated, irrespective of the final plasma volume.

A slight excess of $CaCl_2$ is employed to ensure rapid and thorough clotting, but the serum cannot then be stored with a high calcium level without the danger of protein precipitation. The removal of excess calcium by a cation-exchange resin gives a product which can be handled and stored with no more problems than fresh serum (*Table 14*). The plasma is diluted about 1:8 upon collection into a blood bag, a little is lost in the fibrin clot and a small dilution occurs from the saline surrounding the resin. The decalcified serum should always be re-tested for specificity and titre to check the effects of processing.

After $CaCl_2$ treatment the plasma calcium can rise to over 30 mmol/litre. A single de-ionization step will reduce it to $6-10$ mmol/litre and two cycles give a level of $3-4$ mmol/litre, just above normal plasma calcium levels.

The resin which is supplied stained with an amber dye should be washed with large volumes of water until the supernatant is colourless. It should then be neutralized, if necessary, with a little NaOH to a stable pH of 7.2 (21). After use the resin can be re-cycled by thoroughly washing it free of all traces of serum followed by regeneration in 1.8 M NaCl.

5.5 Sodium azide preservation

HLA sera are widely exchanged between laboratories. Mailing frozen on dry ice is successful provided the CO_2 vapour cannot penetrate the container and acidify the serum, but it is expensive. A simple alternative is to add 10 μl of a 10% (w/v) solution of sodium azide to 1 ml of serum, giving a final concentration of 1/1000 (15.4 mmol/litre). The serum is mailed by first class post at room temperature. On receipt the serum can be frozen, stored and used normally.

Sodium azide is not without hazard since it is a dangerous poison and can form explosive metal azides on contact with copper and brass (not forgetting metal sink wastes and fittings). The 10% solution is best stored at 4°C clearly labelled in a plastic container and handled with plastic equipment.

6. EVALUATION AND SELECTION OF RABBIT COMPLEMENT

Some firms are willing to supply samples of rabbit complement for evaluation before the purchase of a large supply (see Appendix of Suppliers).

Table 14. Recalcification of plasma and cation removal.

Preparation of ion-exchange resin[a]

1. Place 30 g of resin in a 400 ml glass bottle, fill with distilled water, swirl for a few seconds, allow resin to settle, decant stained wash fluid. Repeat until wash fluid is clear.
2. Add 50 ml of water and one drop of 1% (w/v) nitrazine yellow to resin, add 1 M NaOH dropwise, if necessary, swirling until indicator turns blue (pH 7.2). Leave overnight to check for acid leaching, re-adjust pH to 7.2.
3. Wash resin in 0.85% (w/v) NaCl until supernatant is colourless, decant all liquid from last wash, fit rubber septum and cap, autoclave at 121°C for 20 min.

Recalcification

1. Add 3 ml of 25% (w/v) $CaCl_2$[b] to a 'single unit' donation of citrated plasma (usually 200−220 ml in volume) in a glass bottle. Adjust volume of $CaCl_2$ if donation collected into a non-standard volume (i.e. <63 ml) of anticoagulant.
2. Incubate at 37°C until a firm clot has formed (20−40 min), free clot from bottle wall and allow to contract for 30 min.
3. Drain serum overnight at 4°C into a sterile bottle of ion-exchange resin, retaining the fibrin clot on a fine mesh sieve.
4. Pack a loose plug of cotton wool into the quill connector of a plasma transfer set (Terumo 505 Coupler) to retain the resin. Force the quill through the septum of the serum/resin bottle, invert the bottle to form a resin bed, clamp bottle upside-down.
5. Place the other needle into a second bottle of resin fitted with an air bleed. Open clip and adjust to allow serum to drain into the second bottle at a rate of 2 ml/min.
6. Mix serum and resin and repeat the de-ionization, collect the serum in a clean container, take samples for titre and specificity tests. Freeze below −30°C.

[a]Duolite C225 (Na), standard grade, 14−52 mesh (BDH).
[b]50 g of $CaCl_2 \cdot 6H_2O$, H_2O to 100 ml.

Suppliers of rabbit complement collect fresh blood in the abbatoir in large pools from 2 – 80 litres in volume. The separated serum is snap frozen in litre volumes, or in the final containers, and stored at −80°C prior to issue in small volumes frozen or freeze-dried.

Blood collected from stock laboratory animals is allowed to clot, the serum rapidly separated, pooled and snap frozen directly in small aliquots. Individual samples from each rabbit are retained for assay.

The cell death seen at the completion of a microcytotoxicity test is a result of complement activation triggered by two antibodies acting synergistically. One antibody present in variable quantity in individual rabbits is a rabbit anti-human xeno-antibody; it is produced in response to environmental stimuli in the form of foodstuffs, gut organisms and other natural immunogens. The other is an allo-antibody, the human anti-HLA typing serum. The sensitivity of the cytotoxicity test is dependent on the strength, avidity and interaction of these two independent antibodies and on the activity of the native complement components in the rabbit serum. It is crucial that a batch of complement is thoroughly tested before introduction into routine work. It may be said that the quality of an HLA typing laboratory could well be judged by the care taken in the evaluation and selection of complement batches.

The selected complement must be sufficiently active to allow the detection of known examples of weak antibody; a regional external quality assessment scheme will often set the standard and help compare the overall sensitivity of the CDC test with that of other participants.

A complement must not be toxic to the target cells in the absence of HLA antibody. Few complement batches are suitable for use with all types of target cell, especially with prolonged incubation times. The prudent course is to reserve complement batches for use in the technique for which they are most suited; this approach has the advantage that changes of complement in any one technique are less frequent and this ensures long periods of stable test conditions.

6.1 Complement evaluation procedure

The following section describes a three-part complement evaluation procedure in use in the United Kingdom Transplant Service (UKTS) laboratory. The activity is measured by a checker board titration, followed by an assessment of the natural rabbit cytotoxins, and finally, a period of parallel testing comparing the current batch and its chosen successor.

(i)   A wide selection of complement samples is obtained to give the best possible chance of finding an acceptable batch. The primary screen for complement activity is a checker board titration by microcytotoxicity using the same antibodies and target cells to ensure comparable results. The test antibodies, an anti-HLA-A2 and an anti-HLA-B12 with titres between 1/4 and 1/8, are complement-fixing IgGs [judged by the failure of dithiothreitol (DTT) to destroy the lytic activity, Section 9.3]. The target cell is cryopreserved in liquid nitrogen or obtained fresh for the assay; it reacts with both standard antibodies. A standard freeze-dried complement is tested at the same time as the new complement samples in order to define the standard of acceptable activity. The detailed procedure and

Table 15. Chequer board titration for complement activity.

1.	Bleed and isolate target lymphocytes or recover from liquid nitrogen storage (*Table 4*) and standardize at 2.0×10^6/ml.
2.	Double dilute (in volumes of 200 μl) two standard antibodies from neat (1/1) to 1/16 in RPMI 1640 medium supplemented with 10% (v/v) FBS (RPMI−10% FBS).
3.	For each complement under test, prepare a pair of oiled trays containing all the dilutions of the two antibodies as follows: arrange the trays with the long axis horizontal, place 1 μl of each dilution in all 10 wells of a single row, 1/1 serum in row F, 1/2 in row E and so on, placing the 1/16 dilution in row B. Inert AB serum (1 μl) is pipetted into all the wells of row A.
4.	At 3 min intervals add 1 μl of the standard target cell to all the wells of a pair of trays. Incubate at 22°C for 30 min.
5.	Add required number of drops (each ∼20 μl) of CFT buffer to a row of test tubes according to the scheme below, prepare one row for each complement under test.
6.	Follow the chart (below) and prepare direct dilutions of complement by adding the appropriate number of drops of complement to the tubes a few minutes before the dilutions are required. Keep on melting ice.

Dilution chart

Tube number		1	2	3	4	5	6	7	8	9	10
Number of drops of CFT buffer (20 μl)		0	2	3	4	6	9	8	10	12	14
Number of drops of complement (20 μl)		10	8	6	4	3	3	2	2	2	2
Dilution	1+	0	1/4	1/2	1	2	3	4	5	6	7

7.	After precisely 30 min incubation take the first pair of trays and add 5 μl of the 1 + 7 dilution of the first complement to all the wells of column 10 of both trays. Expel surplus complement and refill the syringe with 1 + 6 complement without washing it between dilutions, add 5 μl to all the wells of column 9, and so on, through all the dilutions, finally filling the wells of column 1 with 5 μl of undiluted complement.
8.	Take the second pair of trays, add dilutions of the second complement after 30 min incubation as before, and so on, for all complement batches.
9.	Stain and fix the trays after 1 h incubation with complement at 22°C. Read and record results in the usual manner.
10.	Select for further tests any complement which matches or surpasses the established standards.

instructions for preparing the direct complement dilutions are shown in *Table 15*. Examples of acceptable and unacceptable titrations are shown in *Table 16*.

(ii) Complement batches which have been shown by titration to have acceptable activity are then screened for natural cytotoxic antibody (*Table 17*). A hierarchy of complement uses can be established; a complement is allocated to the most appropriate purpose on the results of the toxicity tests. The most demanding conditions for complement are found when testing Mabs. A 3 h incubation with human B cells suspended in culture medium in the absence of any human serum is a reliable screening test to find a non-toxic complement. Serum collected from rabbits less than 30 days old is often a source of such reagents. A complement might be toxic in medium alone but be perfectly satisfactory, even in extended incubation with B cells, when inert human AB serum is present in the test. A batch with these characteristics is reserved for B cell typing with allo-antisera. For use in routine HLA-ABC typing, a complement must show no toxicity after a 1.5 h incubation in the presence of inert human serum.

Table 16. Examples of satisfactory and poor complement.

Cell no. 16		Recovered, frozen normal peripheral lymphocytes
HLA type		A2,A23;B44,27
Tested		12/5/87

Tested by CB

Anti-HLA-A2

Complement dilutions	Neat	5/4	3/2	1/2	1/3	1/4	1/5	1/6	1/7	1/8
Antibody dilutions										
Neat	8	8	8	8	8	8	6	6	.	.
1/2	8	8	8	8	8	6	2	.	.	.
1/4	8	8	8	6	6	.	.	.	.	.
1/8	6	8	8	4	.	.	.	.	.	.
1/16	.	.	2	.	.	.	.	.	.	.
AB serum	.	.	.	.	.	.	.	.	.	.

Complement batch 110

	Neat	5/4	3/2	1/2	1/3	1/4	1/5	1/6	1/7	1/8
Neat	8	8	8	8	4	.	.	.	.	.
1/2	8	6	6	4	.	.	.	.	.	.
1/4	4	4	2	2	.	.	.	.	.	.
1/8	.	.	.	.	.	.	.	.	.	.
1/16	.	.	.	.	.	.	.	.	.	.
AB serum	.	.	.	.	.	.	.	.	.	.

Anti-HLA-B12

Complement dilutions	Neat	5/4	3/2	1/2	1/3	1/4	1/5	1/6	1/7	1/8
Antibody dilutions										
Neat	8	8	8	8	8	8	6	6	4	.
1/2	8	8	8	8	8	8	4	2	.	.
1/4	8	8	8	8	6	2	.	.	.	.
1/8	8	8	6	6	.	.	.	.	.	.
1/16	2	2	2	.	.	.	.	.	.	.
AB serum	.	.	.	.	.	.	.	.	.	.

Complement batch 215

	Neat	5/4	3/2	1/2	1/3	1/4	1/5	1/6	1/7	1/8
Neat	8	8	8	8	8	4	4	2	.	.
1/2	8	8	6	6	6	2	.	.	.	.
1/4	8	8	8	4	4	.	.	.	.	.
1/8	2	2	2	2	.	.	.	.	.	.
1/16	.	.	.	.	.	.	.	.	.	.
AB serum	.	.	.	.	.	.	.	.	.	.

Complement batch 110

Complement batch 10B

Neat	8	8	8	8	8	8	8	6	4	.
1/2	4	6	8	8	8	8	8	8	2	.
1/4	.	6	6	8	8	8	6	4	.	2
1/8	.	.	4	6	8	6	2	.	.	.
1/16	.	.	2	2	2	2	.	.	.	.
AB serum	.	.	.	.	.	.	.	.	.	.

Complement batch B1/2

Neat	8	8	8	8	8	8	8	6	4	.
1/2	8	8	8	8	8	8	8	8	4	.
1/4	8	8	8	8	8	8	6	6	.	.
1/8	8	8	8	8	6	6	2	.	.	.
1/16	6	6	6	4	2	.	.	.	.	.
AB serum	.	.	.	.	.	.	.	.	.	.

Neat	8	8	8	8	8	8	4	6	.
1/2	4	6	8	8	8	8	6	6	.
1/4	.	6	8	8	8	6	4	.	.
1/8	.	.	2	6	4	2	.	.	.
1/16	.	.	.	.	.	.	.	.	.
AB serum	.	.	.	.	.	.	.	.	.

Neat	8	8	8	8	8	8	8	8	4
1/2	8	8	8	8	8	8	6	6	6
1/4	8	8	8	8	8	6	6	2	.
1/8	8	8	8	6	6	2	.	.	.
1/16	4	6	2	.	.	.	.	.	.
AB serum	.	.	.	.	.	.	.	.	.

Interpretation

8,6,4,2 = positive cytotoxicity scores; . = negative.

Comments

Batch 215   is the standard complement.
Batch B1/2   is equally active and selected for further acceptance tests.
Batch 10B   fails assay because of unacceptable prozone with undiluted complement.
Batch 110   is substantially inferior.

Table 17. Tests for complement toxicity.

1.	Fill columns 1−5 of an oiled 60-well microwell tray with 1 μl of RPMI 1640 supplemented with 10% inert FBS and remaining wells (columns 6−10) with inert human AB serum.
2.	Add 1 μl of standardized B cells at a concentration of 2×10^6/ml in CFT buffer to the first column of each diluent (i.e. to columns 1 and 6). The remaining columns are filled with four different B cells in a similar manner. Incubate for 1 h at room temperature.
3.	Add 5 μl of each complement to two rows of tests, thus three complements may be screened in duplicate on one tray.
4.	Re-incubate at room temperature for 2 h, stain with eosin, fix and read the trays for cytotoxicity.
5.	In a similar manner, five peripheral lymphocyte samples can be tested on diluent trays, and if applicable, five lymphoblastoid cell lines, using a 1.5 h total incubation period.
6.	Decide on the basis of the activity, and the natural toxicity, the technique for which each complement is best suited and proceed to parallel testing.

(iii)   Finally, before ordering large stocks and switching from a proven complement batch to its selected replacement, a short period of parallel testing should be implemented to confirm that the new batch is virtually indistinguishable from the old in operational use. If laboratory rabbits are bled for complement, the details of the activity and toxicity are entered on the bleeding records and unsuitable donor rabbits replaced with new stock.

7. AUTOMATED READING TECHNIQUES

The fatigue of reading cytotoxicity trays on a manually operated microscope can be eased by the use of a microcomputer-controlled microscope stage. The operator of these semi-automated systems assesses the cell death by eye and enters the result into the computer by means of a keypad. On data entry the computer moves the stage to position the next well directly above the objective. The method of testing and reading the trays is unchanged from the standard manual procedure. The electronically coded data can now be handled by a variety of sophisticated software packages which can store, display, sort and analyse the results at the user's instruction.

Automatic reading systems (22) have been developed to the point where the wells are scanned and the raw data recorded automatically. The cell death in each well is calculated by reference to cytotoxicity controls. The results are displayed on a screen and printed out on a plate map for interpretation; the data is stored for later analysis and investigation.

The NIH test method is modified for automated tray reading; cell death is detected by quantitation of the light emitted by fluorescent labels rather than phase-contrast microscopy. A red or green fluorescent label is used singly or in combination.

Carboxy-FDA (CFDA) is used to label living cells prior to the CDC test. It penetrates the intact cell membrane and is converted by cellular esterases into the active fluorescent derivative carboxy-fluorescein. On excitation in blue light, viable cells appear as discrete points of green light which are detected by the photomultiplier. The carboxy-fluorescein escapes through the ruptured membrane of dead cells and disperses through the medium giving an even light of low intensity. To prevent this background signal affecting the quantitation, a 'quench' solution of 4 mmol haemoglobin is added to absorb the background energy and permit good discrimination between negative and positive test results.

Table 18. HLA typing by double fluorescence for automated reading.

1.	Select a batch of 72-well microtest trays which give the lowest background fluorescence in the automated system in use.
2.	Prepare a typing serum set (*Table 2*), reserving the positions allocated in the machine manual for calibration controls. Do not add phenol red or any other dyes to the sera.
3.	Use inert AB serum and 0.5% (w/v) saponin solution in the control wells to set the background cell death and the maximum possible positive value.
4.	Oil the trays and dispense sera in the usual manner (Section 3.1). Centrifuge the trays at 150 *g* for 3 min to centre the serum in the wells. Store the trays frozen at below −30°C.
5.	Separate lymphocytes from whole blood and wash free of platelets (*Table 6*) or recover cells from liquid nitrogen storage (*Table 4*).
6.	After the third wash remove all the supernatant carefully and leave the cells in a pellet; resuspend in 1 ml of CFDA solution and incubate at 37°C for 15 min.
7.	Wash twice in CFT buffer, proceed with B and T cell separation and typing by conventional methods (*Tables 7−9*). It is crucial that the cells are dispensed into the trays accurately—select the most reliable repeating dispenser.
8.	When complement incubation phase is completed add 5 μl SSQ (*Table 19*) to the wells instead of eosin formalin, or add 40 μl of PI to 2 ml complement before use and after 1 h incubation add 5 μl 3% ink/EDTA.
9.	Store the trays undisturbed at 4°C for at least 15 min before evaluation in the scanner. Follow the calibration and operating instructions provided with the equipment.

Table 19. Reagents used in automated double fluorescence method.

Saponin: 0.5% (w/v) in AB serum.

CFDA: Store powder at −20°C or lower.
   Stock solution: 10 mg of CFDA, 2 ml of acetone (BDH Analar). Store in dark at 4°C.
   Daily working solution: 10 μl of stock solution, 2.5 ml of PBS.

Propidium iodide (PI) (Sigma) stock solution: 10 mg of PI, 10 ml of PBS. Store in dark at 4°C.

Ethidium bromide (EB) (BDH) stock solution: 10 mg of EB, 10 ml of PBS. Store in dark at 4°C.

Bovine haemoglobin (Hgb) (4 mmol): add 27.2 g of Hgb (Sigma), 500 mg of disodium EDTA·2H$_2$O, to 100 ml of PBS for 1−2 h at 37°C, mix occasionally. Store frozen in 10 ml quantities.

Higgins calligraphy ink (Faber−Castell Corp., USA): 3% ink working solution. Add 0.3 ml of ink to 9 ml of PBS, add 0.5 ml of 30% bovine serum albumin, 50 mg of disodium EDTA·2H$_2$O.

SSQ solution with haemoglobin: 400 μl of EB working solution, 10 ml, 4 mmol of Hgb/EDTA.

SSQ solution with ink: 200 μl of EB working solution, 10 ml of 3% ink/EDTA.

Ethidium bromide and propidium iodide become intercalated with double-stranded nucleic acids and emit a red fluorescence when excited. The dye cannot penetrate a living cell but is able to enter a dead cell through the damaged membrane and becomes concentrated in the nuclear debris. When suitably excited a dead cell appears bright red; a living cell is not fluorescent and is hardly visible. The stains are added at the end of the test period in a mixture which also contains the quench solution and EDTA, to stop further complement-dependent cell death, or are added with the complement.

A technique using a single fluorescent label is vulnerable because of the imprecision caused by the variation in the number of lymphocytes pipetted into each well. A high level of skill and attention is required to achieve reproducible results. With a double fluorescent technique every cell, living or dead, will fluoresce in one colour or the other. The proportion of living to dead cells can therefore be estimated automatically and the well-to-well variation in the cell numbers discounted in the calculations (23).

Table 18 outlines a procedure for labelling and testing lymphocytes in a double fluorescence system for automated reading and *Table 19* details the reagents required.

Automated microscopes (Leitz, Saxon Orak, Carl Zeiss) detect the fluorescence in each well using computer-controlled changes of the excitation and emission filters to discriminate the intensity of the two colours. The Astroscan 2100 detects both colours simultaneously and discriminates the two signals by means of a divided fibre optic bundle.

An even distribution of cells over the whole of the base of the well is essential for reliable automated reading. The initial centrifugation of the trays before the addition of the cells eliminates beading and ensures an even depth of serum in all the wells. An accurate 'shooting' technique (Section 3.6) is used to add the labelled lymphocytes. The subsequent reagents are added by a 'soft-drop' technique to avoid disturbing the carpet of settled cells.

In this 'soft-drop' method, the reagent is gently dispensed to form a bead on the tip of the needle, the needles are then gently lowered into the wells until the reagent just touches the surface of the oil and the drop is removed by surface tension effects. It is most important in avoiding carry-over to ensure that the needle tips do not come into contact with the reaction mixture. The haemoglobin quench solution is so viscous that it will damage a close lapped metal piston in a glass syringe barrel. This problem does not arise in syringes with polytetrafluoroethylene (PTFE) seals on the piston. Another approach is to substitute artists' waterproof black ink for the haemoglobin quenching agent. A 3% (v/v) solution of Higgins Calligraphy ink (Faber−Castell) is suitable, it seems as good a quenching agent as haemoglobin. Not all artists' inks are satisfactory, some Indian inks are fluorescent themselves!

The EDTA in the quench solution prevents further specific cell death by chelating the calcium ions needed for complement-dependent lysis. Since the cells are not fixed chemically, they continue to die off spontaneously and give a progressively higher background of cell death. For this reason the trays should be stored in the dark at 4°C for a maximum of 24 h, if storage is unavoidable.

The specificities of a few of the HLA typing sera can be slightly different in automated systems from those found by the NIH method. Ethidium bromide crosses the membrane at an earlier stage of cell death and the method seems a little more sensitive. The typing sera reactions with the first few hundred cells need to be examined carefully to establish the 'automated method' specificities.

The CFDA powder is unstable at room temperature; it is stored frozen below −30°C. Ethidium bromide and propidium iodide are potentially hazardous mutagens; gloves must be worn when handling them in powder form or in solution.

8. HLA TYPING BY ELISA TECHNIQUES

The CDC test has gained universal acceptance for HLA typing with human antisera and there seems little place for methods exploiting allo-antibodies which do not fix complement. This is not the case with mouse hybridoma reagents, where antibodies which fail to activate complement can be found in significant numbers when the clones are screened for activity. The potential value of unlimited supplies of rigorously standardized reagents is self evident.

The exploration of the range and character of murine responses to HLA proteins demands the use of antibody binding assays: ELISA is the most convenient of these techniques—the principles and methods of which are described in detail in Chapter 4.

In HLA investigations both fixed and fresh cells have been used successfully. The traditional approach is to immobilize the target antigen, usually whole cells, by adherence to poly-L-lysine (PLL)-treated trays followed by a short fixation in glutaraldehyde solution. The flat bottomed 8×12 microtitre tray is the usual carrier, fitting in with the wide range of tray washers and readers manufactured to this format. The test volume of 50 μl is not usually a constraint when screening supernatants against a single cell, but it does not allow much scope for panel work when the total volume of a culture supernatant might be only 250 μl. It is also difficult to imagine HLA typing using a microtitre tray of fixed cells requiring the addition of 50 μl of a full range of 96 Mabs of different specificities.

The 72-well microwell tray ELISA method, using conventional PLL coupling and a 15 min fixation with 0.0125% (v/v) glutaraldehyde is useful in screening microlitre volumes of human monoclonal reagents against human cell line targets (R.T.J.Hancock, personal communication). The peroxidase-linked anti-Ig conjugate and the 2,2'-azino-bis(3-ethylbenzylthiazoline-6-sulphonic acid substrate were selected so that the results could be read photometrically in the microEIA reader which was under evaluation in the 10th International Histocompatibility Workshop. The microEIA system, using fresh lymphocytes with no fixation or immobilization on a solid surface, is carried out on 72-well microwell trays. This development was part of the investigation of mouse monoclonal anti-HLA in the 10th workshop; it employs regular microwell dispensers and syringes compatible with the CDC assay. A microEIA reader has been developed for the test by Genetics Systems of Seattle.

In this method, 1 μl quantities of antibody are dispensed under paraffin oil into the trays; this has the great advantage that the trays can be prepared in advance in batches in the conventional manner (Section 3.1). The target cells are added with a conventional 1 μl repeating syringe; the technique is therefore as economical as the CDC test itself. The cells are not immobilized on a solid surface so a delicate washing process is necessary to prevent loss of cells and consequent loss of signal. The washing is very demanding; it involves multiple centrifugation steps and an abrupt inversion to throw off the wash fluid. The colour intensity is measured, through the tray, in the microEIA reader giving a rapid and objective value to the amount of antibody bound to the cells that remain in the tray.

The microEIA method could become the trigger to release the full potential of Mabs into routine HLA phenotyping but first, a more acceptable system must be developed to surmount the considerable difficulty found in washing lymphocytes which are not attached to a solid support. By eliminating rabbit complement as a reagent in the assay the technique is much more amenable to standardization, the readings are also objective: it is a serious challenge to the CDC test.

Table 20. Platelet fluorescence CDC test.

Preparation and CFDA labelling of platelets

1. Centrifuge 10 ml of citrated whole blood at 200 *g* for 10 min, separate platelet-rich plasma (PRP). Centrifuge PRP at 800 *g* for 10 min, discard supernatant plasma, add 20 ml of PBS/citrate (*Table 6*), resuspend cells. Alternatively, collect platelet-rich PBS/citrate usually discarded after the first wash of lymphocytes separated on density medium.
2. Centrifuge at 300 *g* for 5 min, harvest supernatant of pure platelets, discard button of leukocytes and red cells.
3. Centrifuge platelet-rich supernatant at 800 *g* for 10 min, discard supernatant, suspend platelets in 1% (w/v) ammonium oxalate solution, allow to stand for at least 15 min, centrifuge at 800 *g* for 10 min, take off all supernatant.
4. Add 1 ml of PBS/CFDA (*Table 19*), resuspend platelets, incubate at 37°C for 20 min.
5. Wash labelled platelets twice in CFT buffer at 800 *g* for 10 min. Adjust platelet count to $1.5 - 2.0 \times 10^4/\mu l$, check viable platelet count on microwell tray with UV illumination, adjust if necessary.

Platelet fluorescence CDC test method

1. Reserve space on the microwell tray for the control sera. Use a multispecific anti-HLA and an anti-Pl^{a1} for cytotoxicity positive controls, saponin (*Table 19*) for dye/quenching system control and AB serum to estimate the viable fluorescent platelet count in each sample.
2. Add 1 μl of CFDA-labelled platelet suspension to 1 μl of test antiserum in duplicate wells and to the control sera, in an oiled microwell tray, using good microcytotoxicity technique (*Table 7*).
3. Incubate tray at 37°C for 30 min.
4. Place tray at 22°C for 10 min to cool, add 5 μl of rabbit complement to each well, incubate for 90 min at 22°C.
5. Add 5 μl of 3% Higgins ink working solution containing no added stains (*Table 19*) to each well, leave for 15 min to settle.
6. Examine for fluorescence with UV illumination and the fluorescein filter set. Compare with the platelet count seen in the inert AB serum negative control.
   An equivalent platelet count to that seen with AB serum = negative
   Fewer platelets to that seen with AB serum = doubtful positive
   No platelets seen = positive
7. Confirm that platelets are indeed present in every positive test by switching on the phase-contrast illumination when no platelets are seen under UV.

9. FURTHER APPLICATIONS OF COMPLEMENT-DEPENDENT CYTOTOXICITY

9.1 Detection of platelet antibodies by the CDC method

Most cytotoxic HLA antibodies are capable of lysing platelet suspensions in a microwell tray in the presence of complement, but it is difficult to distinguish viable and dead platelets with routine eosin staining and phase-contrast microscopy. However, the CFDA fluorescence method (*Table 20*) gives very good discrimination. The viable platelets appear as bright green points of light when viewed under UV illumination with the fluorescein filterset in the lightpath. The carboxy-fluorescein escapes from dead platelets and is present as a free label in the supernatant. The addition of calligraphy ink quenches this diffuse fluorescence and the well appears to be completely free of small fluorescent particles.

The platelet fluorescence CDC (PFCDC) or thrombocytotoxicity test (24) relies on an assessment of the green light emitted from each well. It is obviously important to ensure that each well has an adequate number of platelets present. The platelet carpet is easily visible in a negative test, but in a positive test no fluorescence is seen under UV illumination. The wells in which the platelets have apparently been lysed must therefore be checked for the presence of platelets by phase-contrast microscopy. The PFCDC method fits in naturally with routine lymphocytotoxicity testing, the equipment and reagents are familiar and readily to hand.

Platelets previously frozen in DMSO can also be recovered and tested by PFCDC. The usual higher background cell death seen with recovered platelets is not a problem, as the dead cells are simply not visible under UV. The initial count can be checked in a preliminary tray and adjusted to take account of the number of viable platelets.

The PFCDC is a convenient method for testing large panels of fresh and previously frozen platelet suspensions to establish a panel of Pl^{a1} negative donors. The green fluorescence can be detected and quantitated by those automated scanning devices (Section 7) which have programs tailored for single-colour CFDA fluorescence.

The PFCDC method can be useful in screening the sera of patients who have suffered from febrile transfusion reactions or who fail to show a platelet increment after platelet transfusion. Pure platelet and lymphocyte suspensions may be tested independently, or 100 μl of the donor's lymphocyte suspension can be added back to 1 ml of the platelet suspension prior to CFDA labelling. The test wells can then be read manually under UV microscopy for the simultaneous presence of lymphocytotoxic and thrombocytotoxic antibodies.

Some clinically significant anti-platelet antibodies might not potentiate direct complement-dependent cell lysis; it is recognized that the PFCDC test will fail to detect these cases. In these circumstances an antibody binding method should be employed: the platelet immunofluorescence test (25,26), or a platelet ELISA test (27) may well detect antibodies of this nature.

9.2 Monitoring of humoral activity in renal patients

One of the most important uses of the CDC test is to detect antibody in the serum of potential transplant recipients directed against antigens present in the potential donor's tissues. The procedure for this test, the cross-match, is detailed in Section 9.3.

9.2.1 Regular pre-graft HLA antibody screening tests

The regular monitoring of the serum of the potential transplant recipient permits the specificity and characteristics of any HLA antibody present to be accurately defined. This information will then form an integral part of the selection procedure to prevent the patient from being considered for inappropriate tissue.

Another advantage of regular screening is that the laboratory scientist performing the cross-match (often alone—as dawn is breaking!) is fully aware of the patient's history of sensitization; subsequent decisions are then taken in an informed manner.

Serum should be collected at 3 monthly intervals while patients are on the transplant waiting list. This interval allows peaks of antibody to be detected and reveals all but the most transient sensitization episodes.

The serum should be tested for class I antibodies against a panel of normal peripheral lymphocytes selected to contain examples of all the HLA antigens found in the population—a panel size of 30 will usually suffice. The tests should be incubated at 22°C to provide maximum sensitivity while avoiding the detection of antibodies with a thermal optimum of 4°C. A word of caution—'cold' antibodies can be clinically significant if the transplanted kidney is still cold at the moment when blood flow is re-established.

Duplicate tests incubated at 37°C identify antibodies with a large thermal amplitude. The methods detailed in *Tables 2* and *7* are appropriate for antibody screening using a recovered frozen cell panel (*Table 4*); such screening panels can also be frozen on trays (9).

Antibodies directed against class II targets are detected by the use of selected recovered B cell panels (*Table 6*) using 15 or more members in a test with a 3 h extended incubation.

If class I antibodies are present in a serum then B cells bearing the appropriate target antigen will also be killed. Exhaustive platelet absorption (*Table 13*) of 50 μl volumes of serum removes the class I antibody and permits identification of class II specificities.

Screening on randomly selected panels gives the proportion of donors that might be expected to give positive reactions in the cross-matching tests. This frequency is often referred to as panel reactive antibody (PRA). When PRA levels reach 80−90% severe difficulties arise in finding suitable donors. Special schemes are needed to overcome these problems (Section 9.2.2).

When the PRA is at a low or moderate level, screening tests allow more precise definition of HLA specificity. This specificity is entered in the patient's records and kidneys with this phenotype are censured in matching and offering procedures.

HLA antibodies can be stimulated by pregnancy, blood transfusion and after a failed kidney graft. The additional exposure to HLA by pregnancy inevitably results in more women than men becoming highly sensitized.

Another important function of the screening tests is to differentiate IgM and IgG anti-HLA antibodies. This can be achieved by Cleland's reagent DTT. IgM antibodies are susceptible to reduction and consequent inactivation by DTT (29) while IgG antibodies are unaffected. The DTT is in turn inactivated by the addition of cystine to prevent the reduction of complement components. *Table 21* gives a method for the DTT treatment of serum (30). The procedure is carried out *in situ* in the microwell tray.

The biological relevance of antibody class distinction is that IgM antibodies do not seem able to bind K cells (killer cells or cytotoxic effector cells) *in vivo* and fail to give positive results in antibody-dependent cellular cytotoxicity (ADCC) tests. IgM anti-HLA seem ineffective *in vivo* and are not a barrier to transplantation (31).

It is advisable to characterize the DTT-resistance of anti-HLA antibodies in a patient's serum as part of the regular screening programme while the patient is on the transplant waiting list, rather than attempt DTT treatment of a serum for the first time as part of the final cross-match procedure.

It is important that the serum samples are filed in a deep freeze after the antibody screening is completed particularly if the sample shows an increase in PRA. In general the higher the PRA the greater the amount of serum that should be stored, to a maximum volume of 5−10 ml. Filed samples will be recovered for use in selecting potential donors and in the final cross-match tests. With highly sensitized patients many more tests will be needed.

Table 21. Dithiothreitol treatment of serum in the CDC test.

1.	Suspend lymphocytes at 2×10^6 in DTT/CFT[a] solution and in CFT buffer alone.
2.	Add 1 μl of lymphocytes in DTT/CFT to 1 μl of antiserum in duplicate wells of an oiled microwell tray.
3.	Add 1 μl of lymphocytes in CFT buffer alone, to 1 μl of antiserum, in duplicate, to serve as the untreated control.
4.	Incubate tray at 22°C for 30 min.
5.	Add 1 μl of cystine/CFT[b] to wells, leave for 5 min, add 5 μl of rabbit complement.
6.	Incubate for 60 min at 22°C. Stain, fix and read in the usual manner.

Include known DTT-sensitive and DTT-resistant sera, with appropriate target cells, as controls on the DTT activity.

[a]16 mg of DTT in 10 ml of CFT buffer, make up fresh weekly.
[b]240 mg of cystine in 10 ml of CFT buffer, shake to dissolve, centrifuge at 400 g for 5 min, use saturated supernatant.

9.2.2 *Highly sensitized patients (HSPs)*

When the PRA level is 80% or greater, specificities defy analysis. At this level, a simple list of the phenotypes of the panel cells which do not react with the patient's serum should be documented. These 'windows of compatibility'—that is, 'safe' antigens to which the patient has yet to form antibodies, give an indication of acceptable mismatches. A selected panel of 100 individuals will reveal the majority of these 'windows'.

Greater precision can be achieved by the use of cell panels individually tailored for each patient. Each cell selected differs from the patient's own HLA phenotype by only one antigen; an extremely large frozen cell panel is required to cover every conceivable patient, a panel of 5000 or so typed cells covering most eventualities.

Special screening panels often reveal that HSPs do not become sensitized to their own, or their mother's non-inherited HLA antigens (J.J.Van Rood, personal communication), failure to react being explained by tolerance acquired *in utero*. Another feature of HSPs is a tendency towards homozygosity for HLA-A, -B antigens.

If 'safe' antigens can be determined they can be incorporated as 'allowable mismatches' in the kidney placement routines operated by the various national organ exchange organizations and given high priority, the objective being to secure that elusive cross-match negative donor for the HSP from the larger national pool of kidney donors.

9.2.3 *Identification of auto-antibodies*

Renal patients occasionally develop autoreactive cytotoxic antibodies which lyse their own lymphocytes and the majority of random donor lymphocytes in the routine CDC test, thus giving the impression that the patient has an allo-antibody with a high reaction frequency and could be falsely classified as an HSP.

The presence of an auto-antibody is not a contra-indication to transplantation (28), whereas an IgG allo-antibody in a recent serum sample directed against lymphocytes of the potential donor most certainly is. Autoreactive antibodies are detected by testing the patient's own lymphocytes against own serum, most conveniently during the panel screening tests. Two other techniques can help to pinpoint auto-antibodies. One test to detect autoreactive antibodies is to use a panel of lymphocytes collected from patients suffering from CLL. CLL cells are arrested at an early stage of differentiation and fail to express the 'auto-antigen', although HLA expression is quite normal. Hence,

Table 22. HLA antibody tests of increased sensitivity.

1.	Extending the standard incubation time to a total of 3 h.
2.	Use of ethidium bromide nuclear stain instead of eosin and formalin after the routine CDC method.
3.	Use of magnetic beads to isolate the target cells (*Table 11*) and adding bead−lymphocyte clusters in the test trays for the standard incubation time.
4.	Adding a wash step to remove antibody/diluent prior to the addition of complement in the CDC test.
5.	Enhancing the antibody toxicity after the first stage incubation by suitable wash steps followed by the addition of rabbit anti-human IgG prior to the addition of complement in the CDC test.
6.	Use of antibody binding assays using fluorescent anti-IgG and quantitation by FACS analysis.
7.	Radionuclide labelling (^{51}Cr) of the target lymphocytes and estimation of the ^{51}Cr released after a CDC test.

negative reults with a CLL panel in a CDC test with the serum of a patient with a high frequency PRA suggests an auto-antibody. Another aid to identification is the fact that autoreactive antibodies are usually IgM and thus sensitive to reduction by DTT (*Table 21*).

9.2.4 *Alternative tests for screening for HLA sensitization*

The sensitivity of the cytotoxic test in its ability to detect all graft damaging antibodies is often questioned. Antibodies in sera which give negative results in the routine CDC test may be detected by the alternative tests listed in *Table 22*. The use of control sera known not to contain anti-HLA is of importance in establishing a negative baseline when tests of great sensitivity are contemplated.

9.2.5 *Post-graft screening*

Test for HLA antibodies should continue at regular 3 monthly intervals at least for the first year post-grafting. The range of tests should be similar to those done prior to grafting. Regular screening will detect antibodies that may become important prognosticators of graft failure. If rejection is suspected sequential screening may reveal a rapidly rising level of PRA. This is a poor prognostic sign. If a graft fails due to immunological rejection peak samples should be collected immediately and every 2 months after graft failure. Highly reactive PRA can be found after graft failure when immunosuppression is withdrawn or after nephrectomy when the failed tissue is removed and circulating antibody is no longer absorbed by the tissue.

Large serum samples from these critical periods should always be stored for future tests. They are irreplaceable as reference material in the definition of the patient's immune profile, and a starting point in the quest for replacement grafts.

9.3 **Cross-matching for allografts**

As a result of regular antibody screening (Section 9.2) a complete record of a series of filed serum samples should be available on all patients awaiting transplant. These records must be readily available in the laboratory for inspection in the event that a suitably matched kidney becomes available. When this happens the ABO blood group and HLA phenotype of the offered kidney are checked against recent records to ensure that the patient has not inadvertently been offered an inappropriate kidney (this process can be greatly facilitated by a personal computer) then it is ensured that the virology

Table 23. Preparation of lymphocytes for cross-match tests.

Lymphocyte preparation from lymph node

1. Three to four lymph nodes usually obtained by the surgical team are supplied in a bottle of saline or irrigation fluid.
2. Take one lymph node and drop into a bottle of clean CFT buffer to wash off blood, fat, etc.
3. Place the node in a small clean plastic tray (Petri dish), hold with forceps and with caution prick the node several times with a sharp needle.
4. Fill a syringe with 5 ml of CFT buffer, hold the node in the forceps and spear it with the syringe needle. Inject the buffer moving the needle around in the node allowing all the cells to be flushed out into the dish.
5. Wash the lymphocytes twice in CFT buffer, standardize for use as an unseparated suspension or process to separate T and B cells.

Lymphocyte preparation from spleen

1. The spleen is usually sectioned into 2 cm cubes by the theatre team and supplied in a sterile bottle of isotonic fluid.
2. Place the spleen in a sterile dish, hold in forceps and strip as many free cells as possible from the capsule and internal membranes by firmly stroking it with a dissecting set angled seeker.
3. Wash the free cells into a sterile 30 ml bottle with CFT buffer. Mix cells and diluent and stand for 5 min.
4. Layer the free cells from the top of the bottle onto sterile density medium, centrifuge and separate as in *Table 5* avoiding if possible the heavy platelet layer above the lymphocytes and the aggregated material which may lie directly at the interface.

tests, especially HIV, cytomegalovirus (CMV) and HBsAg, are in order, or in progress, and the stage is set for the cross-match.

9.3.1 *Preparation of lymphocytes*

Peripheral blood lymphocytes collected from donors supported on respirators are acknowledged to be difficult material for use in cross-matching tests. The donor may have received blood transfusions and any number of drugs in life-saving efforts. The peripheral blood lymphocytes may be blast-like or generally unreactive. Separation and washing of lymphocytes (*Table 5*) followed by incubation at 37°C for $1-2$ h to allow *de novo* synthesis of HLA antigens should be attempted if difficulties are experienced in obtaining a typeable cell suspension.

A more reliable approach and one which is certainly much quicker (time is of the essence to reduce the period during which the kidney is in chilled storage) is to harvest viable cells from a lymph node or a sample of spleen collected by the surgical team at donor nephrectomy. *Table 23* outlines the procedures to separate viable cells from these tissues for use in HLA typing and the cross-match. Around $2-5\%$ of the cells from a lymph node will be B lymphocytes; they may be separated from the T cells by SBRC rosetting as detailed in *Table 6*. The lymphocytes separated from spleen may contain up to $50-60\%$ B cells; this is often high enough to permit HLA-DR typing with no further B cell enrichment. When unseparated spleen cells are used in the cross-match it must be remembered that antibodies reactive only against B cell antigens may give a high cell death which may need experienced interpretation. Spleen lymphocytes can be fractionated into T and B cells by the usual methods.

It is generally acknowledged that a kidney is at greater risk the longer it is chilled on ice, this period is known as the cold ischemia time. The introduction of magnetic bead separation can dramatically reduce the HLA typing and cross-matching times on transplant material, the method may even give greater sensitivity in the cross-match resulting in better graft survival as well as improvements related to the reduced cold ischemia time. The methods given in this section are traditional, tried and tested. The methods for the use of magnetic beads are presented in *Table 11*. When a body of data is available, comparing graft survival with traditional or rapid cross-match methods, then the appropriate system should be employed.

It is convenient to confirm the HLA phenotype of the offered kidney at the same time as the cross-match test if it has been transported from another centre. The number of HLA antigens shared by the donor and the recipient may influence whether the offered kidney is acceptable. The donor centre may have interpreted a type performed on peripheral blood only. With the superior results expected with lymph node or spleen lymphocyte preparations extra antigens which will alter the match grade may well be found.

9.3.2 *The cross-match procedure*

While the lymphocytes are being prepared from the donor samples a citrated blood sample should be obtained from the nominated recipient and processed at the same time to yield unseparated B and T cells for control and reference purposes. The patient's lymphocytes are especially useful if auto-antibody has been previously detected in the screening history. A fresh clotted sample obtained for the cross-match as the patient arrives at the transplant centre is a guarantee that very recent sensitization is not overlooked.

The patient's fresh serum is plated out in 1 μl volumes on oiled microwell trays in replicates of 10. The appropriate historic samples selected by reference to the patient's screening records are treated in a similar manner with replicate rows of inert AB serum separating one serum from another. Six or more identical trays are prepared to allow for different target cells. *Table 24* shows a plan for a cross-match which allows the patient's fresh serum and two stored sera to be tested in quintuplicate against three cell preparations of the donor at temperatures of 22 and 37°C. The left hand side of the tray is the cross-match and there is provision for auto-control cells on the right.

The multiple rows of AB negative controls have two purposes. They separate critical sera from each other, eliminating carry-over as a cause of error and permit a repeated examination of the background cell death while the search is made for small increments of cytotoxicity in the wells with patients' serum.

The T cell and unseparated lymphocyte cross-match trays are incubated for 30 min before the addition of complement and for 1 h afterwards. The B cell cross-match tests have a total of 3 h incubation, 1 h before the addition of complement and 2 h thereafter.

When IgM antibodies have been detected in the regular screening tests, extra trays should be tested at 22°C using cells suspended in DTT (*Table 21*) to confirm that the antibody is indeed DTT-sensitive and that IgG antibody has not developed since the last screen.

If all the cross-match tests give a negative result, the phenotypes are as stated and the HIV, CMV and HBsAg virology tests are satisfactory, then the surgical team are

Table 24. Example of a form for recording the results of lymphocytotoxicity cross-match tests.

| United Kingdom Transplant Service |

FINAL CROSS MATCHES	UNSEPARATED CELLS	B CELL ENRICHED	T CELL ENRICHED
	Pre XM Viability %	Viab. % Purity %	Viab. % Purity %
Source (delete N/A)	PBL/Spleen / L.Node	PBL/Spleen / L.Node	PBL/Spleen / L.Node
Date:	Times	Times	Times
Set up			
Complemented			
Read			

Sera	Lab.No.	DONER CELLS 22°C AUTO	DONOR CELLS 22°C AUTO	DONOR CELLS 22°C AUTO	
Historic 1.					F
AB serum	–				E
Historic 2.					D
AB serum	–				
Fresh serum					B
AB serum	–				A
		37°C	37°C	37°C	
Historic 1.					F
AB serum	–				E
Historic 2.					D
AB serum	–				C
Fresh serum					B
AB serum	–				A

SUMMARY

Final Crossmatches	22°			
	37°			

DONOR TISSUE TYPE FOUND.   HLA | A   B   Cw   DR   DQ

Match Grade | A | B | DR | confirmed/different to that given

Reported to: by: Date & Time:

informed that there is no immunological reason why the kidney should not be transplanted.

While the transplant is underway, or if there is time during the incubations, the surplus donor and recipient lymphocytes should be carefully frozen in DMSO (*Table 4*) and all the recipient serum samples stored in the deep freeze for future reference and research.

In recent years evidence has emerged to suggest that clinically relevant anti-donor allo-antibody must be of IgG class and directed towards HLA mismatches on the donor cells (31). Antibody directed towards auto-antigens and IgM antibody to HLA appears innocuous in terms of hyperacute rejection although an exception must be made with regard to cold antibodies (32). Allo-antibody directed towards non-HLA targets, especially those confined to B cells, also seems irrelevant (33).

Current informed opinion suggests that a transplant may proceed if negative results are obtained in the cross-match after treatment of the serum with DTT.

IgG antibodies in the fresh serum directed against HLA targets present on B cells are probably harmful, therefore a positive cross-match directed against B cell antigens which is resistant to DTT treatment is a contra-indication to transplantation. Similarly an antibody in a fresh serum which is resistant to DTT treatment and which reacts with HLA targets on separated donor T cells is almost certain to damage the kidney with a high risk of hyperacute rejection and consequent graft loss.

9.3.3 *Peak positive—current negative*

The PRA levels of anti-HLA may slowly decline with time after the last immunological challenge. This decay can produce a cross-match with a negative result with fresh serum but positive results with a stored historic serum. With suitable immunosuppressive regimens many patients with an antibody profile of this character have received successful grafts (34). However, the impression gained is that a positive cross-match in any serum in a patient receiving a regraft should be respected (35).

Difficult cases of this nature need full discussion between the immunologist and the surgeon to take account of factors like the patient's clinical condition, access sites for dialysis, etc. to help reach a decision on transplantation.

If the transplant does not proceed and the kidney is to be offered to a better matched patient elsewhere, then lymphocyte or tissue samples must accompany the organ for cross-matching tests. A kidney distributed with no samples for cross-match tests is almost always wasted.

As a courtesy to the receiving centre the donor's cell suspension tubes should be carefully labelled with the donor name, hospital and date; the cell type (B, T, etc.) and the tissue of origin (blood, spleen, etc.). The samples should then be packed with all the unused spleen samples or lymph nodes and despatched with the kidney. The receiving laboratory will save several hours preparation time by this thoughtful act and the organ will be transplanted that bit quicker.

10. ACKNOWLEDGEMENTS

I am indebted to Godfrey Laundy, Ian Roberts and Karin Yousaf for details of techniques developed at UKTS, and to Ben Bradley for close consultation on transplantation policy in the sensitized recipient and for critical reading of the manuscript. Thanks are also due to Barbara Ray for photographic services and secretarial assistance.

11. REFERENCES

1. Terasaki,P.I. and McClelland,J.D. (1964) *Nature,* **204**, 998.
2. NIH T and I Staff (1976) In *NIAID Manual of Tissue Typing Techniques.* Ray,J.D. (ed.), DHEW Publication No. (NIH) **76**, 545.
3. Bodmer,W.F., Tripp,M. and Bodmer,J.D. (1967) In *Histocompatibility Testing 1967.* Curtoni,E.S., Mattiuz,P.L. and Tosi,R.M. (eds), Munksgaard, Copenhagen, p. 341.
4. Ryder,L.P., Anderson,E. and Svejgaard,A. (eds) (1979) *HLA and Disease Registry* (3rd Report). Munskgaard, Copenhagen.
5. Tiwari,J.L. and Terasaki,P.I. (eds) (1985) *HLA and Disease Association.* Springer-Verlag, New York.
6. Dupont,B.(ed.) (1988) *Immunobiology of HLA, I) Histocompatibility Testing, II) Immunogenetics and Histocompatibility.* Springer-Verlag, New York, in press.
7. Park,M.S. and Terasaki,P.I. (1974) *Transplantation,* **18**, 520.
8. Lamm,L. and Degos,L. (eds) (1983) *Essential Aspects of Tissue-Typing.* Council of Europe, Strasbourg.
9. Sinnott,P.J., Kippax,R.L., Sheldon,S. and Dyer,P.A. (1985) *Tissue Antigens,* **26**, 318.
10. Boyum,A. (1968) *Scand. J. Clin. Lab. Invest.,* **21**, Suppl. 97, 77.

11. Dorn,A.R., Moriarty,C.S., Osbourne,J.P., Schultz,L.C., McCarthy,J.P., Lister,K.A. and Horne,L.A. (1987) *International Clinical Products Review,* **6**(2), 30.
12. Vartdal,F., Guadernack,G., Funderud,S., Bratlie,A., Lea,T., Ungelstad,J. and Thorsby,E. (1986) *Tissue Antigens,* **28**, 301.
13. Longo,A. and Ferrara,G.B. (1980) In *Histocompatibility Testing 1980.* Terasaki,P.I. (ed.), UCLA Tissue Typing Laboratory, Los Angeles, p. 283.
14. Gelsthorpe,K. and Doughty,R.W. (1977) *Tissue Antigens,* **10**, 236.
15. Pellegrino,M.A., Ferrone,S. and Theofilopoulos,A.N. (1976) *J. Immunol. Methods,* **11**, 273.
16. Danilovs,J.A., Ayoub,G. and Terasaki,P.I. (1980) In *Histocompatibility Testing 1980.* Terasaki,P.I. (ed.), UCLA Tissue Typing Laboratory, Los Angeles, p. 287.
17. Van Rood,J.J., Van Leeuwen,A. and Ploem,J.S. (1976) *Nature,* **262**, 795.
18. Kennedy,L.J., Bourel,D., Dejour,G., Fouchet,R. and Bodmer,J.G. (1987) *Tissue Antigens,* **29**, 43.
19. Konoeda,Y., Terasaki,P.I., Wakisaka,A., Park,M.S. and Mickey,M.R. (1986) *Transplantation,* **42**(2), 253.
20. Stinchcombe,V., Jones,T. and Bradley,B.A. (1985) *Tissue Antigens,* **26**, 161.
21. Moghaddam,M., Goldsmith,K.L.G. and Brazier,D.M. (1976) *Vox Sang,* **30**, 315.
22. Bruning,J.W., Claas,F.J.H., Kardol,M.J., Lansbergen,Q., Naipal,A.M. and Tanke,H.J. (1982) *Human Immunol.,* **5**, 225.
23. Van Lambalgen,R. and Bradley,B.A. (1985) *Tissue Antigens,* **26**, 87.
24. Lizak,G.E. and Grumet,F.C. (1980) *Human Immunol.,* **1**, 87.
25. Brand,A., Van Leeuwen,A., Eernisse,J.G. and Van Rood,J.J. (1978) *Blood,* **51**, 781.
26. Von Dem Bourne,A.E.G.Kr., Verheugt,F.W.A., Oosterhof,F., Von Riesze,E., Brutel de La Riviere,A. and Englefriet,C.P. (1978) *Br. J. Haemat.,* **39**, 195.
27. Taaning,E. (1985) *Tissue Antigens,* **25**, 27.
28. Ting,A. and Morris,P.J. (1977) *Lancet,* **ii**. 1095.
29. Pirofsky,B. and Rosner,E.R. (1974) *Vox Sang.,* **27**, 480.
30. Kruyer,H., Van Dam,M. and Welsh,K. (1985) *UKTS Bulletin,* No. 18.
31. Chapman,J.R., Taylor,C.J., Ting,A. and Morris,P.J. (1986) *Transplantation,* **42**(6), 608.
32. Lobo,P.I., Vestervelt,F.B., White,C. and Rudolf,L.E. (1980) *Lancet,* **ii**, 879.
33. Reed,E., Lewison,A., Sucia-Foca,N., Hardy,M., Lattes,C., McCabe,R., Brentsilver,J. and Reemstma,K. (1983) *Transplantation Proc.,* **15**, 1838.
34. Cardella,C.J., Falk,J.A., Nicholson,M.J., Harding,M. and Cool,G.T. (1982) *Lancet,* **ii**, 1240.
35. Kerman,R.H., Flechner,S.M., Van Buren,C.T., Lorber,M.I. and Kahan,B.D. (1985) *Transplantation,* **40**, 615.
36. Nomenclature on HLA. (1988) *Bull. WHO,* in press.

CHAPTER 3

Immunoassays using radiolabels

DAVID CATTY and GERRY MURPHY

1. INTRODUCTION

The use of radiolabelled ligands as a means to quantify small molecules immunologically came about from the demonstration 30 years ago by Berson and Yalow (1) of the extraordinary sensitivity of the measurement of binding of trace amounts of radio-iodinated insulin to antibody. In consequence it was also possible to measure the capacity of very low concentrations of serum insulin to bring about a quantitative inhibition of this binding. The competitive inhibition principle with standard radiolabelled antigen became the adopted strategy, as a fluid phase saturation assay (radioimmunoassay or RIA), to measure a growing range of hormones, drugs and other small molecules. This was assisted by new methods of radiolabelling and the successful preparation of anti-bodies to small immunogenic molecules once attached to larger protein carriers. The theory and practice of RIA has been expertly reviewed (see, for instance, ref. 2). RIA has become an established discipline in medical service laboratories investing largely in commercially prepared kits and dedicated equipment, but new molecules require new assays and guidance in setting up and standardizing an RIA from first principles may be valuable to many. For this reason this chapter includes an account of the critical stages in RIA development and evaluation. The example uses an intrinsic tritium (^{3}H) label in the standard antigen; many assays utilize a chemically substituted foreign radioactive atom, with radioiodine being the usual choice. Radioiodination is describ-ed in Chapter 8.

A preliminary step in RIA is antibody titration against labelled antigen. Where antigens are large and the antibodies polyclonal (polyspecific), precipitation will occur spontaneously over a range of antibody:antigen proportions; where this is optimal all the available antibody is precipitated. At this point, measurement of complexed immunoglobulin determines the antibody content of the serum; this is called the quantitative precipitin test. For anti-carbohydrate antibodies, for example to pure bacterial polysaccharides, the antibody can be determined from the total protein at the maximum protein precipitation point—this was the basis of the first purification and measurement of antibodies by Heidelberger and Kendall (3). For anti-protein antibodies, however, the test required modification by use of radioiodinated antigen and an example test for anti-albumin serum is provided. The test offers an exact measure of serum antibody content not easily obtainable by other means and is a valuable standardization procedure (4). The precipitin test also serves to illustrate the principles of antibody:anti-gen ratios in precipitation and the formation of soluble immune complexes, and to provide an estimate of effective antigen valency. It is an excellent first exercise in preparing radiolabelled antigen and using it safely in tube titrations.

The capacity of RIA to detect ever smaller amounts of analyte increases as the operating amount of antibody is reduced, the limit being dictated in practice by the ability of the signal and the counter to distinguish bound labelled antigen against background, the equilibrium constant of the reaction between analyte and antibody, and the degree of experimental error. With polyclonal antibodies the maximal sensitivity will seldom, if ever, exceed 1×10^{-14} mol/litre (or $\sim 10^7$ molecules/ml) (4). By contrast, an assay using an excess of antibody on a solid phase to 'capture' analyte, and a radiolabelled second antibody to reveal the bound antigen, offers theoretically greater sensitivity down to a single captured antigen molecule. There are reasons why in practice, with radiolabelled antibody, this extreme sensitivity is not achieved (4) but nevertheless the format of immunoradiometric assays (IRMA), especially the two-site (or sandwich) assays, offers certain obvious advantages.

(i)   Greater sensitivity.
(ii)   Use of a solid phase binding principle which allows a simple separation of bound and free antigen by an uncomplicated washing step.
(iii)   It depends on binding of two antibodies to two (often different) antigen epitopes with two opportunities for an analyte-specific reaction, (two-site assay).
(iv)   Monoclonal reagents are ideally suited to the assay as first or second antibodies (or both), as precipitation is not a required feature. Monoclonals afford the potential of both great specificity and high avidity binding characteristics. This is a great advantage in the capture stage.
(v)   Analyte measurement depends on observation of bound labelled antibody with opportunities for use of 'universal' radiolabelled antiglobulins (if the capture antibody is of a different species or isotype to the second).
(vi)   Procedures for the radioiodination of antibodies are well standardized.
(vii)   The approach is simply modified for the detection and measurement of antibody (including antiglobulins) using a solid phase-coated standard antigen. This is an indirect antibody radioassay.

The protocols for performing an antigen-capture IRMA and indirect antibody radioassay (for monoclonal antibody screening) are given in this chapter, with guidance in a number of related tests.

2. THE QUANTITATIVE PRECIPITIN TEST

2.1 Principle

An exact amount of pure antigen [human serum albumin (HSA) in the example] is radioiodinated (^{125}I) and the c.p.m./μg (specific activity) determined for estimation of antigen in precipitates and supernatants. Labelled antigen is then dispensed into small precipitin tubes in the range $2-500$ μg in a volume of 0.3 ml. To these is added a standard volume (0.5 ml) of an undiluted antiserum (sheep or rabbit as example) containing a high titre of specific IgG antibodies. Proportions of antibody to antigen will vary from extreme antibody excess in the first tubes to extreme antigen excess in the last. After mixing and a period of equilibration it will be noted that precipitation has occurred in some tubes, notably in a zone in the middle antigen range. Precipitation is the result of extensive crosslinking of antigen molecules by antibody to form an

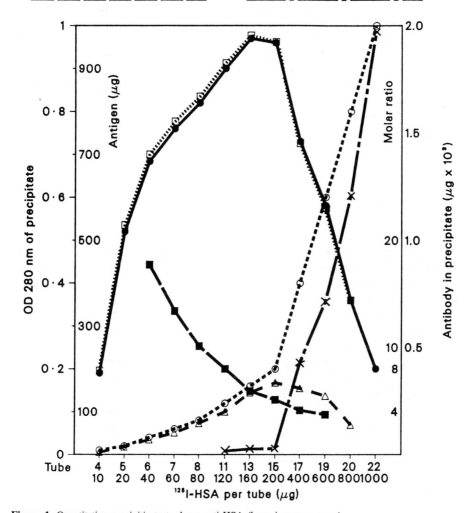

● OD 280nm dissolved precipitate   □ Antibody in precipitate
○ Antigen added   △ Antigen in precipitate
■ Molar ratio antibody: antigen   × Antigen in supernate

Figure 1. Quantitative precipitin test; sheep anti-HSA (hyperimmune serum).

insoluble lattice of complexes, aided by further non-specific aggregation. There are three distinct regions of precipitation in this reaction (see *Figure 1*).

(i)   Antibody excess, where all available antigen and some antibody is precipitated but excess antibody in the supernatant can be demonstrated by the addition of further antigen which leads to more precipitate. The amount of precipitate increases with increasing antigen, with a corresponding reduction in the amount of supernatant antibody. The antibody:antigen ratio in precipitates in antibody excess provides an estimate of the operational valency of the antigen. The antibody excess region moves into the equivalence zone.

(ii) The equivalence zone, which is a region close to maximum precipitation, is where, over several tubes, there is no detectable antigen or antibody in the supernatant. Within the scale of antibody:antigen proportions existing in the zone, an exact equivalence point, or point of optimal proportions occurs in which the available antibody is for the first time fully involved in complex formation.

(iii) Antigen excess: The transition between equivalence and antigen excess may be identified by a stage of maximum precipitation in which all the antibody is found in complexes in the presence of a trace excess of supernatant antigen (5). Analysis of the immune complex components at maximum precipitation can be done by subtracting the amount of precipitated antigen (determined by a radioactivity count) from the total protein to arrive at the antibody content. This value defines the total antibody in 0.5 ml of whole serum. From this point there is a rapid decline in amount of precipitate, with formation of soluble complexes in increasing antigen excess.

2.2 Reagents and equipment

2.2.1 Reagents

(i) *Radioiodinated protein.* Radioiodinated pure protein antigen (HSA in the example, 15 mg) at 3.5 mg/ml in phosphate-buffered saline (PBS), pH 7.2, with a specific activity giving approximately 1000 c.p.m./μg, can be prepared by labelling 100 μg of protein to high specific activity (5$-$10 μCi/μg) and diluting out in unlabelled antigen. For labelling procedure see Chapter 8.

(ii) *Antiserum.* The antiserum used is 20 ml of sheep or rabbit antiserum, complement heat-inactivated at 56°C for 50 min. 10 ml is sufficient if duplicate tubes are not used and less still with fewer steps in the antigen scale in low and high dose regions.

(iii) *Phosphate-buffered saline.* 0.1 M, pH 7.2

    2.7 g $Na_2HPO_4 \cdot 12H_2O$
    0.39 g $NaH_2PO_4 \cdot 2H_2O$
    9.0 g   NaCl

Dissolve in 1 litre of distilled water.

(iv) *Sodium hydroxide solution.* 0.1 M in distilled water.

2.2.2 Equipment

7 × 50 mm diposable clear polystyrene precipitin tubes (1 ml capacity).

Rack for precipitin tubes (ELISA microtitre plates for above tubes).
5 ml glass test tubes and rack.
Micropipettes with disposable tips.
Fine tip Pasteur pipettes with teats.
Washing tray to contain radioactivity.
Absorbent bench paper.
Disposable latex gloves.
Radioactivity disposal bin.
Parafilm.

Hand gamma counter.
Indelible fine tip marker pen.
Refrigerated centrifuge with small tube inserts in angle head rotor.
Incubator at 37°C.
Refrigerator at 4°C.
Gamma counter.
Spectrophotometer (280 nm).

2.3 **Protocol**

2.3.1 *Setting up the tubes*

(i) Prepare a set of precipitin tube reactions according to the scheme set out in *Table 1* using duplicate labelled tubes and following the sequence as indicated. Use gloves to handle the radioactive antigen, and dispose of all contaminated tips in the radiation disposal bin.

(ii) Cover each tube with parafilm and mix using a vortex mixer. Incubate at 37°C for 4 h, observing precipitation in the first hour, and then place at 4°C for a minimum period of 8 h, preferably several days.

2.3.2 *Analysis of reactions*

Tubes are selected that represent critical points in the evolution of precipitate over the antigen range with all tubes taken in the equivalence zone which should be in the middle of the series; include the control tubes for antigen alone (tubes 2, 9 and 21) which monitor dispensed antigen counts at three concentrations, and the no-antigen tube (tube 1) which provides a background reading. Wear disposable gloves for handling radioactive tubes throughout all the following steps.

(i) Centrifuge the selected tubes at 10 000 r.p.m. for 30 min at 4°C and then carefully withdraw each supernatant by fine Pasteur pipette, holding the tubes at an angle with the precipitate uppermost and the pipette tip running to the bottom along the lower inside wall of the tube. Transfer each supernate to a new labelled tube and cover. Use a fresh pipette for each pair of tubes.

(ii) Wash the precipitate (and antigen-alone tubes) in ice-cold PBS (0.4 ml) and centrifuge again. Transfer the washings to a second set of labelled supernate tubes being again careful not to disturb the precipitate. The antigen-alone tubes are discarded. Proceed to step iv with precipitate.

(iii) Cover the supernate tubes, place in counting tubes and count for 1 min in the gamma counter. Add together the counts of the supernate and wash volume of each tube. Mean the results of each pair of tubes. Tubes 2, 9 and 21 represent total added counts for 2, 100 and 1000 μg antigen which are used for reference in calculating the antigen in precipitates and supernatants. This is necessary because of changes in counting efficiency over the labelled antigen range. Prepare a curve relating dispensed antigen to observed counts and use this to determine antigen values. Tube 1 is a no-antigen blank for background which is deducted from other readings. Set the supernate aside for testing for free antibody (see step viii). Place all used pipettes, tips, tubes etc. in the radioactive disposal bin.

Table 1. Quantitative precipitin test. Addition of reagents to tubes.

Tube no. (in duplicate)	1	2	3	4	5	6	7	8	9	10	11	12	13	14	15	16	17	18	19	20	21	22
Reagent (order of addition):																						
1. Antigen-[^{125}I] (HSA) µg/tube	0	2	2	10	20	40	60	80	100	100	120	140	160	180	200	300	400	500	600	800	1000	1000
2. PBS	Add as required to make up to 0.3 ml total volume before addition of 3.																					
3. Antiserum (0.5 ml)	+ 0.5 ml PBS	+	+	+	+	+	+	+	+ 0.5 ml PBS	+	+	+	+	+	+	+	+	+	+	+	+ 0.5 ml PBS	

Total volume of each tube after addition of 3 is 0.8 ml.

(iv)   Wash the precipitates once more, discarding the washings, then dissolve the precipitates by adding to each tube 0.5 ml of 0.1 M NaOH, covering with parafilm and mixing with the vortex.

(v)   Count the radioactivity of the dissolved precipitate for 1 min. DO NOT DISCARD. Mean the counts of duplicate tubes and deduct the background. Then calculate the amount of antigen in each (dissolved) precipitate from the known specific activity of the antigen.

(vi)   Place the tubes back in their rack and prepare pairs of labelled 5 ml glass test tubes to correspond. Carefully transfer the solutions from the precipitin to the glass tubes; add 0.5 ml of NaOH solution to the small tubes and use a pipette (fresh one for each pair) to rinse the tubes up and down and transfer the washings to the corresponding glass tubes. Add 2.0 ml more of NaOH to each larger tube.

(vii)   Read the OD 287 nm absorption of each tube, using 0.1 M NaOH as the blank. Finally discard the radioactive solutions, carefully rinse out the glass tubes and the cuvettes in KCl solution until non-active and wash the cuvettes in distilled water. Dispose of pipettes, tips, gloves and other contaminated materials in the disposal bin and check hands, tray and surrounding area for any contamination, using the hand counter.

(viii)   From the precipitate OD readings select the supernatants in the ascending, antibody-excess zone up to the tube with maximum precipitate. Add to each of these a further 40 μg of radiolabelled antigen. Incubate for 4 h at 37°C and overnight at 4°C. Then centrifuge the tubes as in step i, wash any precipitate (discarding the supernates and washings) and count the tubes. Note the first tube in which no precipitate can be detected. This defines the beginning of the equivalence zone with no free antibody in the supernate. (The other limit of equivalence is defined by the appearance of free antigen in supernate.)

(ix)   Prepare a table with the calculated data for each monitored tube as in *Table 2*.

(x)   Draw up a precipitation curve together with other calculated and observed data for the monitored tubes as shown in the example in *Figure 1*. Mark in the equivalence zone. Normally maximum antibody precipitation occurs in a tube in mild antigen excess and this can be determined from the data. Multiply the weight of maximum precipitated antibody by a factor of two to arrive at the antibody concentration per ml of serum.

2.3.3 *Technical notes*

(i)   It is possible to perform an approximate quantitative precipitin test for antibody without using a radiolabel in the antigen, by using the maximum precipitate tube and assuming that the total antigen of this tube is in the precipitate. This may be inaccurate because maximum precipitation normally occurs in antigen excess.

(ii)   Although the use of radiolabelled antigen allows an improved estimate of antibody, the sensitivity of the test is poor. A large volume of antiserum is required to measure precipitated proteins accurately by OD. The conversion of antigen to OD values is particularly inaccurate. Sensitivity and accuracy are improved by using Folin reagent for protein estimations. An alternative, and the one originally used by Heidelberger and Kendall (5) is to perform microKjeldahl reactions on the precipitates and express the results in units of antibody nitrogen (4).

Table 2. Quantitative precipitin test for antiserum to human serum albumin.

Tube no.	4	5	6	7	8	11	13	15	17	19	20	22
Analysis												
1. Added antigen (µg).	10	20	40	60	80	120	160	200	400	600	800	1000
2. Calculated antigen in supernate (µg) (from counts)[a].	1.1	1.6	2.2	3.6	4.3	7.9	12.8	14.0	213.7	357.0	604.3	986
3. Calculated antigen in precipitate (µg) (from counts)[a]	5.2	17.5	34.9	51.1	72.8	100	145.2	167.5	154.8	137.4	68.5	—
4. Sum of supernate and precipitate antigen.	6.3	19.1	37.1	54.7	77.1	107.9	158.0	181.5	368.5	494.4	672.8	986
5. % Recovery of antigen (4/1 × 100).	63	96	93	91	96	90	99	91	92	82	84	99
6. OD at 280 nm, 1 cm, of dissolved precipitate (3 ml).	0.190	0.520	0.684	0.760	0.820	0.900	0.970	0.960	0.730	0.580	0.360	0.200
7. Calculated contribution to OD of the antigen in precipitate[b].	0.001	0.003	0.006	0.009	0.013	0.018	0.026	0.030	0.028	0.024	0.012	—
8. Calculated contribution to OD of the antibody in precipitate[b].	0.189	0.517	0.678	0.751	0.807	0.882	0.944	0.930	0.702	0.556	0.348	—
9. Calculated weight of antibody in precipitate (µg)[c].	391	1070	1403	1554	1670	1825	1953	1924	1452	1150	720	—
10. Molar ratio of antibody: antigen in precipitate[d]			17.7	13.4	10.1	8.0	5.9	5.1	4.1	3.7		

[a]Counts are converted to absolute amounts of antigen by reference to a constructed curve relating counts to dispensed weights of antigen [see Section 2.3.2(iii)].

[b]An Ig % (w/v) solution of HSA (10 000 µg/ml) has an absorbance at 280 nm (1 cm cell) of 5.32. Thus the precipitate in tube 13 (*Figure 1* and *Table 2*) containing [from the count curve—see Section 2.3.2(iii)] 145.2 µg of antigen, when dissolved in 3 ml for OD reading (48.4 µg/ml) will make an OD contribution for the HSA of 48.5 × 5.32/10 000 = 0.026. As the OD 280 nm of the dissolved precipitate in tube 13 is 0.970, then, by subtraction, the antibody component contributes 0.944. An Ig % (w/v) solution of sheep IgG (10 000 µg/ml) has an absorbance at 280 nm (1 cm cell) of 14.5. Then in tube 13 an OD of 0.944 represents 0.944 × 10 000/14.5 µg antibody/ml = 651 µg/ml. As the precipitate was dissolved in 3 ml the total antibody added in tube 13 was 651 × 3 = 1953 µg. This represents the antibody in 0.5 ml of serum. Thus the antibody concentration of the serum (determined at maximum antibody in precipitate) is 3.91 mg/ml.

[c]The molar ratio of antibody:antigen in a precipitate is determined by dividing the weight ratio of the two components by the quotient of the molecular weights of antibody and antigen (150 000:66 000 = 2.27). Thus in tube 13, at maximum precipitation, the molar ratio is (1953/145)/2.27 = 5.9. Note that as the example reaction moves through equivalence into antibody excess (*Figure 1, Table 2*), so the molar ratio increases. This is the result of some antibodies finding only one available antigen determinant in linking to the complex, and to an effective saturation of determinants. Antigen valency is estimated in antigen excess for this reason.

3. IMMUNORADIOMETRIC ASSAYS

3.1 **Principles and assay design**

The following principles apply to all IRMA protocols.

(i)   They utilize radiolabelled antibody, as opposed to labelled antigen in RIA. This has the major advantage that methods for labelling immunoglobulin to high specific activity with retained specific binding properties are well standardized and easy to perform. The approach also allows the measurement of antigen molecules that are difficult to purify for radiolabelling, are difficult to radiolabel, or lose antigenic properties in the labelling procedure.

(ii)   They utilize a solid phase binding reaction principle which allows for a simple separation of free and bound reagents by one or more washing cycles. The solid phase can be a variety of antigen- and antibody-coated beads, including magnetic beads for easy separation (these are proving popular as a format in commercial kits), plastic tubes, or the wells of flexible plastic microtitration plates which are the most popular form and are convenient for most routine work.

There are several forms of IRMA designed for different tasks; all, in principle, have a corresponding enzyme-linked immunosorbent assay (ELISA) alternative based on the use of enzyme-conjugated antibody with a substrate-generated signal (see Chapter 4). With the commonly used ELISA enzyme − substrate systems there is little difference in sensitivity and required operative skills between ELISA and radiolabel assays— laboratories tend to stay with the latter if committed by equipment. Newly equiped laboratories may well choose ELISA for reasons of economy and safety. The following are the major forms of IRMA.

3.1.1 *Antigen inhibition assay*

This uses a coated solid phase (standard) antigen and a radiolabelled antibody diluted to a concentration at which it can be effectively inhibited from binding to the coated antigen in the presence of free (test) antigen. The assay is rendered quantitative by reference to a standard antigen inhibition curve.

3.1.2 *Antigen-capture (two-site or sandwich) assay*

This uses a solid phase layer of (capture) antibody to bind antigen from solution; the presence of bound antigen is then revealed by use of a second antibody as a labelled probe. The assay has the potential for combined high specificity and sensitivity, especially when exploiting the use of selected monoclonal antibodies with high avidity for antigen. As in the ELISA alternative, the two antibody components are required to bind spatially distant antigen epitopes. The capture and second antibody may both be monoclonal reagents; the specificity and avidity of polyclonal antibody when used is a critical factor. Affinity-purified polyclonal antibody may be needed as the capture layer if high sensitivity is required. Because of the antibody-excess, solid phase antigen-capture principle, this assay is theoretically much more sensitive for antigen detection than RIA. However, the nature of radioiodine decay is such that with monoiodinated antibody as the probe, and a counter efficiency of 50%, a signalling rate of about 1 c.p.m./250 000 molecules only can be obtained; this means that to achieve a count significantly above background over a few minutes, about one million labelled antibodies are required to bind to captured antigen (6). The only amplification resource that is available is to use a labelled antiglobulin reagent. This demands a separate species of antibody (or different isotype) for capture and second layer and scrupulous absorption of the antiglobulin, and specificity testing, to ensure binding only to the second layer. Additional steps are involved with a risk of increased background. The ELISA alternative of this assay format has greater practical sensitivity because the enzyme amplifies the signal by reacting with many substrate molecules.

3.1.3 *Indirect antibody radioassay*

This is equivalent to the indirect antibody ELISA (see Chapter 4) and has the same range of applications. It uses a coating of standard antigen, to which test antibodies are applied. The binding of antibody is revealed by a radiolabelled antiglobulin. The assay is a valuable screening method for detecting monoclonal antibodies in hybridoma culture supernatants, where a 'universal' anti-mouse Ig labelled probe can be used. Positive wells can also be screened with labelled anti-isotype reagents to determine the antibody class of the secreted monoclonals. However, the short half-life of the label is a major disadvantage in applying the radioassay to routine work.

3.1.4 *Specific immune complex radioassay*

This, as with the ELISA method, detects preformed antigen−antibody complexes in serum by using an antigen-capture coating antibody (usually a monoclonal) and a labelled antiglobulin probe to reveal the bound antibody component of the complex. The antiglobulin must be species-specific.

3.1.5 *Serum antibody competition test (SACT)*

A radiolabelled monoclonal antibody to an antigen epitope of diagnostic importance is titrated against coated antigen (which need not be a purified molecule) and a dilution then used which can be inhibited from binding to the solid phase antigen by the presence of antibody in test sera mixed with the labelled reagent.

3.2 **General protocol for IRMA**

As the principles of IRMA methods differ from ELISA only in the nature of the antibody label, the protocols for performing the assays are virtually identical as are all elements of standardization. Refer to Chapter 4 for further details of methodology. Special considerations of methods applying to radioassay are given in the Technical notes in Section 3.2.5.

3.2.1 *Equipment and reagents*

Flexible round-bottomed 96 well plastic microtitration plates (e.g. Dynatech; Flow Labs—see Appendix of Suppliers).
Coating antigens and standard inhibitor antigens, as appropriate.
Coating antibodies—affinity purified IgG fractions, or monoclonal as required.
Radioiodinated antibody (IgG preparation) antigen-specific or antiglobulin, as appropriate—specific activity about $10-20$ $\mu Ci/\mu g$ IgG.

Reference positive and negative antigen or antibody samples, as appropriate.

Coating buffers as for ELISA (Chapter 4).

Washing and diluting buffer—PBS−Tween 20 with 1% (v/v) fetal calf serum (FCS).

Quenching buffer and labelled antibody dilution buffer—PBS with 3% (w/v) bovine serum albumin (BSA), or 2% (w/v) ox haemoglobin, or 5% (w/v) FCS.

Micropipettes, including multichannel and repeater-dispenser models as helpful options.

Scissors or cutters for separating plate wells for counting, or heated nichrome wire.

Radioactivity work tray.

Radioactivity disposal bin.

Disposable latex gloves.

Gamma counter and counting tubes.

Hand gamma counter.

3.2.2 *The antigen-capture IMRA*

(i)   Coat plates with 5−10 μg/ml of affinity-purified polyclonal antibody or monoclonal antibody using 50 μl per well, by incubation overnight at 4°C. Use normal immunoglobulin in control wells.

(ii)   Wash plates in washing buffer and quench in quenching buffer 1−2 h at room temperature (see Technical notes i and iii).

(iii) Titrate standard antigen by preparing a set of dilutions in PBS−Tween 20, dispensing 50 μl to antibody-coated and control wells and incubate for 1−2 h at 37°C.

(iv)   Wash plates and add to each well 50 μl of diluted labelled antibody (see Technical note iv). Incubate for 1 h (or longer), remove the well contents, wash and dry the plates. Cut up the plates into wells and place in labelled tubes for counting.

(v)   Draw a standard antigen binding curve and determine an appropriate range of standard concentrations for future reference.

(vi)   Perform a test with standard positive and negative samples to determine background values and required dilutions to ensure that test samples fit the scale.

(vii) Run tests for unknowns concurrently with the standard antigen and include dilutions of standard positive and negative controls.

(viii) Measure test antigen concentrations by relating counts to the standard curve. Counts are proportional to the amount of antigen bound.

3.2.3 *The antigen inhibition assay (7)*

(i)   Coat plates with 5−10 μg of antigen [less may be optimal as determined by trial (see Technical note i)], as in Section 3.2.2(i).

(ii)   Wash and quench as necessary.

(iii) Titrate radiolabelled antibody against the coated antigen using 50 μl per well and incubating for 1−2 h as necessary.

(iv)   Draw a titration curve of bound antibody counts against dilution and select an antibody dilution giving about 50% binding (see Technical note iv).

(v)   Pre-mix a range of standard antigen dilutions with the labelled antibody at its determined dilution for inhibition and add the mixture to the wells. Incubate for 1−2 h, remove the labelled well contents, wash the plates, dry, divide and count the wells.

(vi)   Draw a standard antigen inhibition curve, calculating % inhibition as

$$\% \text{ inhibition} = \left(1 - \frac{\text{c.p.m. label} + \text{inhibitor}}{\text{c.p.m. label only}}\right) \times 100$$

(vii)   Repeat the test with standard positive and negative samples to determine useful dilutions.

(viii) Run the full assay with standard antigen, positive and negative controls and test samples.

(ix)   Measure test antigen concentrations by relating % inhibitions to the standard inhibition curve prepared for the assay.

3.2.4 *The indirect antibody radioassay*

(i)   Coat plates with antigen, using 50 μl of 1−20 μg/ml (determined by trial).

(ii)   Wash, and quench as necessary.

(iii)   Apply reference monoclonal antibody dilutions in diluting buffer (irrelevant monoclonal as negative control) in the log range 1:10−1:10 000 (50 μl per well). Apply the test monoclonal culture supernates, initially diluted 1:2, to other wells. Incubate for 1 h at 37°C and wash in washing buffer five times.

(iv)   Add to each well 50 μl of radiolabelled anti-mouse Ig reagent, diluted in the diluting buffer, adding approximately 50 000 c.p.m. per well.

(v)   Incubate for 1 h at 37°C, then wash in PBS with 1% (v/v) FCS, dry and separate the wells for counting.

(vi)   Observe the counts in the negative control wells and the range of counts in the reference antibody wells. An approximate measure of monoclonal antibody titre in positive test wells is gained from comparing counts with those of reference reagent. Further quantitation is achieved by titration of strongly positive test samples in repeat assays.

3.2.5 *Technical notes*

(i) *Coating plates*. Antigens and antibodies are used in the range 1−30 μg/ml for coating overnight at 4°C. After washing the wells may require quenching with FCS or haemoglobin in PBS−Tween 20 for 1−2 h at room temperature. Different makes of flexible plate can be tried to find a manufacturer's brand that gives good binding with low background and low well variation for the particular coating preparation.

(ii) *Intermediate antigen or antibody addition steps*. The quantities of reagent are determined in preliminary titrations using standard reagents. Incubation times should be determined by trial. 50 μl per well is used throughout.

(iii) *Washing steps*. These should be done with great care, to reduce non-specific binding effects. Radioactive fluids should be withdrawn using a fine nylon tube attached to the tip of a pipette, to avoid damage to the well and removal of bound reagent. Active material should be collected and disposed of by an accepted method and not tipped into a general sink. This applies also to the first washings.

(iv) *Radiolabelled antibodies*. These should be diluted to give approximately 50 000−100 000 c.p.m./50 μl. Specific activity should be such that optimal working dilutions for performance of the assay will give counts in this range. 50 μl of antibody is used in assays. Labelled antibody solutions are usually prepared in PBS containing a protein solution to reduce non-specific binding to plastic. The inclusion of 0.05% Tween 20, as in ELISA, is also helpful. To aid antibody binding a 2% (w/v) final concentration of polyethylene glycol (6000 mol. wt) can also be added to the buffer. This may reduce incubation time to 30−60 min (7,8)—the optimal incubation times are determined by trial.

(v) *Replicate wells*. As with other immunoassays all reactions should be performed in a minimum of duplicate samples.

4. RADIOIMMUNOASSAYS OF LOW MOLECULAR WEIGHT MOLECULES

4.1 **Introduction**

This section describes the performance of RIAs for small peptides and other molecules (usually hormones) of low molecular weight that are not usually immunogenic *per se* (9). The ways in which reagents peculiar to this technique are prepared are first discussed with emphasis given to practical considerations; the establishment of a 'typical' RIA is then described by means of a specific example.

RIA (9) is a saturation assay technique (10). As conventionally performed it utilizes a radiolabelled standard antigen (ligand) and a specific antibody (binder); both are adjusted in concentration such that when standard volumes are mixed together and allowed to equilibrate, the bound labelled antigen, as a separated complex, provides a substantial level of radioactivity that can be counted over a few minutes. A quantitative inhibition reaction is then performed using unlabelled standard antigen over a range of concentrations—this is based upon the ability of the antigen to quantitatively compete with labelled ligand for binding to the limited amount of antibody. The distribution of labelled ligand between bound and unbound compartments can then be measured as a function of the amount of unlabelled standard antigen present. An inhibition curve is drawn. In the assay, labelled antigen and antibody are incubated with test samples— the presence of antigen in these is indicated by reduced labelled antigen binding and the degree of inhibition plotted on the standard curve to give a quantitative result.

4.2 **Steps towards a radioimmunoassay**

The essential components of an RIA are as follows.

(i)   Specific antibody.
(ii) Labelled tracer ligand (standard antigen) in purified form.
(iii) Unlabelled standard antigen competitor.
(iv) Reagent for physical separation of bound and unbound ligand (usually an antiglobulin, but can be ammonium sulphate or some other enhancer if free ligand is soluble in the solution).

4.2.1 *Preparation of specific antibody*

For RIA there is a critical requirement for both a high degree of specificity and high affinity of the antibody. The production and quality control of polyclonal antisera is considered in Volume I, Chapter 2, and of monoclonal antibodies in Volume I, Chapter 3. Molecules of molecular weight less than about 5000 are not usually sufficiently immunogenic to be used for immunization without conjugation to a carrier protein. Methods for hapten conjugation to protein carriers is reviewed in Volume I, Chapter 2. Bovine serum albumin is a popular carrier for raising anti-hormone antibodies to both peptides and steroids. The orientation of the conjugated hapten is clearly of importance in determining specificity and this must be considered in choosing a conjugation method. Density of conjugation is also important. Although there are about 60 free amino acid groups in albumin it is recommended that the hapten—albumin molar ratio should not exceed 12 in preparing the immunogen (11). There may be advantages also in using conjugation methods that avoid chemical denaturation of the carrier; for example in the mixed anhydride technique, side reactions and heat can be avoided by performing the conjugation at 4°C (12). Cholecystokinin-33 has been successfully conjugated to albumin for antibody production using the carbodiimide method (13); in this case no separation preceded injection, but others have used dialysis to purify conjugates prior to injection (14). Novel approaches to the production of specific antisera for RIA have included pre-treatment of animals with a cross-reacting steroid coupled to a large molecular weight carrier, a procedure which apparently inactivated cross-reacting antibody-forming precursor cells (15). There are also reports that conjugation of small peptides to protein carriers is unnecessary and reaction with simple organic compounds can provide a suitable complex to produce antibodies (16). In some cases (e.g. angiotensin), physical adsorption to carbon particles may be a sufficient preparation to generate specific antibodies in high titre (17).

4.2.2 *Labelling techniques for ligand*

The use of a radiolabel for ligands offers some definite advantages over other labelling principles, especially in reliability and precision of assays and in sensitivity in saturation tests. Some hormones can be intrinsically labelled so that, for instance, a carbon or hydrogen atom of the molecule is replaced constitutively by ^{14}C or ^{3}H during synthesis. The example RIA described below (Section 4.3) used a glyco[^{3}H]chenodeoxycholic acid as labelled ligand. A more popular way of obtaining a labelled ligand of high specific activity is by an extrinsic labelling procedure, of which the most universally applied is radioiodination and, in particular, the use of ^{125}I. This has many advantages; the labelling procedures are relatively simple, it has a high specific activity with a half-life of 60 days, its counting efficiency is in the order of 50−70% and gamma counting does not require a sample preparation step. The methods of radioiodination are extensively reviewed in Chapter 8 of this volume and will not be considered further here. They are not without problems, however, in some cases, particularly with small molecules where the inclusion of an iodinated radical may affect the antigenic reactivity compared with the original or native antigen. The smaller the antigen the more likely will it be that the iodination procedure itself will act to oxidize the molecule. The oxidation which occurs when the Chloramine-T method is used to iodinate cholecystokinin decreases its immunoreactivity by between 70−100% (18). The use of solid phase reagents has been promoted to provide a gentler method to achieve radioiodination (19). An alternative strategy is to use a radiometric assay for antigen using a labelled antibody (20). Section 3.2 provides a protocol for the IRMA.

4.2.3 *Procedures for separating bound from free ligand*

The final step in an RIA is to determine the distribution of labelled ligand between the bound and free compartments. This subject has received much attention; one of the earliest reviews is the most comprehensive (21). Several methods can be used; in every case, however, it is essential to ensure that, whatever the approach, the efficiency of separation does not vary over the range of volumes or dilutions of test plasma or serum that are incorporated in the test [see Section 4.3.3(ix)].

Methods of separation will vary in different assays—the primary consideration being the relative solubility of the free and bound labelled ligand. The principle behind many approaches is to bring the antibody−antigen complex out of solution, leaving behind the unbound labelled moiety or, as an alternative, to adsorb unbound ligand onto a solid phase. Some popular approaches to achieve this separation are as follows.

(i)   Chemical precipitation by ethanol, ammonium sulphate or polyethylene glycol—this depends on differences in solubility between immune complexes (or immunoglobulin *per se*) and unbound ligand.

(ii)   Use of an antiglobulin reagent which produces, under conditions of optimal proportions, an insoluble precipitate of all immunoglobulin of the specific antiserum including antigen-bound complex coupled in a lattice to divalent antiglobulin molecules. This is an efficient method but requires a second incubation step. The rate and efficiency of precipitation can be enhanced by the use of polyethylene glycol (8,22).

(iii)   The use of solid phase antibodies. This approach has many attractions, in particular, the use of the specific antibody adsorbed as a coating (antigen-capture) layer onto polystyrene plates or tubes. In this format the RIA has close similarities to the competitive antigen form of ELISA (see Chapter 4). It achieves a simple means of separating bound from free antigen by a washing step, but care is needed (as in ELISA) to ensure the minimum of non-specific labelled antigen binding to the solid phase.

4.3 **Setting up a radioimmunoassay**

As an example, an assay for conjugated chenodeoxycholic acid is given.

4.3.1 *Preparation of glycochenodeoxycholic acid−albumin conjugate for immunization*

Bile acids are steroid carboxylic acids. In man they may be conjugated with either glycine or taurine and differ only by the number of hydroxyl groups on the steroid nucleus. In preparing a hapten−protein immunogen for a specific antibody it is essential that these differences are retained in the conjugation process. The method used to prepare the bile acid conjugate was the mixed anhydride technique (12). The conjugation method is described in Volume I, Chapter 2 (Section 3.1.2) (23). This yields an average of 12 hapten molecules per albumin molecule.

4.3.2 *Preparation of antisera*

Three adult New Zealand White rabbits were injected with 5 mg of conjugate in Complete Freund's Adjuvant in the thigh muscle. This was repeated in the other leg 10 days later. Booster doses were given intradermally in saline (100 μg each time), starting 2 weeks later, and repeated every 4−6 days until a strong Arthus reaction followed injection some 10 weeks after the first injection. The binding activity of trial bleeds taken after the fourth intradermal injection, and after all subsequent injections, revealed a rising titre of anti-bile acid antibodies. The animals were exsanguinated 3 days after the sixth intradermal injection.

4.3.3 *Assessment of antisera*

(i) *Preparation of 'working' labelled ligand solution.*

(1)   Prepare a stock solution of radioactive glyco[^{3}H]chenodeoxycholic acid (New England Nuclear) in absolute ethanol to provide an activity of 10 μCi/ml.

(2)   Dilute further (1:80) in a phosphate buffer solution containing

13.4 g	KH_2PO_4
5.71 g	Na_2HPO_4
9.0 g	NaCl
1.0 g	NaN_3
1.0 g	BSA
0.125 g	Porcine gamma globulin

in 1 litre of distilled water. Adjust to pH 7.5.

This constitutes the *'working' labelled bile acid (ligand) solution* (25 pmol/ml).

(ii) *Titrating the antisera against labelled ligand to find the 'working' titre.*

(1)   Prepare the antisera in a doubling dilution series in test tubes using the phosphate buffer solution.

(2)   To 0.3 ml of each dilution in duplicate add 0.1 ml of labelled bile acid (2.5 pmol). A control of labelled ligand and 0.3 ml of buffer solution is used to determine total added radioactivity.

(3)   Add a further 0.1 ml of phosphate buffer to each tube, mix (by vortex mixer) for 10 sec and allow to stand at room temperature for 2 h.

(4)   Add saturated ammonium sulphate in distilled water at room temperature (0.5 ml) to all tubes (0.5 ml of phosphate buffer solution to the control 'total' tube). Mix the solutions for 10 sec as above and allow to stand for 15 min.

(5)   Centrifuge the tubes at 3000 g for 20 min at 4°C.

(6)   Add 0.3 ml of each supernatant to 10 ml of NE 260 scintillation fluid (New England Nuclear) in a liquid scintillation vial.

(7)   Allow the vials to dark-adapt and equilibrate within the counting chamber prior to counting.

(8)   Adjust the counter settings to provide sufficient counts per sample to hold counting errors to less than ±2% at 95% confidence limits.

(9)   By comparing the counts in the series of antibody tubes (mean of each pair) with that of the total added count control, calculate the effect of antibody in reducing supernatant counts as a percentage of labelled ligand bound. Draw curves of these data against antiserum dilution (see *Figure 2*).

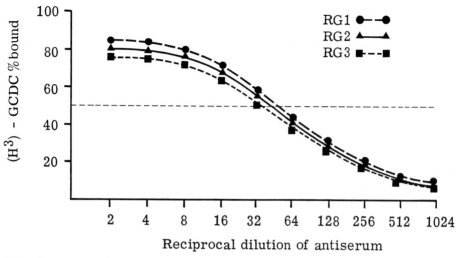

Figure 2. Assessment of antisera. RG1, RG2 and RG3 are antisera of three rabbits to glycochenodeoxycholic acid.

(10)   From the curves determine the *working titre* of each antiserum as that original dilution, when reacted in the above conditions, that binds about 50% of labelled ligand. At this range of dilution the inhibition of antibody binding to labelled ligand by unlabelled standard ligand is most sensitive. *Figure 2* gives the titration results of the three prepared rabbit antisera, taken from trial bleeds 7 weeks after the initial injection. It can be seen that the binding curves for all three rabbits are very similar, but rabbit 1 antiserum is superior and this rabbit was selected as the source for the subsequent working antibody reagent.

(iii) *Setting up a competitive inhibition reaction with unlabelled standard ligand.*

(1)   Dilute non-radioactive glycochenodeoxycholic acid (Weddel Pharmaceuticals Ltd) and taurochenodeoxycholic acid from stock in phosphate buffer solution in the range 8−250 pmol/0.1 ml.

(2)   Add 0.1 ml of the standard ligand dilutions to 0.3 ml of antiserum (diluted 1:500 to working titre) in duplicate tubes. Prepare controls for zero inhibition (to give maximum binding of added labelled ligand—set at 50%, using antiserum at 1:500) by adding 0.1 ml of buffer to the antiserum.

(3)   Add 0.1 ml of labelled ligand to each tube, (including control tubes with no antibody for total added counts).

(4)   Allow the assay to proceed as in (ii) above.

(5)   Calculate the percentage free labelled ligand at each point in the inhibition series from the supernatant counts and draw curves plotting these data against amount of unlabelled ligand added. Clearly, with no competitor the expected 50% of free labelled ligand will be found, but as competitor is introduced and increases so more labelled ligand will be unbound. This is illustrated in *Figure 3*. The standard inhibition reaction, as illustrated, forms the basis for the quantitative assay of hormone in test serum samples. It will be noted that the effect of taurochenodeoxycholic acid is indistinguishable from that of glycochenodeoxycholic acid.

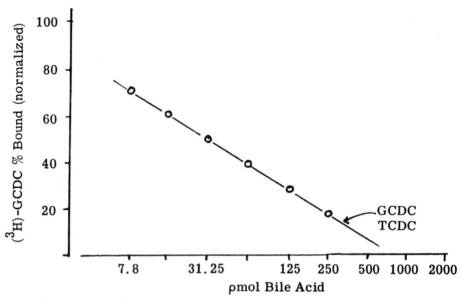

Figure 3. Competitive inhibition with unlabelled standard ligands of taurochenodeoxycholic acid (TCDC) and glycochenodeoxycholic acid (GCDC) which give superimposed results.

(iv) *Testing the specificity of the competitive inhibition assay.* This is a critical step in quality control of an RIA, the essential point being to demonstrate under the working conditions of the assay that no related molecules (i.e. other members of the hormone family with similar antigenic structure) are capable of producing significant levels of displacement of the homologous labelled ligand from the antibody. This is usually calculated as the relative amount of other antigens required to produce a 50% displacement of the homologous ligand. The assay is performed as in (iii) above, substituting other antigens for the unlabelled standard (homologous) ligand and using a wide range of concentrations. The results of such an analysis calculated on 50% displacement of glyco[³H]chenodeoxycholic acid is shown in *Table 3*. No cross-reactivity is detectable with aetiocholane, androsterone, epi-androsterone or cholesterol (data not shown). It can be seen that conjugated bile acids exhibit greater cross-reactivity than the corresponding free bile acids and the degree of interference from the latter appears to be a function of the number of nuclear hydroxyl groups present.

(v) *The quantitative assay for antigen in test serum samples.* For bile acids it is necessary to perform an initial serum extraction.

(1) Precipitate serum proteins by addition of 1 vol. of serum to 19 vols of methanol – ethanol (5:95 v/v) containing 0.1% ammonia solution. Heat the mixture under reflux for 15 min.
(2) Allow the suspension to cool and then centrifuge at 3000 *g* for 15 min at 15°C.
(3) Evaporate the supernatant to dryness under reduced pressure and dissolve the residue in 2 vols of methanol.

Table 3. Cross reactivity with different bile acid species. Published with permission of Marcel Dekker Inc. from ref. 23.

Bile acid	Amount required to produce 50% displacement [^3H]GCDC (pmol)
Glycochenodeoxycholic	30
Taurochenodeoxycholic	30
Glycocholic	300
Taurocholic	300
Glycodeoxycholic	3000
Taurodeoxycholic	3000
Chenodeoxycholic	300
Cholic	1200

No cross reactivity was detected with deoxycholic acid, any of the lithocholate fractions or the 4 common 3α-SO_4 bile acids

The assay is performed in parallel with a standard competition assay, using extracted serum samples diluted to at least 1:5 in the phosphate buffer solution. Quantitation of test antigen is gained by comparing the percentage of free labelled ligand in the test assay tubes against the standard inhibition curve.

(vi) *Testing cross-reactivity under running conditions.* This is frequently neglected in RIAs but should be an essential final step in quality control of any assay. The principle is to test known antigen-positive samples under conditions of excess potential competitors for antibody. A useful approach in the chenodeoxycholate acid assay, as an example, is to run test samples of the serum-conjugated molecule in the presence of a range of concentrations of the free unconjugated acid. With the antiserum used, the degree of inhibition achieved with conjugated ligand is unaltered in the presence of free acid at lower concentrations, but when the concentration of the latter exceeds 18 μmol/litre (~ 10 times the concentration of conjugated chenodeoxycholate in the original sample) the errors in the estimation of conjugated ligand become considerable (23).

(vii) *Determining precision of the assay.* A measure of assay precision is achieved by comparing the standard inhibition curves obtained on a number of successive occasions and calculating the coefficient of variation at the lowest, intermediate and highest standard ligand concentrations. In a succession of 20 curves generated in the conjugated chenodeoxycholate assay, precision was 5% (lowest), 11 − 12% (intermediate) and 14% at the 250 pmol level. A further estimate of between-batch precision is gained by analysis of the same test sample placed in different batches. With this protocol for 10 batches, between-batch precision was 6% (3.8 ± 0.23; mean ± SD). Within-batch precision can be estimated from duplicate results of a large number of test samples run at varying dilutions so that at least two dilutions fall within the standard range. In the example assay, with duplicates of 200 test samples, the within-batch precision was 2%.

(viii) *Determining the sensitivity of the assay.* An estimate of the sensitivity of an assay is gained from determining the minimum amount of inhibiting ligand that can be added to the mixture of antibody and labelled ligand to reduce the amount of bound label by a statistically significant amount. This is influenced by the precision of the assay. In the example assay, the addition of only 8 pmol of glycochenodeoxycholate to the incubation mixture reduced the amount of bound label achieved with zero inhibitor by 1500 d.p.m. (coefficient of variation at zero = 5.5%, n = 20). In consequence an assay of 0.1 ml of extracted undiluted serum would enable bile acid concentrations as low as 0.06 pmol/litre to be measured.

(ix) *A check on recovery of antigen during serum extraction.* In assays requiring a serum extraction step it is necessary to examine the efficiency of this procedure. A guide to this can be gained by exposing the labelled ligand to extraction. The recovery of glyco[^{3}H]chenodeoxycholic acid was 94 ± 3% ($n = 3$). A second test is then to add the labelled ligand standard concentrations to normal sera and to determine its recovery rate. This should not be significantly different and in the above example was 92.8 ± 4.6% ($n = 5$).

5. ACKNOWLEDGEMENTS

Our special thanks to Dudley Sampson for expertise in bile acid radioimmunoassay and to Mrs F.O'Reilly for preparation of the manuscript.

We are also grateful to the Publishers of *Analytical Letters* for allowing us to reproduce *Table 3*, originally published in ref. 23.

6. REFERENCES

1. Berson,S.A. and Yalow,R.S. (1958) *Adv. Biol. Med. Phys.*, **6**, 349.
2. Parker,C.W. (1976) *Radioimmunoassay of Biologically Active Compounds.* Prentice-Hall Inc., New Jersey.
3. Heidelberger,M. and Kendall,F.E. (1929) *J. Exp. Med.*, **50**, 809.
4. Maurer,P.H. (1971) In *Methods in Immunology and Immunochemistry*, Vol. III. Williams,C.A. and Chase,M.W. (eds), Academic Press, New York, Chapter 13, p. 1.
5. Heidelberger,M. and Kendall,F.E. (1935) *J. Exp. Med.*, **62**, 697.
6. Ekins,R. (1981) In *Immunoassays for the 80s.* Voller,A., Bartlett,A. and Bidwell,D. (eds), MTP Press, Lancaster, England, p. 5.
7. Hole,N.J.K., Catty,J.P. and Catty,D. (1987) *Mol. Immunol.*, **24**, 75.
8. Catty,D. and King,T.D. (1974) *Immunochemistry*, **11**, 615.
9. Yalow,R.S. and Berson,S.A. (1958) *J. Clin. Invest.*, **39**, 1157.
10. Ekins,P.P. (1974) *Br. Med. Bull.*, **30**, 3.
11. Teale,J.D. (1978) *Radioimmunoassay 2. Scientific Foundations of Clinical Biochemistry.* Chapter 19, Williams,D.L. and Marks,V. (eds), Heinemann Medical, p. 279.
12. Erlanger,B.F., Borek,F., Beiser,S.M. and Leiberman,S. (1957) *J. Biol. Chem.*, **228**, 713.
13. Byrnes,D.J., Henderson,L., Borody,T. and Rehfeld,J.F. (1981) *Clin. Chim. Acta*, **111**, 81.
14. Murphy,G.M., Edkins,S.M., Williams,J.W. and Catty,D. (1974) *Clin. Chim. Acta*, **54**, 81.
15. Takeishi,K., Hamaoka,T., Suguira,N., Hanaihara,C. and Yanaihara,N. (1981) *J. Immunol. Methods*, **47**, 249.
16. Borek,F., Stupp,Y. and Sele,M. (1965) *Immunology*, **98**, 739.
17. Boyd,G.W. and Peart,W.S. (1968) *Lancet*, **I**, 129.
18. Rehfeld,F.J. (1978) *J. Biol. Chem.*, **253**, 4016.
19. Guenther,J.G. and Ramsolen,H. (1984) *Biotech. Lab.*, **38**.
20. Woodhead,J.S., Addison,G.M. and Hales,C.N. (1974) *Br. Med. Bull.*, **30**, 44.
21. Ratcliffe,J.G. (1974) *Br. Med. Bull.*, **30**, 32.
22. Bolton,A.E. (1981) In *Immunoassays for the 80s.* Voller,A. Bartlett,A. and Bidwell,D. (eds), MTP Press Ltd, Lancaster, England, p. 69.
23. Sampson,D.G., Murphy,G.M., Cross,L.M. and Catty,D. (1979) *Anal. Lett.*, **12**, 927.

CHAPTER 4

ELISA and related enzyme immunoassays

DAVID CATTY and CHANDRA RAYKUNDALIA

1. INTRODUCTION

In the early 1970s, the search for simple sensitive methods for detecting and quantitating antigen and antibody that did not rely upon particle agglutination or radiolabelled reagents led to the development of solid phase enzyme-coupled reagent assays (1,2). In principle (*Figure 1*), the labelling by chemical conjugation of an enzyme to either antigen or antibody allows detection of immune complexes formed on a solid phase, as the fixed enzyme, once washed free of excess reagents, on subsequent substrate interaction can yield a coloured product which can be visualized and/or measured by optical density. The approach has many of the properties of an ideal immunoassay; it is versatile, robust, simple to perform, uses stable reagents economically and achieves, by use of the solid phase, a simple separation of bound and free moieties. Various methods of enhancing and amplifying the substrate signal (for instance by using luminescence and enzyme cascade systems) have brought the sensitivity of some enzyme immunoassays to within the range of the hormone radioimmunoassay. Non-competitive antigen-capture assays can theoretically achieve a sensitivity capable of detecting a single bound antigen molecule. Because of their combined simplicity and sensitivity, solid phase enzyme immunoassays can be used reliably for large number screening of small volume test samples in the simplest of laboratory environments. This technical advance has had the greatest impact in epidemiology and in the diagnosis of infectious diseases (3 – 13), but the assays are also used routinely for screening monoclonal antibodies, for detection and measurement of hormones and drugs, for the determination of specific antibody isotypes and immune complexes, and for many other applications. In essence, problems of specificity are no different from, and no greater than, those of other immunoassays and, in the same way as in these assays, can be brought to a minimum by the use of quality-controlled reagents and standardized procedures. Use of monoclonal antibodies with defined specificity and homogeneous affinity has led to the recent development of many new tests—some commercially available such as those for pregnancy testing and for AIDS virus antibody. A variety of solid phase surfaces has been exploited; the earliest tests relied on plastic tubes but these have been largely replaced by plastic microtitration plates with flat, optically clear, well bottoms to allow easy *in situ* optical density measurement with special enzyme-linked immunosorbent assay (ELISA) readers. Recent modifications include solid phase reactions on micropegs, dip-sticks and beads, and 'dot-ELISA' assays on protein-binding membranes such as nitrocellulose.

Although, as technology advances, ELISA plate assays may eventually be replaced by homogeneous 'dip-stick' types of procedure, the microplate systems will for many

(i) Antibody or antigen is chemically coupled to an enzyme

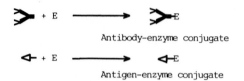

Antibody-enzyme conjugate

Antigen-enzyme conjugate

(ii) Antigens or antibodies are coated onto ELISA plate wells or other solid phase

antigen
coating

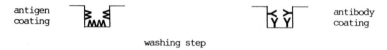

antibody
coating

washing step

(iii) One or more layers of immune complex are formed on the solid phase

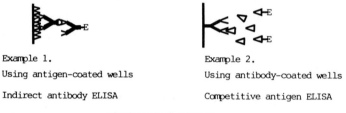

Example 1.

Using antigen-coated wells

Indirect antibody ELISA

Example 2.

Using antibody-coated wells

Competitive antigen ELISA

washing steps between
complex layers

(iv) Reaction between fixed enzyme and substrate leads to coloured product

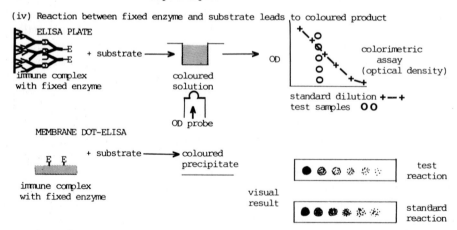

ELISA PLATE

immune complex
with fixed enzyme

+ substrate →

coloured
solution

OD

OD probe

colorimetric
assay
(optical density)

standard dilution +—+
test samples OO

MEMBRANE DOT-ELISA

immune complex
with fixed enzyme

+ substrate → coloured
precipitate

visual
result

test
reaction

standard
reaction

Figure 1. Principle of ELISA and related immunoassays.

years remain the most amenable format for most research and routine applications. It is this format which is used here to describe the principle of enzyme immunoassays, protocols for quality control of reagents and performance of specific tests.

2. PRINCIPLES OF ELISA

The performance of ELISA and related solid phase assays depends on four major principles (see *Figure 1*).

Table 1. Popular enzyme and substrate systems for ELISA.

Enzyme	Conjugation method (ref.)	Soluble substrates (ref.)	Reading wavelength (nm)	Insoluble substrates
HRP	1. Two-step glutaraldehyde (1)	O-Phenylenediamine dihydrochloride (OPD)	492	Diaminobenzidine (DAB)
	2. Sodium m-periodate (2)	Tetramethylbenzidine (TMB)	450	4-Chloro-1-napthol (CNP)
	3. N-Succinimidyl-3-(2-pyridyldithio) propionate (SPDP) (3,4)	2,2'-Azino-di(3-ethyl)benzthiazoline sulphonic acid (ABTS)	650 (405 after stopping) (7)	3-Amino-4-ethyl carbazole (AEC)
		5-Aminosalicyclic acid (ASA) (8)	450	
AP	Glutaraldehyde one-step method (5)	N-p-nitrophenyl alkaline phosphate (PNPP) (9)	402–412	Naphthol As-mx phosphate +Fast Blue BB salt (NAPFB) Naphthol As-mx phosphate +Red BB salt (NAPR) 5-Bromo-4-chloro-3-idolyl phosphate (BCIP)
β-Galactosidase (β-G)	m-Maleimidobenzoyl-N-hydroxy-succinimide ester (MBHS) (6)	O-Nitrophenyl β-D-galactoside (ONPG) (6)	420	
Urease	Glutaraldehyde one-step method (7)	Bromocresol purple (BP)	588	
Penicillinase G (PG)	Glutaraldehyde one-step method (5)	Iodine and starch (IS) (10)	visual (blue to colourless)	

References for *Table 1.*
1. Avrameas,S. and Ternynck,T. (1971) *Immunochemistry*, **8**, 1176.
2. Nakane,P.K. and Kawaoi,A. (1974) *J. Histochem. Cytochem.*, **22**, 1084.
3. Nilsson,P., Bergquist,N.R. and Grundy,M.S. (1981) *J. Immunol. Methods*, **41**, 81.
4. Pain,D. and Surolia,A. (1981) *J. Immunol. Methods*, **40**, 219.
5. Avrameas,S. (1969) *Immunochemistry*, **5**, 49.
6. Kato,K., Hamaguchi,Y., Fukui,H. and Ishikawa,E. (1975) *J. Biochem.*, **78**, 423.
7. Chandler,H.M. Cox,J.C., Healey,K., MacGregor,A., Premier,R.R. and Hurrel,J.G.R. (1982) *J. Immunol. Methods*, **43**, 187.
8. Matsuda,H., Tanaka,H., Blas,B.L., Nosenas,J.S., Tokawa,T. and Ohsawa,S. (1984) *Jap. J. Exp. Med.*, **54**, 131.
9. Engvall,E. and Perlmann,P. (1971) *Immunochemistry*, **8**, 871.
10. Geetha,P.B., Ghosh,S.N., Gupta,N.P., Borkar,P.S. and Ramachandran,S. (1978) *Hind. Antibiot. Bull.*, **21**, 11.

(i)   A variety of enzymes, including horseradish peroxidase (HRP) and alkaline phosphatase (AP)—the most popular—can be chemically coupled to either antibody or antigen under conditions which retain the biological properties (i.e. substrate interaction, antigen binding, antigenicity) of both components of the conjugate.

(ii)   Most antigens, for example proteins, peptides, polysaccharides and bacterial lipopolysaccharides, bind spontaneously to plastic surfaces such as the wells of polystyrene microtitre plates. Antibodies, as proteins, also attach whilst retaining their antigen-binding activity. Thus antigen- or antibody-coated plates can be prepared as the initial step. Once antigens or antibodies applied to coat or 'sensitize' the solid phase are bound, they become resistant to vigorous washing in detergent buffer whilst excess unbound reagent is simply removed by this process.

(iii) In subsequent steps one or more layers of a solid phase captured immune complex are formed, with unbound entities again efficiently washed away. This affords the basis for high specific to non-specific signal ratio when captured enzyme reacts with substrate.

(iv)   An enzyme conjugate of antibody or antigen when bound in the immune complex leaves the enzyme component available for substrate interaction. Addition of substrate, in the usual form of assay, results in a progressive substrate solution colour change. The reaction can be stopped at an appropriate stage and the colour signal determined by visual comparison with standards or by optical density measurement. Appropriate enzyme—substrate systems are used for this purpose—some popular ones with absorption wavelengths of the soluble substrate products are given in *Table 1*. When test formats require the solid phase itself to show colour change, as in some 'dip-stick' assays and on 'dot-ELISA', the requirement is for the substrate to form an insoluble fixed coloured precipitate. *Table 1* gives a number of such substrates for HRP and AP. *Table 2* gives the concentration and buffer conditions for using a range of substrates with soluble or insoluble product properties.

3. FORMS OF ANTIBODY AND ANTIGEN ASSAY

A number of alternative assay systems can be used for the detection and measurement of antibody and antigen using antigen or antibody solid phase coating principles. Specific immune complexes can also be examined, and for these, and antibody responses to defined antigens, the use of isotype-specific antiglobulins allows the class and subclass composition to be studied; tests can be operated to look for the presence of a specific antibody class of diagnostic value. A range of popular and useful assay systems is illustrated in *Figure 2*. Some notes on the principles and applications of these assays are set out below.

3.1 **Simple-two layer assays**

ELISA plates are prepared by coating with either antigen or antibody and are then exposed to a potentially binding enzyme-labelled complementary antibody or antigen. In assay 1 (*Figure 2*) a test antigen (e.g. a cell extract that may contain a virus, or

Table 2. Solutions for soluble and insoluble substrates in ELISA and dot-ELISA (membrane) assays.

Enzyme[a]	Substrate[a]	Buffer
HRP	OPD	10 mg/25 ml of sodium citrate buffer, 0.15 M pH 5.0; add 5 μl of 30% (v/v) H_2O_2.
	TMB	2.5 mg/250 μl of DMSO[b]; make up to 25 ml with sodium citrate buffer, 0.1 M pH 6.0; add 5 μl of 30% (v/v) H_2O_2.
	ABTS	60 mg/100 ml of sodium citrate buffer, 0.1 M pH 6.0; add 35 μl of 30% (v/v) H_2O_2 (stop with 1.25% sodium fluoride—read at 405 nm).
	DAB	10 mg/20 ml of Tris buffer, 50 mM pH 7.4; filter and add 20 μl of 1% (v/v) H_2O_2.
	CNP	6 mg in 1 ml of methanol; add 10 ml of Tris buffer, 50 mM pH 7.4; filter and add 40 μl of 30% (v/v) H_2O_2.
	AEC	80 mg in 1 ml of N,N'-dimethylformamide + 200 ml of acetate buffer, 0.1 M pH 4.5; filter and add 50 μl of 30% (v/v) H_2O_2.
	ASA	80 mg/100 ml of hot distilled water. Adjust to pH 6.0 with 1 M NaOH and add 10% by vol. of 0.05% (v/v) H_2O_2; stop with 25 μl of 1 M NaOH.
AP	PNPP	5 mg/5 ml of diethanolamine–HCl buffer, 0.1 M pH 9.8 + 1 mM $MgCl_2$.
	NAPFB	(A) 4 mg of naphthol As-mx phosphate/200 μl of dimethylformamide in a glass tube. (B) 10 mg of Fast Blue BB salt/10 ml of Tris buffer, 0.05 M pH 9.2 + 2 mM $MgCl_2$. Mix A and B and filter.
	NAPR	(A) 4 mg of naphthol As-mx phosphate/200 μl of dimethyl formamide in a glass tube. (B) 10 mg of Red BB salt/10 ml of Tris buffer, 0.05 M pH 9.2 + 2 mM $MgCl_2$. Mix A and B and filter.
	BCIP	1 mg/ml in AMP solution (2-amino-2-methyl-1-propanol).
β-G	ONPG	2.5 mg/ml in sodium phosphate buffer, 0.1 M pH 7.0 + 1 mM $MgCl_2$ + 0.1 M β-mercaptoethanol.
Urease	BP	8 mg/1.48 ml of 0.01 M NaOH; make up to 100 ml with de-ionized water; add 100 mg of urea, and EDTA to 0.2 mM. Adjust the pH to 4.8 with 0.1 M NaOH or HCl. Store at 4°C.
PG	IS	Add to each ELISA plate well 25 μl of each of the following reagents in sequence: (i) 1% (w/v) gelatine in 0.1 M PO_4 buffer pH 7.0; (ii) 1% (w/v) starch solution in warm distilled water; (iii) 3.04 mg/ml benzyl penicillin in 0.1 M PO_4 buffer pH 7.0 (5000 U/ml); (iv) 0.01 N iodine in 0.1 M KI stock solution (in dark bottle).

[a]For full definition of abbreviations see *Table 1*.
[b]DMSO, dimethyl sulphoxide.

101

an insect blood meal that may come from man) is used to coat the wells. The presence of the antigen in the coating layer is revealed by the application of a standard antigen-specific antibody—enzyme conjugate (e.g. anti-virus, anti-human immunoglobulin). After exposure to this antibody the wells are washed and enzyme substrate added. If labelled antibody has bound through the presence of antigen in the coating layer (as in control antigen wells), the enzyme—substrate interaction occurs and a colour develops.

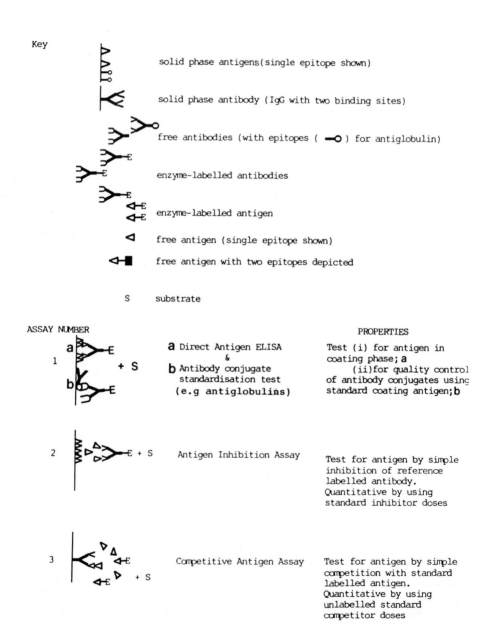

Key

solid phase antigens(single epitope shown)

solid phase antibody (IgG with two binding sites)

free antibodies (with epitopes (—O) for antiglobulin)

enzyme-labelled antibodies

enzyme-labelled antigen

free antigen (single epitope shown)

free antigen with two epitopes depicted

S   substrate

ASSAY NUMBER

PROPERTIES

1

a Direct Antigen ELISA
&
b Antibody conjugate
standardisation test
(e.g antiglobulins)

Test (i) for antigen in coating phase; **a**
(ii)for quality control of antibody conjugates using standard coating antigen;**b**

2

Antigen Inhibition Assay

Test for antigen by simple inhibition of reference labelled antibody. Quantitative by using standard inhibitor doses

3

Competitive Antigen Assay

Test for antigen by simple competition with standard labelled antigen. Quantitative by using unlabelled standard competitor doses

ASSAY NUMBER

PROPERTIES

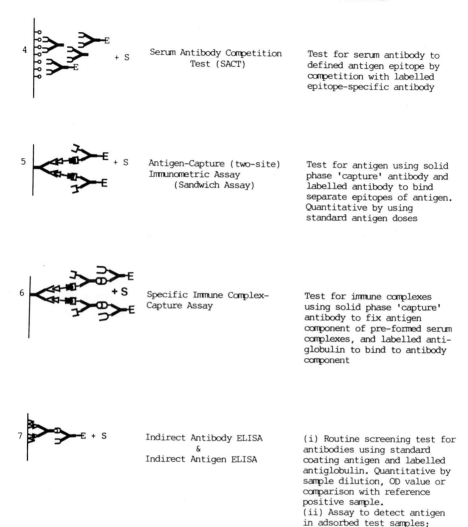

4   + S   Serum Antibody Competition Test (SACT)

Test for serum antibody to defined antigen epitope by competition with labelled epitope-specific antibody

5   + S   Antigen-Capture (two-site) Immunometric Assay (Sandwich Assay)

Test for antigen using solid phase 'capture' antibody and labelled antibody to bind separate epitopes of antigen. Quantitative by using standard antigen doses

6   + S   Specific Immune Complex-Capture Assay

Test for immune complexes using solid phase 'capture' antibody to fix antigen component of pre-formed serum complexes, and labelled antiglobulin to bind to antibody component

7   E + S   Indirect Antibody ELISA
&
Indirect Antigen ELISA

(i) Routine screening test for antibodies using standard coating antigen and labelled antiglobulin. Quantitative by sample dilution, OD value or comparison with reference positive sample.
(ii) Assay to detect antigen in adsorbed test samples; uses reference antigen-specific first antibody and labelled antiglobulin

Figure 2. Enzyme immunoassays for antibodies and antigens.

Negative controls are wells coated with samples of similar provenance but known to be specific antigen-free. The reactions are stopped when positive controls are optimally developed. Assay 1 is also used for the quality control (i.e. tests for specificity and titre) of antibody−enzyme conjugates. In this case the wells are coated with specific antigen or other molecules to which the antibody may cross-react. The conjugate is titrated against the antigen and compared with a reference antibody conjugate for both titre and specificity.

Two simple ways of determining and measuring antigen in solution are as follows.

103

In assay 2 (*Figure 2*) a standard antigen is used to coat the wells. An antibody−enzyme conjugate is diluted out, as in assay 1, to give optimal binding when applied to the antigen layer. Optimal binding is usually defined as that giving an optical density reading of approximately 1.0 on measurement of substrate reaction. The conjugate diluted to this point is easily and quantitatively inhibited (i.e. its binding sites are blocked) by trace amounts of free antigen in test samples. Thus when the diluted conjugate is pre-incubated with dilutions of antigen-positive test samples, and the mixture then applied to the wells, the free test antigen quantitatively blocks antibody binding and there is a gradation of subsequent substrate interactions according to the degree of antibody inhibition. The assay is calibrated by using dilutions of standard antigen inhibitor. Antigen-negative samples are included to provide the background reading.

In assay 3 a principle of antigen competition is utilized instead of antibody inhibition. In this form of simple assay for antigen the wells are coated with specific antibody. Enzyme-labelled standard antigen is then titrated on the antibody to determine an optimal dilution which is easily competed for by free antigen. Standard free antigen dilutions are then used in competition with the same labelled antigen to construct a standard antigen competition curve. Test samples are then pre-mixed and incubated with the labelled antigen. Where samples are antigen-positive there is competition for binding to antibody, the amount of enzyme indirectly binding to the antibody is quantitatively reduced and this is reflected in the degree of subsequent substrate reaction over a given time. In this assay the enzyme−antigen conjugate can be used at very low concentrations and offers a correspondingly very sensitive antigen estimation system. Known positive and negative antigen sample controls are incorporated into each run.

The competition principle is also applied in a simple form of antibody test illustrated in assay 4 (*Figure 2*). Wells are coated with standard antigen and can then be exposed to a previously determined optimum dilution (using assay 1) of a specific reference antibody conjugate which gives a standard degree of substrate reaction over a set time. If this antibody conjugate is mixed with a competing antibody to the same antigen epitope(s) and the two are added to the antigen-coated wells, then there is a quantitative competition for binding and the amount of bound enzyme will be reduced over a wide range of test antigen dilutions. A reference antibody is used for calibration, and controls are known antibody-positive and -negative samples. This test is operationally most successful when using a labelled monoclonal antibody, where competition by test sample antibody is restricted to a single target epitope of the coating antigen. This form of assay is called a serum antibody competition test. It is a simple means by which a monoclonal antibody defining an epitope unique to an infective organism (for instance) can be used to identify a diagnostic antibody specificity of the host.

3.2 Two-site (sandwich) antigen-capture and specific immune complex-capture assays

An assay system favoured for its combined simplicity, specificity and sensitivity, and its easy conversion to 'dot-ELISA' or 'dip-stick' formats, is the so-called sandwich ELISA illustrated as assay 5 in *Figure 2*. Antibody coating the solid phase (often a monoclonal of high affinity) is exposed to test sample (and positive and negative control samples, and standard antigen in dilutions) and, after washing, the complex is exposed further to a diluted reference antibody conjugate to the same antigen. With the restriction that the detected and standard antigen must have multiple epitopes for antibody binding, or a repeating, spatially distant, single epitope (especially where the same monoclonal antibody is used for the coating and conjugate antibody layers), this assay is potentially very sensitive; the use of monoclonal antibodies provides special features of specificity and low background characteristics. Assay 6 is a modification of the sandwich principle in which pre-formed serum immune complexes can be detected by using an antiglobulin−enzyme conjugate as the third layer. The antibody isotypes of the immune complexes can be determined and quantified by using a panel of isotype-specific antiglobulin conjugates on the same test samples in repeated assays.

3.3 The indirect antibody ELISA and indirect antigen ELISA (assay 7)

This assay is the most popular means to screen serum samples for the presence of specific antibody and has played an invaluable role in epidemiological studies of many infections. Antigen (frequently viral-, bacterial- or parasite-soluble extract) is used to coat the ELISA wells. Serum (or other body fluid such as milk, saliva, faecal extracts or CSF) is then applied, and bound specific antibody is revealed by the use of an antiglobulin conjugate. The antiglobulin reagent may be of broad specificity to detect all antibody classes or it may be class- or subclass-specific or directed to secretory component (for instance) to detect specific secretory IgA antibodies in milk or saliva. The assay is commonly used to screen hybridoma clones for specific antibodies (using anti-mouse immunoglobulin conjugates) and to determine monoclonal antibody isotypes. A major advantage of this assay is that it can utilize a 'universal' anti-species (e.g. anti-human) immunoglobulin−enzyme conjugate to test for antibody in any number of human samples. As both the antigen coating and the applied conjugate can be standardized, the performance of the assay is operationally simple and easily controlled. The same assay principle can be used in an indirect antigen ELISA. In this case the first antibody is a specific reference reagent used to detect antigens in coating samples. The use of a first antibody and a labelled antiglobulin gives the assay greater sensitivity than the direct antigen ELISA (assay 1).

4. PREPARATION OF ANTIBODY−ENZYME CONJUGATES AND THEIR QUALITY CONTROL

It is within the competence of anyone with a modest experience of immunochemistry to prepare their own antibody−enzyme conjugates. A good starting antiserum is essential but assuming this has been prepared and tested for specificity and titre (see Volume I, Chapter 2) then the remaining steps are not difficult. Apart from the considerable cost advantage of self-prepared conjugates, it may not be possible to find a conjugate of suitable specificity from commercial catalogues and there is a risk of loss of activity in transit, or if held in Customs, or if delivery is to countries remote from the supplier. Even purchased conjugates will require stringent quality testing under the conditions of the intended assay. For all these reasons it is often preferable to prepare one's own conjugates. Once prepared they can be stored in active condition for years. The most useful conjugates are antiglobulins since they act as universal reagents in many kinds

Table 3. Equipment and materials required for the preparation and storage of conjugates (see Appendix of Suppliers).

Equipment

Spectrophotometer; variable wavelength model
Balance; $0-100$ g in 0.001 g units
pH meter
Magnetic stirrer with small stirring bars, or rotary wheel mixer for 20 ml and 5 ml glass capped
    bottles
Fraction collector with 4 ml glass collection tubes
UV monitor set at 280 nm, and recorder
Gel filtration columns; 1.6×35 cm and 1.6×95 cm
Graduated pipettes
Pasteur pipettes
Hamilton micropipettes; $10-100$ μl range
Refrigerators; 4°C and -20°C (preferably -70°C)
Glass Universal bottles (20 ml)
Glass bijou bottles (5 ml)
Glass vials for freeze-dried conjugates
Small conical plastic refrigerator storage tubes (500 μl) with attached caps
Dialysis tubing
Dialysis flask (2 litres) with large magnetic stirring bar

Chromatography media

Sephadex G25 and G200
Sephacryl S-200
Concanavalin A (Con-A) $-$ Sepharose

Chemicals

Absolute ethanol	KH_2PO_4
Acetic acid	NaCl
Borax	Na_2CO_3
Boric acid	Na_2HPO_4
Dithiothreitol	NaH_2PO_4
Glutaraldehyde	Sodium acetate
Glycerol	Sodium bicarbonate
HCl (5 M)	Sodium borohydride
Lysine	Sodium m-periodate
Methyl-D-mannoside	SPDP
Merthiolate preservative	Tris [Tris-(hydroxymethyl)-methylamine]
KCl	

Enzymes

AP
HRP

Antibodies

Purified IgG fraction of sheep or rabbit antisera (or other species).

Buffers

Phosphate-buffered saline (PBS), 0.1 M pH 7.4
    NaCl   8.0 g
    KH_2PO_4 0.2 g

Na$_2$HPO$_4\cdot$12H$_2$O   2.8 g
KCl   0.2 g
Make up to 1 litre in distilled water.

Sodium acetate 1.0 mM pH 4.4
  Solution A—8.24 g anhydrous sodium acetate in 1 litre of distilled water.
  Solution B—6.005 g glacial acetic acid in 1 litre of distilled water.
  Add one part of solution A to two parts of solution B. Dilute 1:100 in distilled water to give a
  1.0 mM buffer.

Phosphate buffer, 0.1 M pH 6.8
  NaH$_2$PO$_4\cdot$2H$_2$O   15.6 g in 1 litre of distilled water.
  Na$_2$HPO$_4$ 14.2 g in 1 litre of distilled water.
  Mix in equal volumes and adjust to pH 6.8 by addition of monobasic or dibasic salt solution as
  necessary.

Sodium carbonate/bicarbonate buffer 1, pH 9.5
  Na$_2$CO$_3$ 1.59 g (0.015 M)
  NaHCO$_3$ 2.93 g (0.035 M)
  Dissolve together in distilled water to make 1 litre.

Sodium carbonate/bicarbonate buffer 2, 0.2 M pH 9.5
  Na$_2$CO$_3$ 21.2 g, made up to 1 litre in distilled water.
  NaHCO$_3$ 16.8 g, made up to 1 litre in distilled water.
  Add a sufficient volume of the Na$_2$CO$_3$ solution to the 1 litre of bicarbonate to achieve pH 9.5

Borate buffer, 0.1 M pH 7.4
  Boric acid   24.732 g, made up to 4 litres in distilled water.
  Borax   19.07 g, made up to 500 ml in distilled water.
  Add ~115 ml of borax solution to the 4 litres of boric acid solution and adjust to pH 7.4 by further
  small additions.

Tris−HCl buffer, 0.05 M pH 8.0
  Tris   6.057 g, made up to 1 litre in distilled water.
  Adjust pH to 8.0 by addition of 5 M HCl.

of tests. However, antibodies of all specificities and from any species can be conjugated, including mouse and rat monoclonals, the only limitation being the amount of available immunoglobulin. It is possible, however, to conjugate as little as 100 μg by scaling down the protocols described below. It is also possible to conjugate protein antigens in a manner similar to that for antibody. In this instance ratios of enzyme and linking agents may need to be adjusted to achieve suitable products—this can only be determined on an individual basis by trial and error.

In this section the preparation of antibody−enzyme conjugates is described using sheep or rabbit antibodies. A list of equipment and materials required can be found in *Table 3*. The methods do not differ significantly for other antibody species. Conjugation methods vary according to the selected enzyme (see *Table 1*). The protocols given below are for HRP and AP. The starting material is the purified IgG fraction of the antiserum. This is prepared by sequential ammonium sulphate precipitation and anion-exchange (DE52 cellulose) chromatography as described in Volume I, Chapter 2 (Section 10). The conjugation of urease and β-D-galactosidase to sheep IgG is also described in Volume I, Chapter 2 (Section 3.1.2).

Table 4. The sodium *m*-periodate method.

1. Dissolve 4.0−8.0 mg of HRP (Sigma P8375, activity 285 purpurogallin units/mg of solid) in 1 ml of distilled water.
2. Prepare a fresh 0.1 M solution of sodium *m*-periodate (Sigma) in distilled water and then add 0.2 ml to the HRP solution in a glass bijou bottle—the mixture immediately turns green.
3. Cap the bottle and stir (or rotate) gently for 20 min at room temperature.
4. Dialyse the mixture overnight against a large excess of 1.0 mM sodium acetate buffer pH 4.4 at 4°C.
5. Raise the pH to 9.0−9.5 by addition of 20 μl of 0.2 M sodium carbonate/bicarbonate buffer 2 (*Table 3*), pH 9.5. To this add immediately 10 mg of IgG (antibody) solution in 1.0 ml, previously also dialysed overnight against, in this case, the carbonate/bicarbonate buffer 1, pH 9.5.
6. Stir the mixture gently for 2 h at room temperature on a rotary wheel mixer.
7. Add 100 μl of freshly prepared sodium borohydride solution, made up as 4.0 mg/ml in distilled water. This reduces the free enzyme to block further conjugation. Stand for 2 h at 4°C.
8. Dialyse the conjugate against a large excess of 0.1 M borate buffer pH 7.4, overnight at 4°C, and then separate the enzyme−IgG conjugate from uncoupled materials by passing the reaction mixture down a Sephadex G200 column (1.6 × 35 cm) in borate buffer. Collect the first elution peak that is enzyme- and antibody-active. The column separation step is not essential. Dialysed conjugates may be stored at −20°C or as in step 9, which is recommended.
9. Dilute the conjugate 1:2 in 60% (v/v) glycerol in borate buffer. Add merthiolate to a final concentration of 0.02% (w/v) and then divide into 100 μl aliquots in small capped tubes and store at 4°C. Alternatively (for larger volumes) freeze-dry from buffer solution in glass vials which can be stored at 4°C or −20°C. Conjugates prepared this way and stored as directed will maintain their activity for at least 1−2 years.

4.1 Conjugation of horseradish peroxidase to IgG

The following two procedures can produce high quality conjugates of HRP and antibody.

(i) The periodate method (see *Table 4*) introduced by Nakane and Kawaoi in 1974 (14) and modified by Wilson and Nakane (15). This gives excellent enzyme−antibody (IgG) ratios. It involves the oxidation of peroxidase with *m*-periodate and generates some proportion of conjugate in polymeric form. This does not usually present a problem, however, and the conjugation procedure is uncomplicated and gives reliable results. For this reason it is a recommended procedure.

(ii) The use of heterobifunctional linking reagents such as SPDP (16,17), or *N*-(4-carboxycyclohexylmethyl)-maleimide (18,19). This method (*Table 5*), although substantially more complex to perform, offers more control over the size of the conjugates produced and can yield a predominance of monomeric couplets of IgG and enzyme.

4.2 Conjugation of alkaline phosphatase to IgG by the one-step glutaraldehyde method

(i) Dialyse 10 mg of IgG in 2 ml against a large excess of 0.1 M phosphate buffer pH 6.8, at 4°C for 24 h and transfer to a glass bijou bottle.

(ii) Add 50 mg of AP in 2 ml of the phosphate buffer to the dialysed IgG and mix thoroughly without frothing using a magnetic stirrer.

(iii) Add slowly dropwise, 10% aqueous glutaraldehyde solution with constant stirring to a final concentration of 0.2% (80 μl) and leave gently mixing at room temperature for 2 h.

(iv) Saturate unreacted groups by addition of 200 μl of 1 M lysine solution in

Table 5. The SPDP method.

1.	Dissolve 10 mg of HRP in 2.0 ml of PBS. Add to this 400 μg of SPDP, dissolved in 0.5 ml of absolute ethanol, dropwise with stirring.
2.	Allow the mixture to react for 30 min at room temperature with occasional further stirring.
3.	Remove the excess SPDP and the reaction product *N*-hydroxysuccinimide from the 2-pyridyldisulphide-substituted enzyme by gel filtration through a 1.6 × 35 cm Sephadex G25 column using PBS as the buffer. The substituted HRP is eluted as the first protein peak.
4.	Perform an identical reaction between IgG (antibody) and SPDP, using 10 mg of IgG in PBS and, in this case, less SPDP (20−15 μg) in 0.2 ml of ethanol. The substituted antibody is again harvested from a Sephadex G25 column.
5.	Reactive thiol groups on the substituted HRP molecules are then generated by reduction of the 2-pyridyldisulphide groups. This is done by adding dithiothreitol to the substituted enzyme solution to a final concentration of 0.05 M, at room temperature with mixing.
6.	Remove excess reducing agent, pyridine-2-thionine, by gel filtration using again Sephadex G25.
7.	Mix together the thiol-containing peroxidase and the 2-pyridyldisulphide-substituted antibody in equal (w/w) proportions and stand at 4°C for 18 h.
8.	Apply the reaction mixture to a freshly prepared Con-A−Sephadex column using PBS as the buffer. Wash the columns through thoroughly in PBS and then elute the Con-A-bound HRP−antibody conjugate using PBS containing 10 mM methyl-D-mannoside. The eluted protein peak is both antibody- and enzyme-active.
9.	Further separate the eluted peak into conjugate and uncoupled, treated, enzyme by passage through a Sephacryl S-200 column (1.6 × 95 cm) at a flow rate of 6−10 ml/cm^2/h using PBS. The first (enzyme-active) peak contains the conjugate, which has a predominant molecular weight component of about 200 kd.
10.	Dilute the conjugate 1:2 in 60% (v/v) glycerol in borate buffer, add merthiolate (1:10 000) and store in small volumes at 4°C, or freeze-dry from buffer solution and store in sealed glass vials.

phosphate buffer and after a further 2 h set up the mixture to dialyse against a large excess of PBS overnight at 4°C.

(v) Separate the antibody- and enzyme-active conjugates from other components in the dialysed material by passing through a Sephacryl S-200 column.

(vi) Add to the stock conjugate 1% (w/v) BSA; add merthiolate (1:10 000) and store in small volumes at 4°C.

4.3 Testing the properties of antibody−enzyme conjugates

Before a prepared conjugate can be used routinely for assays it is advisable to check its composition and properties, and to test it adequately as a reagent under controlled conditions. The features of a good conjugate are:

(i) high antibody titre and avidity so that the conjugate can be used at high dilution to give minimal non-specific binding effects;

(ii) adequate specificity at a working dilution;

(iii) a high proportion of monomeric couplets of antibody and enzyme (polymerized conjugates tend to stick to plastic and coating proteins, and in consequence give high background readings which cannot be eliminated by blocking/quenching strategies applied to the test);

(iv) optimal enzyme−antibody molar ratios (generally a mean ratio of one enzyme per antibody molecule offers the best conjugate performance);

Table 6. Properties of HRP−sheep antibody conjugates prepared by the periodate technique at two HRP−protein weight ratios.

Specificity (sheep anti-)	Conjugation ratio HRP:IgG (mg)	OD ratio 403:280 nm	Dilution in ELISA giving OD = 1.0[a]	Background OD (BSA-coated wells)
human IgG	4:10	0.14	1:4000	<0.1
	8:10	0.30	1:17 000	<0.1
human IgA	4:10	0.17	1:1060	<0.1
	8:10	0.31	1:3650	<0.1
human IgM	4:10	0.09	1:285	<0.2
	8:10	0.22	1:925	<0.2

[a]Conjugates were each adjusted to a starting concentration of 1 mg/ml sheep IgG. OD readings are for reactions using orthophenylene diamine substrate, read (after stopping) at 492 nm.

Table 7. Equipment and materials required for the direct ELISA.

Equipment
Incubator at 37°C.
ELISA plate reader (manual or automated) with appropriate filter (492 nm for HRP with OPD, using stopping solution).
Micropipettes with disposable tips; 5−100 μl range, including one variable volume multichannel pipette).
Graduated pipettes: 2 ml or 5 ml with pipette aid (Pi pump) or bulb attachment.
ELISA plates: polystyrene or polyvinyl chloride [see Section 4.3.3(iii), Technical note 1].
Damp ELISA plate storage boxes (~20 × 15 cm, and 10 cm deep) with lids, containing damp filter paper.
Refrigerator at 4°C.
Aluminium foil.
Paper towels and filter papers.
Wash bottle with fine nozzle.
5 ml glass test tubes and test tube rack.
5 litre storage bottle for washing solution.
1−2 litre glass bottles for other buffers and solutions.
20 ml glass Universals with caps, or small conical flasks, for substrate solutions.
Plate washing dish (~30 × 20 cm, and 10 cm deep), for soaking plates.
Marker pen—fine tip, water resistant.

Chemicals
Citric acid
Hydrogen peroxide
OPD (substrate for HRP)
Tween-20

Immunological reagents
Relevant to quality control of conjugates to human immunoglobulins:
    purified human IgG, IgA, IgM, $\varkappa$ light chain, λ light chain[a];
    reference HRP conjugates (if available)[a];
    bovine serum albumin (BSA)—pure grade.

Buffers and solutions
Coating buffer—carbonate/bicarbonate 0.05 M pH 9.6
    Na_2CO_3 1.59 g (0.015 M)
    $NaHCO_3$ 2.93 g (0.035 M)

Dissolve both salts in 1 litre of distilled water; adjust pH by addition of monobasic or dibasic salt solution at same molarity.
Prepare fresh buffer every few days.

Diluting/incubation buffer (PBS−Tween or PBS-T)
  PBS, 0.1 M pH 7.4 (*Table 3*) containing 0.05% (v/v) Tween-20.

Washing solution (saline−Tween)
  0.9% (w/v) saline with 0.05% (v/v) Tween-20.

Substrate buffer—for OPD: citrate buffer, 0.15 M pH 5.0
  Citric acid   7.3 g
  $Na_2HPO_4 \cdot 2H_2O$ 11.86 g
  Dissolve both in 1 litre of distilled water; adjust pH with acid, or dibasic salt at the same molarity.

Substrate (OPD) solution
This must be made up freshly each time (just before use) as it is rapidly inactivated in aqueous form. It is also light-activated, so wrap the container completely in aluminium foil as soon as prepared. Use scrupulously clean glassware and avoid rubber cap liners to bottle tops. Use a clean container on each occasion and clean utensils for handling.
WARNING: USE DISPOSABLE GLOVES TO HANDLE OPD IN POWDER FORM
  1. Dissolve OPD to a concentration of 40 mg/100 ml of substrate buffer.
  2. Add 20 μl of undiluted H_2O_2 [or 5 ml of 30% (v/v)] immediately before use and mix.

Notes: (a) Each complete ELISA plate uses 10 ml of substrate solution.
        (b) For alternative substrates for OPD and other enzyme systems see *Tables 1* and *2*.

Stopping solution
HCl 2.5 M.

---

[a]For developing countries small samples of these reagents are available for reference and standardization purposes from the World Health Organization Collaborating Centre for Production and Quality Control of Immunological Reagents, c/o The Director, Dr D.Catty, Department of Immunology, Medical School, University of Birmingham, Birmingham B15 2TJ, UK (Tel. 021-414-4077).

(v)   adequate coupled enzyme activity. This is influenced by conjugation conditions and the degree of coupling achieved. Under- and over-coupling can produce poor results.

  Features (i), (ii) and (iii) are assessed by the performance of the conjugate in a direct ELISA protocol (assay 1 of *Figure 2*) as used in quality control exercises. This involves the coating of ELISA plates with appropriate antigens, titration and specificity testing of the conjugate and an evaluation of background properties. Feature (iv) can be determined spectroscopically using the absorption maxima wavelengths for the enzyme and IgG, and feature (v) is determined by a direct substrate test with conjugate in solution at a standardized IgG concentration. The protocols for conjugate testing are set out below. The examples given relate to HRP conjugates of sheep antibodies to human immunoglobulins but the principles apply to any enzyme conjugate.

4.3.1 *Determining HRP−antibody absorbance ratios*

The protein concentration of a conjugate sample is first adjusted in PBS to give an optical density (OD; 280 nm; 1 cm cell) reading of approximately 1.45 (equivalent to 1 mg/ml IgG). A suitable dilution of conjugate is then measured for OD at both 403 nm and 280 nm, the absorption maxima for HRP and IgG, respectively. The ratio of these two readings offers a guide to the amount of enzyme conjugated which is an important element in determining conjugate performance. The difference in working titre of conjugates prepared by different starting weight ratios of HRP and antibody is clearly seen in *Table 6*. Generally, OD ratios (403:280) for HRP conjugates in the range 0.3−0.5 offer high enzyme activity without prejudice to antibody titre, and have low background characteristics.

4.3.2 *Measuring enzyme activity of HRP conjugates*

(i)   Dilute the conjugate in PBS to a concentration of 1 mg/ml IgG (see Section 4.3.1).
(ii)   Further dilute to 1:1000 in PBS (1 μg/ml IgG).
(iii) Add 20 μl of diluted conjugate to 3.0 ml of freshly prepared OPD substrate solution (prepared in substrate buffer, see *Table 7*) in a 3.0 ml glass test tube. Incubate, wrapped in foil, at room temperature.
(iv)   Remove 200 μl aliquots serially at 0, 5, 10, 15, 25 and 30 min and transfer to wells of an ELISA plate, adding immediately, at each time point, 25 μl of 2.5 M HCl as stopping solution. Cover the plate between sample applications, and when the series is complete read the reaction at 492 nm in an ELISA reader.
(v)   Plot the OD readings against time as shown in *Figure 3*. In general, conjugates diluted to 1 μg/ml IgG that achieve an OD of 1.0 in 10−15 min in the test, and a final OD of 1.5 or greater within 25−30 min have suitable enzyme activity for ELISA tests. These properties are easily attained with most HRP conjugates that have enzyme:protein OD 403:280 nm ratios of 0.3−0.5. In *Figure 3* conjugates prepared with inadequate amounts of HRP to give 403:280 nm absorption ratios for the conjugate of about 0.1 do not have adequate enzyme activity. The same three antibodies (to human IgG, IgA and IgM), reacted with twice as much HRP for conjugation, yield conjugates with excellent enzyme properties and higher working titres (*Table 6*).

4.3.3 *The direct ELISA for quality control of HRP antibody conjugates and the basic methodology of ELISA and related tests*

A list of equipment and materials required (in addition to those mentioned in *Table 3*) are listed in *Table 7*.

(i) *Assay principle.* Standard antigens are coated onto wells of an ELISA plate and the test conjugate applied to these, followed, after washing, by substrate. Titre is determined by dilution to endpoint (background of non-antigen wells), and specificity by use (as appropriate) of related antigens and/or molecules which might complicate specific tests with the conjugate. For isotype-specific antiglobulin conjugates, as exemplified below, purified classes of immunoglobulins and light chains are used. The test conjugate can be compared with a reference reagent for performance in all aspects of the quality control assay. Working dilutions of conjugates are determined from the titrations against homologous antigen. The protocol of the assay for class-specific anti-human immunoglobulins is given in *Table 8*.

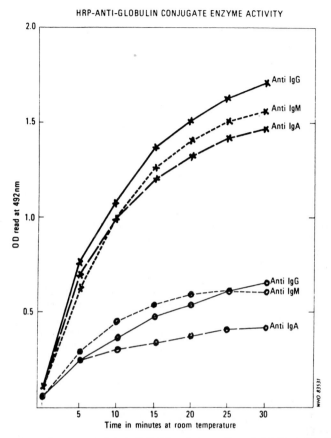

Figure 3. Comparison of enzyme−substrate interactions between the antiglobulin conjugates with optimal HRP:IgG ratios (×) and with less than optimal ratios (○). The same three sheep antibodies, to human IgG, IgA and IgM, were prepared by conjugation procedures which differed only in the amount of HRP used (see *Table 6*). Reactions were performed at a dilution of 1:1000 for each conjugate after adjusting IgG concentration to 1 mg/ml. OPD was used as substrate, and the reactions were measured in an ELISA plate reader using a 492 nm filter. (Reproduced from ref. 57.)

(ii) *Interpretation of results.*

(1)   Good conjugates should titre out to an endpoint greater than 1:10 000 dilution; this is determined by the last dilution giving an OD of higher value than the background OD of conjugate in the BSA wells. Background reactions in the BSA-coated control wells should dilute to minimal values (<0.15) before absorbance in the specific antigen-coated wells begins to dilute out.

(2)   Antisera adequately absorbed on solid phase adsorbents should show a minimum of cross-reactivity with other tested antigens (as conjugates) and any residual reactivity observed with these should have diminished the background readings well before the working dilution is reached with the specific antigen in the dilution series.

(3)   The working dilution of the conjugate is set in the linear part of the OD dilution curve (see *Figure 4*). Where this begins at an OD above 2.0, a dilution of

Table 8. The direct ELISA; basic methodology (example for class-specific anti-human immunoglobulins).

Coating plates with antigen

1. Prepare solutions of purified antigens (human IgG, IgA, IgM, κ chain, λ chain) in coating buffer at $1-5$ μg/ml [see Section 4.3.3(iii), Technical notes 1 and 2 regarding plate-binding properties and optimal coating levels].
2. Prepare also a BSA coating solution at 100 μg/ml.
3. For each conjugate to be tested mark out two ELISA plates below every third row across the plate using the marker pen. Label each section for one antigen. Apply 100 μl of each antigen to duplicate rows (wells $1-12$) and apply the BSA to each third row of the set.
4. Stack the two plates, place a cover on the top one, and place in a damp storage box with lid at 4°C overnight (16 h).

Washing plates

1. Fill a wash bottle with washing solution (saline$-$Tween).
2. Shake out each plate's contents vigorously over a sink and then running along the rows, carefully squirt a stream of solution into each well. Shake out the plate again and bang the inverted plate several times onto a pad of paper towelling.
3. Immerse the plate in washing solution in the washing dish and soak for at least 3 min.
4. Remove, shake out, bang to near dryness and repeat the soaking cycle at least twice more. The saline$-$Tween washing works both to remove excess uncoated (unbound, in later stages) reagent and to prevent (role of detergent) further protein from being adsorbed onto the plastic [see Section 4.3.3(iii), Technical note 4 regarding plate washers].
5. Finally rinse the plate and bang-dry thoroughly. Use the coated plates immediately to apply the conjugate, or store them briefly in covered, damp condition at 4°C [see Section 4.3.3(iii), Technical note 7 regarding long-term storage of antigen-coated plates].

Applying the conjugate

1. Dilute each conjugate in diluting buffer (PBS-T) to 1:100 from the stock (1 mg/ml IgG) preparation; 40 μl in 4.0 ml will suffice for two plates. Then using test tubes prepare a 2 ml double dilution series of conjugate over 23 tubes from 1:100 using PBS-T.
2. For each conjugate, starting from column 1, apply 100 μl of 1:100 conjugate to each well *down* the two plates, repeat for the 1:200 for column 2, etc.
3. Incubate the covered plates in a damp box at 37°C for 1 h and then eject conjugate and wash plates as given above. Apply substrate immediately—do not allow plates to dry out at this stage.

Applying the substrate

1. Prepare the substrate solution as detailed in *Table 7* .
2. Add 100 μl to each well, cover plates and incubate *in the dark* at 37°C for $10-30$ min [see Section 4.3.3(iii), Technical note 4].

Stopping the reaction

When optimally developed [see Section 4.3.3(iii), Technical note 5], stop the reactions by adding 25 μl of stopping solution to each well. Cover plates to avoid evaporation if there is a delay before reading.

Reading the plates

1. The plates are first read by eye, checking that background reactions in the control (BSA-coated) wells afford a sharp contrast to the specific antigen-coated wells. On this basis score the intensity of the colour reactions on a scale of, for example 4 to zero, defining the endpoint titre as the dilution (for each antigen) that gives a perceptibly higher colour than controls (or any colour if controls are blank). Assessment by eye may provide a totally adequate form of quality control where the background properties of test conjugates are low.

2. For more sensitive scoring of plates the reactions are read on an ELISA reader with the appropriate filter setting [492 nm for OPD (see Section 4.3.3(iii), Technical note 6 on ELISA readers]. This has the great advantages of supplying OD data from which the performance of conjugates and assays can be accurately plotted, and duplicate well data can be measured for greater accuracy. Where a reader is not available, duplicate well contents can be transferred to cuvettes of a spectrophotometer set at the appropriate wavelength.

Calculating and plotting data

Results of reference and test conjugates (mean of well duplicates) against the antigens and control (BSA) wells are plotted with absorbance versus dilution (see *Figure 4*).

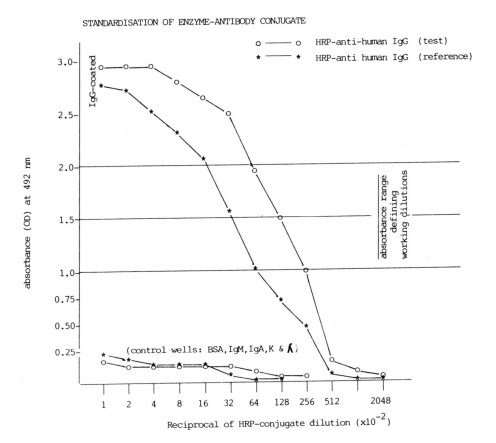

Figure 4. Titration of HRP conjugate of a test anti-human IgG, compared with a reference conjugate. Specificity is tested in wells coated with IgG (positive reaction), IgM, IgA, $\varkappa$ and λ chain (control reactions), all at 1 µg/ml, and background with BSA-coated wells. Both reagents are specific to IgG and give low background. The test conjugate is superior in titre and has a working dilution (for OD 1.5) of 1:12 800. In comparing the conjugates they were first standardized to 1 mg/ml IgG before dilution.

conjugate giving 1.5 − 2.0 can be used, assuming an ELISA reader that measures accurately at this colour intensity, and assuming that background readings have diminished to minimum values at this point—otherwise a compromise between

OD values generated by antigen and BSA has to be made. Background readings should not exceed 0.15 and ideally the ratio of positive signal to background at working dilution should be 10:1 or greater. An OD reading of 1.0 is acceptable in defining working dilutions of conjugates where backgrounds are 0.1 or less at this point. *Figure 4* illustrates the titre, specificity and background properties of an anti-human IgG-specific HRP conjugate compared with a reference conjugate. The test conjugate shows adequate specificity for IgG, has an endpoint titre of 51 200, a working titre (at OD 1.5) of 12 800 and an OD signal-to-background ratio of 15. These values define a conjugate with excellent performance properties that exceed the reference reagent.

(4)   For ELISA tests that are to rely on visual assessment only, it is essential to use conjugates under conditions that afford maximum discrimination between positive and negative results. To achieve this, conjugates may need to be used at relatively higher concentrations than is needed where reader facilities exist. This places special demands on conjugates in relation to background properties.

(iii) *Technical notes.*

(1)   ELISA plates and antigen-coating properties. Polystyrene and polyvinyl chloride plates produced by different manufacturers may offer quite different intrinsic coating properties and there may also be batch variation. It is essential to use good quality plates marketed specifically for ELISA work where 'edge' effects, plate and batch variation are reduced to a minimum and the optical properties of the wells gives efficient reading. It is still worthwhile checking the properties of plates for the desired tests from a number of sources before selecting a suitable brand for regular purchase. It is a simple matter to compare plates by coating several of each brand with a standard antigen dilution, and with BSA for background, and then, in direct ELISA, titrate the antibody conjugate across the wells. Plates with highest antigen adsorbing properties will give the highest OD values; such plates may, however, give unacceptably high background readings. In addition any brand of plate that gives coefficients of variation between replicate wells, rows and plates in excess of 10% is undesirable, as such properties deny both sensitivity and reproducibility to tests. A figure of 5% or less is to be aimed for.

(2)   Optimal antigen coating level. It is very important to ensure that enzyme—antibody conjugates are titrated against their antigen at an optimal antigen coating level so this should constitute a preliminary step in conjugate quality control once a brand of ELISA plate has been selected. Less than adequate coating of the solid phase will reduce sensitivity and afford opportunities for the conjugate itself to bind to the plastic. This will lead to high backgrounds and obscure the properties of the reference and test conjugates alike. Over-coating of the solid phase may lead to non-specific trapping of conjugate (20). The protocol in *Table 9* should be adopted on assessment of any new conjugate—antigen system, when using a new batch of plates or a new supplier, and for every new stock of prepared antigen.

(3)   Quenching and properties of conjugates. High signal (positive)-to-noise

Table 9. Protocol to determine optimal antigen coating level.

1. Coat two rows of wells each with a series of antigen concentrations from 0.1 to 10 µg/ml (or greater for some systems) using BSA at 100 µg/ml for control wells.

2. Follow the rest of the direct ELISA protocol as given in *Table 8*, plotting absorbance against conjugate dilution for each antigen-coating concentration and for controls.

3. Choose for subsequent assays the lowest antigen-coating concentration that gives a combination of optimal dilution curve with low background readings. *Figure 5* shows the effects of human IgG antigen coating concentration on the performance of an HRP−anti-IgG conjugate; optimal conjugate dilutions are achieved with 1.0−2.0 µg/ml coating antigen but minimum background is given only in the 1.0−1.5 µg/ml antigen range, and 1 µg/ml was selected for this stock of antigen, using the same brand and batch of plates.

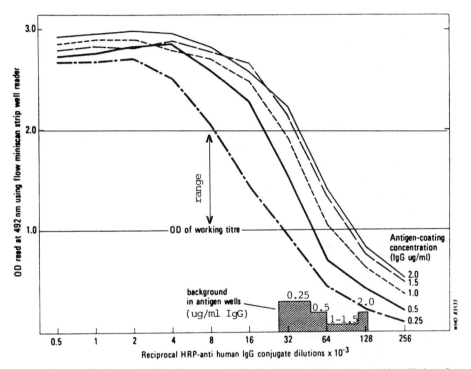

Figure 5. Interaction between IgG coating concentration for ELISA wells and the working dilution of an HRP−anti-human IgG conjugate. 1 µg/ml of IgG is chosen as the optimal coating concentration. Background binding of conjugate to wells increases with antigen-coating concentrations of less than 1 µg/ml, and with 2 µg/ml. (Reproduced from ref. 57.)

(background) ratios are required for good sensitivity in all ELISA tests and the use of BSA controls helps to eliminate conjugates with intrinsically high non-specific binding properties that reduce this ratio. The cause of high backgrounds is usually related to the size of enzyme−protein polymers and it may be necessary, if poor results are obtained, to prepare a new conjugate with differing reagent proportions or to use an alternative technique. In some cases, however, it is possible to reduce the background by quenching antigen-coated wells with a weak protein solution in coating buffer. BSA is usually also used for this strategy, applying this in up to 3% (w/v) concentrations (determined by trial) using 100 μl per well at room temperature for $1-2$ h. The plates are then washed and the assay proceeds.

(4) Plate washers. A range of manually-operated and automated plate washers with buffer reservoirs are available (see Appendix of Suppliers). These are useful where there is a large daily throughput of assays in a laboratory. The technique described in *Table 8* is entirely adequate, however, for small numbers of plates.

(5) Substrate properties and reaction endpoints. OPD as the substrate for HRP is light-sensitive and a yellow colour will develop spontaneously if the OPD $-$ H_2O_2 mixture is left exposed to bright light. For this reason the substrate is prepared just prior to use and wrapped in foil. Plates filled with substrate should be placed in the dark immediately (incubator or box or wrapped in foil). Where reaction time to optimum substrate colour development has not been standardized, it is necessary to observe development frequently. The plate reactions should be stopped when positive controls (i.e. reference conjugates) give optimal readings. A compromise between these two events often needs to be made. A note of the exact time to stopping and the temperature conditions assists future standardization. With conjugates with high enzyme activity, room temperature development may be desirable for better control. A recommended form of endpoint standardization is to monitor positive control reactions on the ELISA reader (using the filter for the stopped colour), stopping one pair of replicate control wells at a time, and stop the entire plate when these achieve a pre-determined value. This has the benefit of allowing strict quantitative comparisons of test reactions with positive controls.

(6) ELISA readers. Many forms of ELISA reader are available commercially (see Appendix of Suppliers). The best are automated with built-in variable filter systems for different substrates and which print out the results. The most modern machines are programmable and have computer software facilities for plate evaluation and quantitative scoring of results. Most readers measure in the OD range 3.0 to zero and give reasonable linear results within these parameters. Some readers give higher values but the linearity is often not as good in the higher absorbance range so the benefits may be minimal. Some manual readers are not as reliable, as demonstrated by greater variation in repeated readings of the same plate. Investment in a well proven automated reader is essential for routine quantitative ELISA work.

(7) Storing antigen-coated plates. For some antigens, after coating and washing, plates can be taken to dryness in a desiccator and then stored in sealed air-tight sachets with some silica gel granules. Antigens vary in stability as dry, coated molecules. Human IgG (myeloma protein)-coated plates have been tested and appear to store for long periods in this state. Every antigen needs testing before consigning large numbers of coated plates to storage. Bring stored plates into use by rinsing in PBS-T.

5. ALTERNATIVE REAGENTS, STRATEGIES AND SOLID PHASES

5.1 Choice of enzymes and substrates for plate ELISA (see *Tables 1* and *2*)

5.1.1 *HRP conjugates*

HRP catalyses the reduction of H_2O_2 with the concurrent oxidation of another substrate. In standard colorimetric assays this is used to produce an optically measurable colour change but fluorophotometric and chemiluminescent assays are also available with this enzyme. OPD, BTS and ASA are the most commonly used chromogenic hydrogen donor substrates. ABTS and OPD show excellent sensitivities. OPD has gained universal popularity and is the substrate of many commercial ELISA tests.

TMB can be recommended for routine assays and could become the substrate of choice because its metabolites are non-mutagenic and non-carcinogenic. The blue colour generated after stopping gives excellent contrast with background and accordingly gives a high sensitivity to assays, especially those interpreted by eye; endpoint determinations are often superior to those obtained with OPD.

The protocol for TMB is as follows (21).

(i)   Dissolve TMB (3,3',5,5'-TMB) in DMSO to a final concentration of 42 mM (10 mg/ml). Dilute 1:100 in sodium citrate buffer, 0.1 M pH 6.0 by dropwise addition of substrate with shaking.

(ii)   Just prior to use add H_2O_2 to a final concentration of 1.3 mM (20 μl of 30% H_2O_2/100 ml).

(iii)   Add 100 μl of TMB$-H_2O_2$ per well and incubate the plates at room temperature for 60 min (or less).

(iv)   Stop the reactions with 25 μl of 2 M H_2SO_4.

(v)   Read the reactions at 450 nm.

5.1.2 *Alkaline phosphatase conjugates*

AP conjugates are extremely stable on storage and resistant to the action of bacteriostatic agents. There are a number of colorimetric and fluorescent substrates and AP is used widely in commercially available immunoassay kits. PNPP is the usual chromogenic substrate, while methyl umbelliferyl phosphate is useful as a fluorescent substrate.

The protocol for using PNPP is as follows.

(i)   Prepare 0.1 M diethanolamine$-$HCl buffer by adding 97 ml of diethanolamine to 800 ml distilled water. Add 1 M HCl to bring to pH 9.8 and make up the volume to 1 litre with distilled water.

(ii)   Dissolve PNPP in buffer to 1 mg/ml.

(iii)   Add 100 μl of substrate solution to each well and incubate plates at room temperature for 30$-$60 min.

(iv)   Stop reactions by the addition of 50 μl of 3 M NaOH.

(v)   Read reactions at 402$-$412 nm (i.e. a filter of 405 nm is usual).

5.1.3 *β-D-galactosidase conjugates*

β-D-galactosidase (β-D-galactoside galactohydrolase from *Escherichia coli*) catalyses the hydrolysis of β-D-galactoside to galactose and alcohol. The recommended chromogenic substrate for colorimetric assays is ONPG. Ultra-sensitive assays have been developed with fluorogenic substrates that can measure macromolecular antigens and antibodies in the femtomole to attomole sensitivity range. A substrate for such assays is 4-methyl-umbelliferyl β-D-galactopyranoside.

The protocol for using ONPG in colorimetric assays is as follows.

(i)   Make up the substrate solution by dissolving 2.5 mg/ml ONPG in 0.1 M sodium phosphate buffer pH 7.0, containing 1 mM $MgCl_3$ and 0.1 M β-mercapto-ethanol.

(ii)   Add 100 μl of substrate solution to each well and incubate for $30-60$ min at 37°C.

(iii)   Stop the reactions with 25 μl of 2 M Na_2CO_3.

(iv)   Read the reactions at 420 nm.

5.1.4 *Urease conjugates*

The use of this enzyme offers important advantages.

(i)   It provides a simple means to obtain a clear titration endpoint that is readily visible.

(ii)   There are no problems of substrate instability that may be encountered with HRP and AP.

(iii)   There is no urease in mammalian tissues, which can be a problem with HRP and AP.

Urease catalyses the hydrolysis of urea to CO_2 and NH_3. The production of NH_3 can be detected readily by a pH shift which can be simply utilized to produce a change in colour of an indicator. The most suitable pH indicator for detection of urease activity in routine plate ELISA is BP which is converted from its yellow colour at acid pH to a strong purple colour on generation of NH_3. This provides the basis for a clear, vivid and linear colour change with a sharply defined visual endpoint—positive reactions can also be read at 588 nm.

Plate ELISA using the urease−BP system has a sensitivity comparable to those employing AP and HRP with chromogenic substrates. Urease conjugates have found a wide use in immunoassays where a sensitive rapid qualitative or semi-quantitative test is required, and antibody−urease conjugates have recently become available commercially. The advantages in the simplicity of urease−BP systems have enabled the development of simple enzyme assay kits including one prepared and field-tested for rapid identification of Australian snake venoms in clinical specimens using an adsorbent column principle (see Section 5.3.6 and ref. 45).

The protocol for use of BP indicator in plate assays is as follows.

(i)   Dissolve 8 mg of BP powder in 1.48 ml of 10 mM NaOH and make up to 100 ml with de-ionized water. Add 100 mg of urea and then EDTA to a final concentration of 0.2 mM to chelate any heavy metal ions which might inhibit the urease, and to provide a slight buffering. Adjust the pH to 4.8 using 0.1 M NaOH or 0.1 M HCl and keep the solution at 4°C until required.

(ii)   Add 100 μl of substrate solution to each well and incubate at 37°C for 2 h.

(iii)   With positive test dilutions observe the gradation from strong purple to yellow and determine the endpoint. For a more accurate determination read the plates at 588 nm.

5.1.5 *Penicillinase conjugates*

Enzyme assays using penicillinase (β-lactamase) conjugates have been used for estimation of some protein hormones and antibodies. Results show good correlation with radioimmunoassay. The enzyme is cheap to purchase and the substrate is readily available. The enzyme provides a simple iodometric assay based on the enzymatic decomposition of penicillin to penicilloic acid, the subsequent reduction of iodine in a starch – iodine solution being detected as a colour change from blue to clear (23). The assay has been modified to a micromethod suitable for ELISA plate assays (24). The order of addition and volume of reactants is given in *Table 2*. The assay, as for urease, is best suited for qualitative tests.

(i)   After addition of reactants incubate the plate at room temperature for up to 1 h.

(ii)   Complete or near-complete decolorization denotes a positive reaction.

5.2 **Signal enhancement and amplification systems**

5.2.1 *Features of assays controlling sensitivity*

Enzyme immunoassays performed using a solid phase fall into three categories which vary in intrinsic sensitivity. Where high sensitivity is a stringent requirement (i.e. to detect and measure molecules with a sensitivity in excess of 10^{-12} to 10^{-14} mol/litre), the choice of assay design becomes critical.

(i) *Competitive assays.* In these assays an antibody or antigen analyte competes with homologous labelled competitor molecules for binding to a limited amount of solid phase reagent (antigen or antibody). Sensitivity (i.e. the minimum detectable amount of analyte) is determined by a combination of the affinity (binding constant) of the antibody (whether this is the solid phase capture element or the fluid phase competitor), and handling errors. Sensitivity for antibody detection and for large antigens seldom exceeds about 1 ng/litre and this is not substantially influenced by signal intensity.

(ii) *Inhibition assays.* In these assays analyte is allowed, in an initial step, to occupy the sites on a labelled free binder, thus quantitatively inhibiting the latter from binding in the next step to solid phase target molecules. Sensitivity is governed by the same features as (i) above.

(iii) *Immunometric assays.* These assays depend on the ability of a capture reagent to extract the analyte efficiently onto the solid phase as a complex. The complexed analyte is revealed quantitatively by the binding of a labelled second reagent, the signal generated from the label being proportional to the amount of analyte complexed to the solid phase. The capture and second reagent are in excess. Antigen-capture tests in this format which use high affinity antibodies are theoretically capable of detecting one bound antigen molecule; in practice, sensitivity is dictated by a combination of label (enzyme) specific activity, signal intensity and the sensitivity of signal detection. Strategies that can improve these features, such as enhanced and amplified signal systems, have more chance of increasing sensitivity in immunometric assay formats than in the other systems. Immunometric (i.e. antigen-capture/sandwich) assays, if used to measure complex antigens, require high avidity antibodies restricted to specific epitopes of the antigen. These requirements are met exceptionally well by monoclonal antibodies whose homogeneity and unlimited supply allows both easy antibody purification, and opportunities for assay standardization.

5.2.2 *Improved enzyme immunoassays—the avidin—biotin system*

There are a number of new approaches designed to reduce the loss of antibody and enzyme activity on conjugation. An important strategy has been the linkage of a low molecular weight co-enzyme to the antibody. An enzyme that binds to the co-enzyme is added to the assay once the antibody—antigen complex is formed. As co-enzymes are small in relation to antibody structure there is less risk of steric interference with the binding site than is possible with larger coupled enzymes. Linkage chemistry in the coupling of co-enzymes to antibody can avoid the use of highly reactive cross-linking agents and the excess of small molecules can be removed by dialysis. The most convenient and widely used co-factor system is the avidin—biotin complex (25). The biotin co-enzyme (mol. wt 244) can be linked to antibody using biotinyl-*N*-hydroxysuccinimide. Enzyme is brought into the solid phase assay by using enzyme-coupled avidin or a complex consisting of unlabelled avidin with attached enzyme-labelled biotin. Since the affinity of avidin for biotin is high, the avidin—enzyme conjugate binds efficiently to the antigen—antibody—biotin complex (26). In addition since one molecule of avidin can bind with four molecules of biotin the multilayer labelled biotin system offers increased sensitivity (25).

a

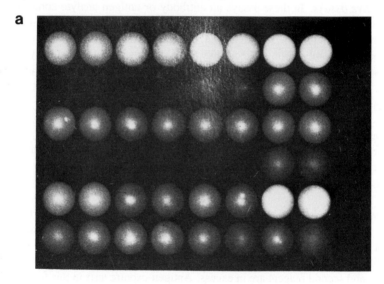

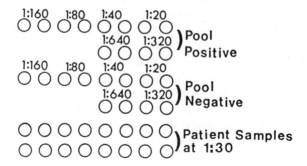

122

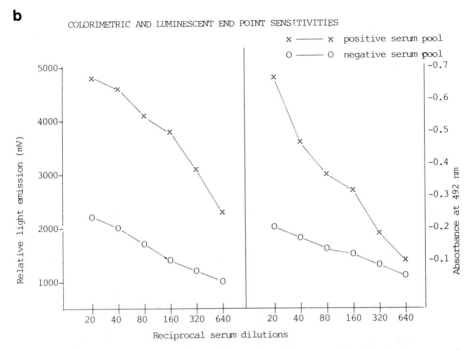

Figure 6. (a) High-speed Polaroid film endpoint record of an enhanced chemiluminescent immunometric enzyme assay for specific immune complexes in *Schistosomiasis mansoni* patients. The test has included serum dilutions of a reference positive sample pool, a reference negative (control European) pool and a series of patients' samples at 1:30 dilution. All samples are in row duplicates. The brightest wells are the strongest (positive) reactions. The assay is using the firefly luciferin-enhanced chemiluminescent system (see text). (b) Titration curves for the same immunometric assay for specific immune complexes using the colorimetric (absorption 492 nm) and enhanced chemiluminescent (luminometer-light emission mV) endpoints for comparison. The assay is using a reference positive serum pool of schistosomiasis patients, and normal European serum pool as a negative control. Note the superior sensitivity of the luminescent endpoint.

5.2.3 *Amplified enzyme linked immunoassays*

Sensitivity in enzyme immunoassays has also been increased by using enzyme amplification systems in which a primary coupled enzyme produces a regeneratable substrate for a secondary enzyme system (27−29). The secondary system can be either a substrate cycle or a redox cycle. In the substrate cycle approach both fructose-6-phosphate and fructose-bisphosphate have been used for the secondary system with both compounds acting as catalysts in a substrate cycle driven by the two enzymes phosphofructokinase and fructose bisphosphatase. The enzyme labels in the immunoassay can be phosphoglucoisomerase or aldolase and the phosphate produced by the cycle can be measured colorimetrically.

In a redox amplifier the enzyme label (AP) is used to catalyse the dephosphorylation of $NADP^+$; the NAD^+ so formed then catalytically activates a NAD^+-specific redox cycle driven by alcohol dehydrogenase and lipoamide dehydrogenase, with generation of an intensely coloured formazan dye as product. The assays, when applied in immunometric antigen-capture systems with monoclonal antibodies, have very high sensitivity and can be read by visual inspection or spectrophotometrically. They have

123

been applied to measurement of thyroid stimulating hormone, progesterone, and human chorionic gonadotrophin.

5.2.4 *Chemiluminescent enzyme immunoassays*

Small molecules such as luminol emit light on oxidation via chemiluminescent reactions which can be used as a signal in enzyme immunoassays (30). This has been another promising approach that increases assay sensitivity and shortens reaction times; the system has been adopted as a major non-isotopic immunoassay alternative for a range of commercial diagnostic tests (Amerlite system, Amersham International) (31). Most chemiluminescent enzyme assays have been based on conjugates with peroxidase which catalyses the luminescent reaction of luminol with H_2O_2. A major advance in sensitivity was achieved with the demonstration that light emission is enhanced by the addition of firefly D-luciferin (32). Conjugates of HRP also catalyse these enhanced luminescent oxidations and these have been exploited analytically in immunometric assays (33 − 35). The luminescent signal is very stable, it is generated fully in 30 sec compared with 30 min for colorimetric HRP−OPD assays and it is 10 − 100 times more intense than the light emission in the unenhanced luminol−peroxidase assay. Light emission from enhanced reactions is intense enough to develop ultra high speed Polaroid instant film (20 000 American Standards Organization) exposed beneath the microtitre plate. This provides a rapid detection system for multiple samples, giving a permanent visual record (see *Figure 6a*) using simple equipment requiring no external power source. *Figure 6b* compares the sensitivity of an immunometric assay using colorimetric and luminescent principles. The enhanced chemiluminescent assay is more sensitive.

5.3 **Alternative solid phase technologies**

There are at least six technical variations in enzyme immunoassays that relate to the solid phase.

5.3.1 *ELISA microtitre plates*

ELISA microtitre plates are utilized in the conjugate quality control protocol (*Table 8*) which is the recommended format for most simple assay procedures detailed in this chapter. Some manufacturers make ELISA well strips that can be assembled into variable sizes of plates which provides economy (see Appendix of Suppliers). The assembly is read on a conventional plate reader. Plates used for chemiluminescent assays may differ from those used in colorimetric tests.

5.3.2 *The 'peg' modification of plate assays*

In the 'peg' modification of plate assays lids to plates have an aligned set of pegs that reach into the wells; these are antibody- or antigen-coated. The solid phase reaction occurs on the pegs but the soluble substrate reaction usually occurs in the wells which are measured as in conventional plate assays. One application of this system is to monitor hybridoma cell cultures in microwell culture plates to determine immunoglobulin or specific antibody production (36). A further modification is to use an insoluble chromogenic substrate that binds to the pegs to give a simple coloured peg test. Such assays are less amenable to precise quantitation.

Table 10. Sensitivity of cuvette and microplate ELISA solid phase systems in HRP−antiglobulin titrations.

	Dilution of conjugate giving reader absorbance value of 1.0 under standardized conditions[a]	
	Cuvette assay[b]	Plate assay[c]
Antigen coating concentration	1 μg/ml	1 μg/ml
Volume used for coating	200 μl	100 μl
Conjugate specificity		
Sheep anti-human IgG (Fc)	1:17 000	1:6400
Sheep anti-human IgA (Fc)	1:3600	1:1600
Sheep anti-human IgM (Fc)	1:925	1:300

[a]Conjugate concentrations were first standardized to 1 mg/ml sheep immunoglobulin by OD 280 nm readings.
[b]Cuvettes were Gilford EIA cuvettes read on a Gilford manual EIA reader.
[c]Plates were Gibco NUNC ELISA-certified microplates.

5.3.3 *Cuvettes*

Cuvettes have a greater capacity and have optically clear sides for horizontal reading in a specialized reader. Cuvettes, which have excellent binding properties for antigens and antibodies, offer greater sensitivity (see *Table 10*). The range of linear accuracy in OD measurement exceeds the standard ELISA plates. The system is more expensive and, in requiring greater reaction volumes, is less economical of reagents. A major use of the cuvette system is for sensitive one-step homogeneous enzyme assays in which modulation of enzyme activity occurs rapidly when antibody binds to enzyme-labelled standard antigen. Non-separation colorimetric competitive enzyme assays are commercially available for determination of some low molecular weight drugs—such as the 'enzyme-modulated immunotest' (EMIT) developed by Syva Company (30).

Table 10 demonstrates that under standard conditions for performance of cuvette and microplate assays the determined working titres of HRP−antiglobulin conjugates are consistently lower in the plates. This can be related in part to the smaller volumes of antigen and conjugate used and in part to the intrinsically lower antigen-binding properties of the plate solid phase. It is essential that quality control comparisons between reference and laboratory-made (or purchased) conjugates are performed within the same plate or cuvette system. Although plates have, generally, lower binding activity for antigen, their sensitivity, at least for many proteins, is not a critical factor and the smaller volumes of reagents required for plate assays can be an advantage.

5.3.4 *'Dip-stick' and 'dot-ELISA' technologies*

In principle any enzyme immunoassay that works sensitively in standard microplates can be modified to perform on adsorbent membranes or dip-sticks using nitrocellulose or similar surface and insoluble substrate products. High affinity monoclonal antibodies have a major role in the development of such tests. Dot-blots, used routinely for nucleic acid hybridization, are finding an increasing application in enzyme immunoassays as 'dot-ELISA'; one protocol is described in Section 6.5.4, but a wide range of plate assays can be modified to perform this way, the system being very amenable to immunometric assay in particular. The simplicity of the dip-stick method enables qualitative tests to be performed outside specialized laboratories and the commercial value of this has already been exploited in the development of dip-stick pregnancy tests (38) which give visual results in less than 5 min. The assays employ monoclonal hormone-specific antibodies to coat the disposable membrane, sample and reagent delivery systems, and coloured insoluble substrate products. It is anticipated that the dip-stick principle will undergo further technical development in conversion to a homogeneous one-step test. In dot-ELISA as little as 1 μl volumes of antigen can be used, adsorbed as spots or discs to nitrocellulose membrane (39,40). These immunometric assays have proved very useful for the rapid screening of sera in the serodiagnosis of infections (41−43) and for identifying monoclonal antibodies (40).

5.3.5 *'Immunobeads'*

Beads that separate from free reagents by gravity or magnetism have been commercially exploited for enzyme immunoassays using fluorescent and chemiluminescent labels (30,44). They offer the major advantages of large active surface area, rapidity of washing cycles and reduced background and signal scattering.

5.3.6 *Enzyme immunochromatography*

Antibodies can be coupled to a porous matrix and held in a fine calibrated column into which analyte and enzyme−antibody conjugates are sequentially drawn. The height of the developed coloured bar on the calibration scale provides a quantitative test for analyte which requires no instrumentation (45). The approach has also been developed using small columns of anti-venom antibodies to detect the venom species in the blood of snake bite patients in Australia using the urease−BP indicator system (22).

6. PROTOCOLS FOR ANTIBODY AND ANTIGEN PLATE ELISA

In this section a description is given of a range of competitive, inhibition, and non-competitive immunometric enzyme immunoassays performed on ELISA microtitre plates. The assays are explained in principle in *Figure 2* and Section 3. The protocols for them, as offered below, use one brand of polystyrene ELISA plate and HRP conjugates of antibodies and antigens prepared as 'in house' reagents. OPD is used as substrate. It is inevitable that conditions for performing the tests adequately will vary slightly according to the plates used and the antigen−antibody system under study. Exact working conditions can only be determined by pilot experiments. In addition, other enzyme−substrate combinations, as reviewed in Section 5, can be used to perform the assays, with appropriate changes in buffer, etc. The general procedures for the assay protocols, equipment and buffers are as given in Section 4.3.3. This section should be read through before starting any test and referred to in performing the sequence of steps.

6.1 **Direct and indirect ELISA for antigen detection (assays 1 and 7—see** *Figure 2***)**

This is a non-competitive assay that depends, in its simplest format, upon the use of a reference antibody−enzyme conjugate to detect antigen in test samples used to coat the wells. When modified to use a labelled antiglobulin third reagent layer, to enhance sensitivity, it becomes an indirect (antigen) ELISA (assay 7). The tests are similar in function to direct and indirect fluorescent antibody tests for tissue antigens (although the emphasis in ELISA is on antigen detection as opposed to antigen localization); cells, organelles or membranes can be used to coat the plates (e.g. to detect viral antigens) or test samples that may contain intact bacteria, parasites or soluble antigens. Both polyclonal and monoclonal antibodies may be used.

6.1.1 *Protocol*

(1)   Check the specificity and working titre of the antigen-specific antibody (as conjugate in the direct test) by preliminary titrations using a standard purified antigen or known antigen-positive sample (see *Table 8*).

(2)   In indirect tests determine the working dilution of the antiglobulin conjugate by following the protocol in *Table 8* and then check its performance in a pilot indirect test with standard antigen using the working titre of the first antibody.

(3)   Establish the optimal coating concentration for antigen in a known antigen-positive sample and (when available) a purified antigen (*Table 9*) which are used subsequently as positive controls in tests—see Technical note 1 [Section 4.3.3(iii)] on antigen-coating.

(4)   Coat wells with positive control sample(s), negative control samples (of same provenance), BSA (100 μg/ml) and test samples. Purified control antigen (where available) should also be used in a range of dilutions to offer a quantitative test.

(i) *Direct assay.*

(5)   Apply the reference antibody conjugate, incubate and wash.

(6)   Apply substrate solution and incubate again; observe development of positive control reactions and stop when these are optimal [see *Table 8*, and Section 4.3.3(iii), Technical note 5].

(7)   Read the plates using a reader; for OPD the filter should be 492 nm.

(ii) *Indirect assay.*

(5)   Apply unlabelled specific antibody, incubate and wash.

(6)   Apply the labelled antiglobulin conjugate, incubate and wash.

(7)   Follow direct assay steps (6) and (7).

6.1.2 *Interpretation*

(i)   In both forms of assay the negative control sample wells and BSA-coated wells should give minimal OD readings.

(ii)   A panel of (minimally) 8 − 10 negative control samples, applied in duplicate wells, can form the basis for determining the cut-off point between positive and negative tests. Take the mean of the reading of the duplicate negative control wells and calculate the panel mean and two standard deviations (2 SD) of this. Test sample OD readings above this can be assigned as antigen positive.

(iii) Where purified antigen standard dilutions have been used, prepare a dilution versus OD curve. Test samples can be quantitated for antigen against this curve.

The sensitivity of the assay can be defined as the concentration giving a reading above 2 SD of the negative control panel.

6.1.3 *Technical notes*

(i) *Coating plates with antigen.* Antigens vary, particularly between proteins, carbohydrates and lipoproteins, in their capacity to coat different plastics. Solid phase formats that show overall suitability for ELISA should then be tested with the available antigens under investigation using a reference positive antibody. Only those formats that give an absorbance of 1.0 or above, with minimal background (<0.2) will offer enough sensitivity between these values to detect weakly positive samples. This applies in all antigen coating test formats. In some cases it may be necessary to modify the coating procedure to achieve an adequate antigen coating (46−49). This includes the adsorption of poly-L-lysine to which antigens are then coupled chemically, irradiation of plates, treatment with glutaraldehyde, or gelatine 'subbing'. In some cases antigens can be made to adsorb to plates by drying down the coating volume. The stability of antigens dried down this way is variable and may give rise to high backgrounds in some cases. The method applies particularly to cells and particulate antigens.

(ii) *Specificity.* The use of polyspecific (polyclonal) first antibodies may offer considerable specificity problems in detecting a single antigen of diagnostic importance in a complex coating mixture. This can only be resolved by adequate specificity testing of the antiserum and appropriate absorption (see Volume I, Chapter 2). The use of monoclonal antibodies is clearly an advantage in this respect.

It must be appreciated that the labelled antiglobulin in the indirect antigen test may bind to immunoglobulin present in the coating test samples if these are of mammalian source. For instance, faecal or expectorated bacteria may be coated with antibody. Antiglobulins require scrupulous absorption to react only with the species immunoglobulin of the first antibody. A major source of false-positive reactions can be attributed to this problem.

(iii) *Sensitivity.* Although monoclonal antibodies are a major benefit in this test, their restricted binding to a single antigen epitope may be a problem in complex antigen mixtures, as the availability of the epitope may be very limited. A mixture of monoclonal antibody specificities may be advantageous. There is no doubt that under some circumstances the assays can be very sensitive. One example is in the indirect test for the host species in blood meals of haematophagous insects. A recent trial run by WHO (50) showed that with appropriate reagents human IgG could be detected in eluted filter paper spots of mosquito blood meals (used to coat ELISA plates) with a sensitivity approaching 1 ng.

6.2 The indirect antibody ELISA (assay 7)

6.2.1 *General considerations*

Although the indirect antibody ELISA has been used for diagnostic purposes in many fields of research and medicine its main application remains in the diagnosis of human and animal infections through the detection of specific serum antibodies which bind to infection-related antigens prepared and coated on the solid phase. The patients' antibodies, thus bound, are revealed by use of an enzyme − antiglobulin conjugate which itself binds specifically as the third layer. This is the basis of the indirect antibody ELISA test. Under optimal conditions of specificity and sensitivity nanogram quantities of human antibody in infected patients can be detected, whilst sera of uninfected patients give negative results. However, as in all sensitive and complex immunological tests, satisfactory results are obtained only by the most careful standardization of reagents and method. No amount of good practice in the conduct of the tests can compensate for bad reagents. Aspects of the test itself also need very careful attention. Although considered here mainly in the context of antibodies and infection, the indirect ELISA is also a valuable assay in the quality control of animal antisera and in the screening of monoclonal antibodies.

6.2.2 *Choice of antigen*

In assessing the suitability of an antigen for use in the indirect ELISA it is essential to establish its diagnostic relevance. This is relatively easy in situations where simple and well-defined antigens can be used. However, in other situations where the antigenic complexities interfere with the host response (e.g. parasitic diseases), the choice of antigen may be particularly difficult. In this respect the following criteria must take a prominent position:

(i)   specificity for the disease;
(ii) capacity to discriminate between past and present infection via the antibody response;
(iii) intensity of infection (i.e. antigen load);
(iv) regression of antibody titre after successful chemotherapy.

In view of the above stringent demands on useful antigens it is unlikely that crude extracts will be of long-term value. Efforts should be made to acquire purified antigens wherever possible; the advent of monoclonal antibodies for antigen purification and the growing involvement of recombinant DNA technology for large-scale production of single antigen molecules will undoubtedly transform infection serodiagnosis, and the value of ELISA in this respect, over the next few years.

6.2.3 *Standard serum samples*

The value of an antibody ELISA test rests on its capacity to distinguish accurately and reliably between positive and negative patients' sera in respect of single species infections. This cannot be established without reference to external standard positive and negative samples which offer a facility for both external quality control of the test (i.e. the right source of antigen and the right specificity of antiglobulin conjugate) and for selection of internal standards for day-to-day use—see Section 8 for a discussion of quality control.

6.2.4 *Selection of antiglobulin conjugate specificity*

The nature of the indirect antibody test allows the same species-specific antiglobulin conjugates to be used universally whatever the specific antibody test may be. A second property of the test system is that a choice can be made to use a general antiglobulin reagent to all of the test species serum immunoglobulins or to individual classes and subclasses. This allows antibody isotype response profiles to be evaluated which can be informative in the context of both diagnostic and immunity studies. Setting up antibody isotype profile studies needs careful standardization.

6.2.5 Protocol

(i) *Working out the conditions of the test by pilot assay.*

(1)   Determine the optimal antigen coating concentration in a dilution experiment using a control positive serum or (preferably) a positive serum pool and the labelled antiglobulin conjugate at its predetermined working dilution (see *Table 8*). Trial coatings should be in the range of $0.2-10.0$ μg/ml of antigen and for each concentration the positive serum should be titrated out to background.

(2)   Use pooled negative serum as one control, BSA-coated wells (100 μg/ml) as a second control and, as a third, antigen-coated wells with conjugate alone (replacing the positive serum step with PBS-T). These controls apply for each antigen coating concentration.

(3)   Use 100 μl vols of all reagents at each step (except stopping solution), and use duplicate wells throughout.

(ii) *Interpretation of pilot assay.*

(1)   The BSA and antigen-plus-conjugate control wells should be negative. If the BSA wells give a reaction the conjugate is too concentrated or has non-specific binding properties. If the antigen-plus-conjugate controls are positive without the BSA, then conjugate is binding to antigen. The reasons for this may be that:

(a) there is immunoglobulin in the antigen, to which the conjugate cross-reacts;
(b) the antigen is overcoated to give non-specific binding;
(c) the antigen is undercoated or fails to coat adequately, leaving opportunities for conjugate to adsorb;
(d) the antigen, although apparently coating optimally, has non-specific binding properties for conjugate and requires reappraisal as a suitable antigen; quenching with BSA may or may not solve this problem.

(2)   With the positive serum diluted out from left to right across the rows of the plates, and the antigen concentrations increasing with successive pairs of rows down the plates, the positive reactions will increase in intensity downwards and to the left and titrate out to the right. Look for the first pair of antigen rows whose concentration affords no greater reaction intensity or endpoint titration for the antibody. Check whether at this coating the antigen-plus-conjugate control gives high background. If necessary, go back one or two dilutions of antigen to find a coating concentration that gives an adequate endpoint titre with low background for control wells. After reading the plates draw out reaction curves plotting OD against serum dilutions for each antigen concentration to confirm the choice of antigen level for future tests. An example of such an analysis is shown in *Figure 7*.

STANDARDISATION OF INDIRECT ANTIBODY ELISA : TITRATION OF COATING ANTIGEN

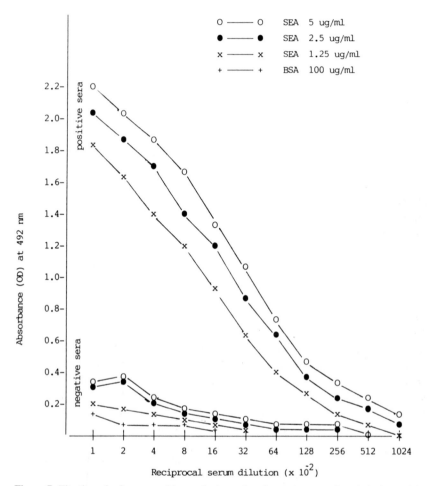

Figure 7. Titration of reference positive antibody pool, and negative control pool, in determining optimal antigen coating concentration for the indirect antibody ELISA. The standardization test shown here is for setting up assays for antibody to the soluble egg antigens (SEA) of *S. mansoni*. Note that the negative control serum gives only low background reading on antigen-coated wells at dilutions where the positive serum provides an OD of 1.0. This point is at two-fold higher dilution using 5 μg/ml coating antigen than using 1.25 μg/ml. The positive serum gives very low readings on BSA-coated wells.

(3)   Using the results of the control positive serum, choose two or three dilutions which, when used for test sera, would identify strongly and weakly positive samples.

Example: If the control serum gives an OD greater than 2.0 at 1:256 and then declines to background at 1:4096, dilutions of test sera of 1:2000 and 1:200 and 1:20 could safely be used to define all positive sera. The 1:20 might be expected to give high background but this can be checked by looking at the result of the control positive serum on BSA wells at around this dilution. Adjust the lowest test dilution as dictated by background reactions.

(iii) *Performing the test for unknown samples.*

(1) Coat plates with antigen at determined concentration, and a column with BSA. Wash the plates.

(2) Prepare the dilutions of test sera, positive control serum pool and a panel of at least eight negative control sera (see Sections 6.2.3 and 8).

(3) Apply the serum dilutions to the plates as follows. For each plate include:

(a) the dilutions of the positive control sera on antigen wells;
(b) the dilutions of the positive control sera on BSA wells;
(c) the dilutions of all eight (or more) negative control sera on antigen wells;
(d) a column of antigen wells without serum (replaced by PBS-T).
Complete the plate with dilutions of test serum samples. *Use duplicate wells* for all serum dilutions.

(4) Incubate the plates and wash.

(5) Apply the labelled antiglobulin conjugate at working dilution.

(6) Incubate the plates and wash.

(7) Apply the substrate solution, incubate again; observe development of positive control reactions and stop when these are optimal.

(8) Read the plates by eye and then on an ELISA reader.

(iv) *Interpretation.*

(1) The dilutions of positive control serum should give a gradation of OD readings upon which test sample reactions can be assigned as strong, intermediate, weak or negative for antibody. By visual assessment these can be graded from 4 to zero and this may be an adequate analysis for some samples.

(2) Borderline results (i.e. weakly positive to negative) are best assigned by reference to the negative control readings at the same dilution. Mean the duplicate OD values and then mean the panel values and calculate 2 SD above the mean. Test results above this value (duplicate well means) can be assigned as positive. *Figure 8* gives an example of such an analysis prepared as a scatter diagram (see also Section 7 on assay standardization).

(3) Positive control serum on BSA wells should be negative, at least at dilutions where test samples are positive.

(4) Antigen-plus-conjugate wells should be negative.

6.2.6 *Quantitation of antibody isotypes by indirect ELISA*

Indirect ELISA can be used as a form of immunometric antibody test run in conditions where the coating antigen is in excess; the proportion of different bound antibody isotypes is then measured. This requires careful standardization. The recommended protocol for human antibody tests is as follows.

(i) *Recommended protocol.*

(1) Prepare purified immunoglobulins of the IgG, IgA and IgM classes and of the

IgG subclasses as required (see Volume I, Chapter 2). The IgG subclass antigens will be myeloma proteins.

(2)   Prepare (or purchase) isotype-specific antiglobulin reagents. For IgG, IgA and IgM these should be enzyme conjugates. For the IgG subclasses (and IgA subclasses) use mouse monoclonal antibodies (see Appendix of Suppliers) and an anti-mouse immunoglobulin enzyme conjugate that binds to all the isotypes of the monoclonal panel and does not react with human immunoglobulins (this can only be achieved by adequate absorption—see Volume I, Chapter 2).

Preliminary for IgG, IgA and IgM quantitations

(3)   Coat duplicate rows of wells with 1 μg/ml of each purified isotype and titrate the specific conjugates to determine the dilution that gives an OD value of 1.5.

(4)   Check by cross-over tests that the conjugates give negative results with the other two isotypes.

(5)   Finally mix the three isotype antigens together so that each is at 0.33 μg/ml. Coat rows of wells with this mixture and check that each conjugate at the determined dilution gives a similar OD reading.

(6)   Adjust conjugate dilutions so that each gives the same value (in the range 0.5−0.75).

Preliminary for IgG subclass quantitations

(3)   Coat rows of wells with representative IgG subclass myeloma proteins at 1 μg/ml.

(4)   Titrate anti-subclass monoclonal antibodies against the respective myeloma protein, using a pre-determined working dilution of the anti-mouse Ig enzyme conjugate.

(5)   Select the dilution of each mouse antibody that provides an OD value of 1.5.

(6)   Mix the four subclass antigens together with each at 0.33 μg/ml. Coat with this mixture and check that each monoclonal specificity gives a similar OD value. Adjust dilutions so that each gives the same value in the range 0.5−0.75.

Quantitative test

(1)   Run assays as in Section 6.2.5(iii) using the polyspecific anti-Ig conjugate; for positive test sera select the dilution for each that gives just less than its maximum OD performance.

(2)   Repeat the assay at each test serum's assigned dilution using multiple pairs of wells to allow for the set of isotype determinations, using a three layer or four layer protocol according to the isotype test. For the IgG subclass (four layer) test include as additional controls to those in 6.2.5(iii), step 3;

(a) conjugate with antigen-plus-positive control serum, without the monoclonal reagent;

(b) conjugate with antigen-plus-monoclonal, without the positive control serum.

(ii) *Interpretation.* When adequately standardized the above protocols provide excellent quantitative data on antibody isotypes, drawn directly from OD values (51).

(iii) *Technical notes.* Isotype studies can also be performed with sera of other species,

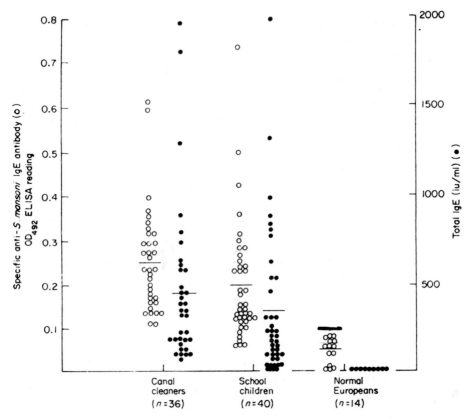

Figure 8. Two forms of enzyme immunoassay used to study features of serum IgE in patients. Scatter diagram of total serum IgE compared with specific IgE antibodies in schistosomiasis patients measured by immunometric (sandwich) ELISA and indirect antibody (isotype-specific) ELISA, respectively. (●), total IgE; (○), specific IgE antibody; *n*, number of samples tested. Two groups of patients are represented. Narrow bars are mean values for each group; broad bar is mean plus 2 SD value of negative control group for IgE antibody which defines the margin for positive antibody titre in the patient groups. From this it can be seen that eight children can be assigned as IgE antibody negative. (Adapted from ref. 51.)

using appropriate antigens for calibrating the assays and isotype-specific reagents. In the mouse and rat a useful strategy for calibration is to use monoclonal antibodies across the isotype spectrum that are directed to soluble antigens that can be used to coat the plates.

Similar studies on isotypes can be performed in immunometric assays for specific immune complexes (assay 6) (52) (see Section 6.7).

6.3 The serum antibody competition test (SACT—assay 4)

Although commonly performed as a radiolabelled antibody test (see Chapter 3), the principle of two antibodies competing for solid phase antigen can also be applied successfully with the reference antibody coupled to enzyme instead of isotope. This form of assay can be a useful means of comparing new specificities of monoclonal antibody with a reference monoclonal, on the assumption that new products blocking reference binding have the same antigen specificity. A further important application is in testing patients' sera (or animal sera) for the presence of a constituent antibody with diagnostic specificity. This can be achieved once a (reference) monoclonal antibody has been produced to an infection-specific epitope, as is the case, for instance, in tuberculosis and leprosy (53,54). A merit of the assay is that it does not require a purified antigen and yet can be a highly specific diagnostic test. The exact conditions of the test will vary considerably according to the nature and complexity of the coating antigen and the binding constant of the reference labelled reagent. In tests where the competing antibodies are both mouse (or rat, or human) monoclonals, it is necessary to run the assay without the benefit of an amplifying labelled antiglobulin step (unless the test antibodies are of isotypes different from that of the reference); good sensitivity may be difficult to achieve under such conditions. Attempts to compete polyclonal antibodies are often unsuccessful because their constituent sets of specificities will not overlap.

The following is a general guide to the steps required in setting up the test with a mouse monoclonal reference antibody and human sera, using an enzyme-labelled anti-mouse immunoglobulin second reagent.

6.3.1 *Protocol*

(i) *Standardizing the antigen and monoclonal antibody.*

(1) Coat plates with duplicate rows of antigen dilutions (suggested range, $1-20$ μg/ml) and every third row with 100 μg/ml BSA.
(2) Titrate the monoclonal antibody against the antigen-coating dilutions across the rows.
(3) Develop the assay with a working dilution of anti-mouse IgG conjugate [see (iii) below], including control wells of antigen and conjugate, and BSA and conjugate (PBS-T replaces antibody).

(ii) *Interpretation.*

(1) Look for the lowest antigen dilution where the monoclonal antibody titrates down optimally to low background OD values. If backgrounds are high this may be reduced by quenching antigen-coated plate with 1% (w/v) or less of BSA.
(2) Check that in this titration set the monoclonal has low background binding to BSA wells, at least in the OD decline region.
(3) Check that the conjugate gives low background values with antigen—alone, and with BSA controls (see Section 6.3.4, Technical note i).
(4) Draw a binding curve of the monoclonal antibody at the selected antigen coating concentration; this should give OD values, with dilution, from approximately 2.0 to less than 0.2.
(5) From this curve select an antibody dilution giving an OD value in the range of $1.5-1.0$ (i.e. in the upper half of the curve but below the plateau). This is the *working dilution of the reference antibody* against which serum antibody can compete and operate sensitively.

(iii) *Standardizing the antiglobulin conjugate.*

(1)   Titrate the conjugate against rows of wells coated with:

(a) mouse Ig at 1 μg/ml;

(b) human Ig at 1 μg/ml.

See *Table 8* for titration procedure and Volume I, Chapter 2 for Ig preparation.

(2)   Choose as *conjugate working dilution* that giving an OD of 1.5—1.0 (against mouse Ig).

(3)   Check that the conjugate does *not* bind to human Ig (see Section 6.3.4, Technical note ii).

6.3.2 *Performing the assay*

(1)   Prepare a six tube dilution series of the reference antibody-positive serum (in doubling or $\log_{10}$ series, and starting at 1:10 or more, as determined by trial).

(2)   Dispense 100 μl of each dilution to pairs of wells on plates coated with antigen at the determined concentration along two half rows (A and B) and then repeat the series to complete the two rows—this provides two sets of positive serum dilutions to be used as different controls.

(3)   Prepare an identical dilution series with the normal serum (negative control) and dispense these samples also into pairs of wells along two half rows (C and D). Do not, however, repeat the dispensing in this case but complete the rows C and D with PBS-T (100 μl) as another control.

(4)   Prepare the same dilution series for each of the test sera and dispense these also into two half rows (i.e. E and F 1—6; 7—12, etc.) and follow on into further plates as necessary.

(5)   Stand the plates at room temperature for 1 h and then add to the well contents 100 μl of the monoclonal antibody for all wells *except rows A and B 7—12* where PBS-T is used (antigen-positive serum-conjugate control).

(6)   Incubate the plate at 37°C for 2 h (with possibly a requirement for overnight reaction at 4°C, determined by trial).

(7)   Wash the plates and develop the competitive test results with the anti-mouse Ig conjugate (100 μl), which is applied to all wells.

6.3.3 *Interpretation*

Table 11 shows the design of control and test sections of the assay. Comparison of OD readings in control series 3 and 4 should reveal both to be high, as negative serum is not expected to have inhibitory activity against the monoclonal antibody (see Section 6.3.4, Technical note iii). Control 3 is the best means to determine the OD representing 100% binding, as the only variable in assay conditions compared with test serum is the possible presence of antibody in the latter. The reactions using the control positive serum dilutions (control 1, *Table 5*) are used to calibrate the competitive action of serum antibody against the monoclonal reagent and to define, by this means, the 0% binding OD value. As the positive serum is diluted out and inhibition depreciates so the monoclonal antibody binding increases. A curve can be drawn of % inhibition against dilution for the positive serum. Results of test sera are expressed as inhibition titres—it is more accurate to calculate the 50% inhibition dilution (ID50).

Table 11. Serum antibody competition test: plate design.

Control series	Rows/wells	Coating antigen	Control reagents			Test serum	Monoclonal antibody	PBS-T	Anti-mouse Ig conjugate	Result (% binding) ≡ enzyme activity
			Positive serum	Negative serum	PBS-T					
1	A and B1–6	+	+				+		+	0^a
2	A and B7–12	+	+					+	+	0
3	C and D1–6	+		+			+		+	100^b
4	C and D7–12	+			+		+		+	100
Tests	E and F1–6 etc.	+				+	+		+	?

Control series: [a]1. Checks that control positive serum competes with the monoclonal antibody, with zero conjugate binding. The minimum OD reading of this control dilution series defines 0% binding (maximum inhibition).

2. Checks that conjugate does not bind to human antibodies.

[b]3. Checks that monoclonal antibody is not inhibited by normal human serum (antibody-negative control). The maximum OD reading of this control dilution series defines 100% binding (zero inhibition).

4. Checks that monoclonal antibody binds to antigen at the expected level for zero inhibition.

6.3.4 *Technical notes*

(i) *Antiglobulin enzyme conjugates and anti-bacterial antibodies.* Animals used for raising antiglobulins will have serum antibodies to common bacterial antigens and these will be present in the conjugate. In assays using bacterial antigens it is always necessary to check that antiglobulin conjugates do not bind the antigen; this is unlikely to occur at working dilutions but it may be necessary to absorb the conjugate against the antigen. One way to do this is to incubate conjugate at 1:100 dilution in antigen-coated wells at 37°C for 1 h and overnight at 4°C.

(ii) *Species cross-reactivity of antiglobulins.* Antiglobulin reagents require extensive absorption against insolubilized immunoglobulins of other species to render them species-specific (see Volume I, Chapter 2). Commercial sources of antiglobulins, although stated to be, for example anti-mouse, will usually cross-react with other species and thus render the assay totally invalid. All purchased conjugates must be scrupulously tested before use.

(iii) *Normal sera as negative antibody controls* (see also Section 8). In view of the wide range of specificities of antibody in 'normal' sera (all serum antibodies are specific to some antigen—mostly of microorganisms) problems may be encountered in finding a serum with genuinely negative (background) binding values. However, in clinical tests at least, the purpose of the assay is to separate positive cases from normal values, so the use of the normal serum pool is to remove the normal element of positivity from the assay by, in essence, background subtraction. If 'normal' sera have high background values, then the sensitivity of the assay is lost—this is a major problem in third-world countries with many endemic infections, as exposure is common in the general population. For these reasons it is often necessary to screen a large number of healthy blood donors in the assay and select from these a panel with minimal binding activity as the source of the negative control.

6.4 **The antigen inhibition assay (assay 2)**

The simplest means to estimate antigen in solution by ELISA is to use the test samples to inhibit enzyme-coupled antibody from binding to the same antigen coating the plate. If the antibody is a monoclonal then the coating antigen need not be a purified standard, but this is required if the antibody is polyclonal, as free (test) antigen would not inhibit all binding specificities at the same concentration. The assay is a useful alternative to the antigen-capture immunometric approach (assay 5—Section 6.6) and although not as sensitive it has the potential to determine antigenic molecules of single epitope structure not possible by the capture principle. In addition there is no requirement to prepare antibody for coating plates. The assay is, however, restricted to conditions where no antibody can be present in test samples, as these would interfere with the antigens. In this assay there is little or no benefit in sensitivity by use of an additional enzyme – antiglobulin conjugate step, although the convenience of this indirect approach should be considered when using monoclonals as first antibodies. The protocol given below excludes this additional step. If needed the usual considerations of antiglobulin conjugate standardization should be applied (*Table 8*) and the reagent finally titrated to working dilution under assay conditions without antigen inhibitor present.

6.4.1 *Protocol for standardizing assay*

(i)   Standardize the antigen coating concentration as for previous assays [e.g. Section 6.3.1(i)], using the labelled antibody in a direct binding test. Use some BSA-coated wells as controls here and in (ii) below.

(ii)   With optimal antigen coating, determine the working dilution of the labelled antibody by titration. Draw the dilution curve and choose a (antigen-inhibitable) dilution that has less than maximum (~ 50%) antigen binding. Check at this stage that this conjugate dilution has low background binding activity in BSA-coated wells.

(iii) Perform a standard antigen inhibition titration as follows.

(1) Make serial doubling (or $\log_{10}$) dilutions of standard antigen in PBS-T in tubes.

(2) In a second set of tubes add 100 μl of labelled antibody, prepared one step less diluted than working dilution.

(iv)   Add to the antibody tubes 100 μl of the antigen dilution series, mix, cover and stand at room temperature for 1 h.

(v)   Transfer 100 μl of the mixture in each tube to a pair of wells of an antigen-coated plate, along two complete rows.

(vi)   Add 100 μl of labelled antibody at its working dilution to a further set of six wells (100% binding, antibody alone control).

(vii) Incubate the plate at 37°C for 1 h and perform the usual washing, substrate and reading steps.

(viii) Draw the antigen inhibition curve using the antibody alone OD value as zero inhibition, and the minimum OD (with high inhibitor) value as 100% inhibition.

(ix)   Repeat the assay as necessary with adjusted inhibitor dilutions (and/or labelled antibody dilution) to achieve a convenient inhibition scale, with optimal sensitivity. At this stage include a dilution series of a reference antigen-positive sample to determine a useful range of test dilutions for future assay work.

6.4.2 *The routine assay*

Prepare dilutions of standard antigen, reference positive and test samples and set up the inhibition assays as in Section 6.4.1. Always include the standard assay with test samples on every plate. *Figure 9* illustrates the measurement of an antigen released in culture from *Schistosoma mansoni* transformed cercariae, after irradiation, compared with standard antigen, using a monoclonal antibody to an antigen in turnover on the membrane.

6.4.3 *Analysis*

The standard antigen inhibition curve for each plate is drawn up using the defined 0 and 100% inhibition limits. The antigen in test samples can be determined from dilutions giving 50% binding inhibition (or other points in the linear section of the curve) by referral to the standard antigen inhibition data (see *Figure 9*).

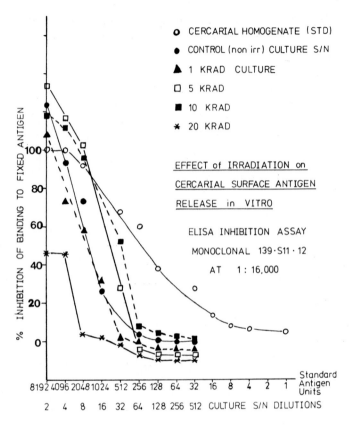

CERCARIAL HOMOGENATE (STD)

CONTROL (non irr) CULTURE S/N

▲ 1 KRAD CULTURE

□ 5 KRAD

■ 10 KRAD

✳ 20 KRAD

EFFECT of IRRADIATION on
CERCARIAL SURFACE ANTIGEN
RELEASE in VITRO

ELISA INHIBITION ASSAY
MONOCLONAL 139·S11·12
AT 1:16,000

Figure 9. Antigen inhibition ELISA (ELISA inhibition assay) used to detect a soluble antigen released from *S.mansoni* transformed cercariae (schistosomula) *in vitro* after irradiation (irr). In this assay a monoclonal antibody is inhibited from binding to coated antigen by the presence of standard antigen or culture supernatant (S/N) over a range of concentrations/dilutions. The 100% inhibition point is determined with standard antigen and the 0% with a blank culture S/N. Cultured parasite-released antigen is more efficient at inhibition than the standard parasite sonicate antigen. Units of standard antigen are ng/ml protein.

6.5 The competitive antigen assay (assay 3)

Competitive assays are as simple to perform as inhibitions and have about the same sensitivity. The form described here depends on antibody coating of ELISA wells, with labelled and unlabelled (standard and test) antigens competing for antigen capture to the solid phase. The assay is rendered quantitative by standard antigen competitor dilutions. Good results can be obtained with polyclonal and monoclonal antibodies which bind remarkably well, in active condition, to the plastic. Affinity-purified antibodies are not required; the IgG fractions of sheep or rabbit serum, or monoclonal ascitic fluid, are adequate preparations. Sensitivity is largely determined by the binding constant of the antibody, as high affinity is reflected in lower concentrations of labelled antigen required to achieve a measurable bound amount; the less labelled antigen involved, the lower the level of competing antigen that can be detected. In analysis of mosquito blood meals 25 ng of the species IgG in the stomach contents can be detected (50).

The assay can be easily modified to a dot-ELISA format, as spotted antibodies bound to nitrocellulose membranes remain active even when stored in dry conditions.

6.5.1 *Protocol for standardizing assay*

(i)   Prepare the IgG fraction of high titre polyclonal antiserum of required specificity (>1 mg/ml specific antibody—see Volume I, Chapter 2), or collect monoclonal ascitic fluid of high antibody content (>1 mg/ml). Prepare also IgG of normal serum of the same coating species, or collect an ascites of irrelevant specificity.

(ii)   Prepare purified standard antigen and use part of this to prepare an enzyme conjugate; the remaining part is used as standard inhibitor. Check the enzyme activity of the conjugate (Section 4.3.2).

(iii)   Measure the concentration of the coating preparations and coat double rows of plates with 1 μg/ml to 10 μg/ml of specific and control Ig.

(iv)   Titrate the conjugated antigen across the Ig-coated rows and select a coating antibody concentration that gives optimal antigen binding titre with a clear negative endpoint (low background). Draw this titration curve and determine the *labelled antigen working dilution*, which should give about 50% maximum binding.

(v)   Check that the labelled antigen does not bind to the non-antibody Ig wells coated at the concentration to be used for the specific antibody.

(vi)   Perform a standard antigen:labelled antigen competition assay as follows.

   (1)   Make serial doubling (or $\log_{10}$) dilutions of standard antigen in PBS-T and place 100 μl of each into test tubes.

   (2)   Prepare labelled antigen to one step less than its working dilution in PBS-T and add 100 μl to each tube of the antigen dilution series. Mix each tube thoroughly.

   (3)   Prepare an antibody-coated plate using the determined antibody Ig concentration and include six pairs of wells coated with non-antibody Ig at the same level (the plate can be prepared over the previous night).

   (4)   Dispense 100 μl of the competition antigen mixture of each tube to a pair of wells of the antibody-coated plate, along two complete rows.

   (5)   Dispense 100 μl of labelled antigen at its working dilution into:
      (a) a further set of six pairs of antibody-coated wells (no competitor control wells);
      (b) the set of six pairs of non-antibody Ig-coated wells.

   (6)   Incubate the plate at 37°C for $1-2$ h (determine by trial).

   (7)   Wash the plate and develop with substrate, following the standard procedure.

   (8)   Stop the reaction when the no competitor control wells reach an OD of 1.0 after stopping (i.e. stop one pair and read—repeat again later as necessary: stop also a pair of non-antibody Ig plus labelled antigen wells).

   (9)   Draw the antigen competition/inhibition curve using the labelled antigen alone (no competitor) control OD value (~ 1.0) as zero inhibition and the minimum OD (with high competitor) value as 100% inhibition.

   (10)   Repeat the assay as necessary with adjusted competitor dilutions and

a

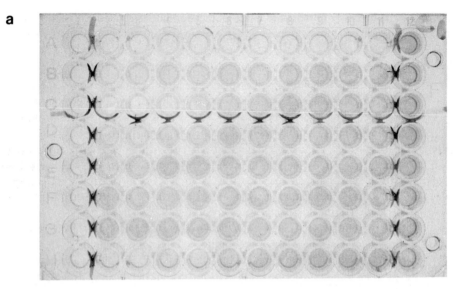

b

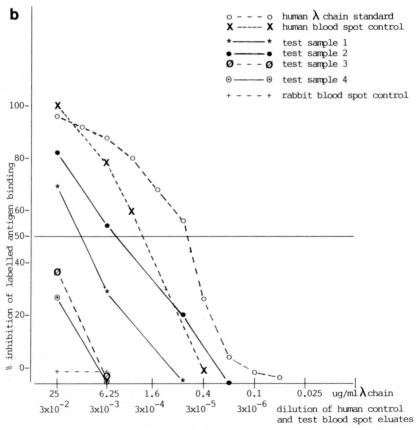

o - - - o   human λ chain standard
X ----- X   human blood spot control

———   test sample 1
●———●   test sample 2
Ø - - - Ø   test sample 3
⊙———⊙   test sample 4
+ - - - +   rabbit blood spot control

labelled antigen dilutions to achieve a convenient competition range with optimal sensitivity. Include at this stage dilutions of a reference antigen-positive sample to determine a useful range of test dilutions for future assay work.

6.5.2 *The routine assay*

Prepare dilutions of standard antigen, the reference antigen positive sample, antigen-negative samples and test samples, and set up the competition assay as in Section 6.5.1. Include the standard competition series on every plate as a reference reaction. [*Figure 10a* shows the competition assay being used to determine human IgG in mosquito blood meals, and *Figure 10b* shows the standard antigen (IgGλ), positive sample and test sample dilution curves.]

6.5.3 *Analysis*

Plot the standard antigen inhibition curve of each plate, using the defined 0 and 100% inhibition limits. Test samples can be quantitated by reference to the standard curve using the 50% binding inhibition titre or another point on the linear section of the curve.

6.5.4 *The dot-ELISA modification of the competition antigen assay*

(i)   Prepare 1 × 2 cm strips of nitrocellulose membrane (see Appendix of Suppliers). Use disposable gloves for handling the membrane.

(ii)   Label each strip with pencil at the top and, in the centre of the lower half, spot 5 μl of antibody, containing 25 μg IgG/ml (0.125 μg per spot) in coating buffer.

(iii)   Dry the spots overnight at room temperature and then quench in 3% (w/v) BSA in PBS-T at 37°C for 1 h. Wash in saline−Tween.

(iv)   Prepare competition mixtures of standard antigen, reference antigen-positive sample, antigen-negative sample and test samples as for the plate assay (Sections 6.5.1 and 6.5.2) but in 400 μl volumes in tubes.

(v)   Incubate the antibody-dotted strips in these mixtures in duplicate in the tubes

Figure 10. (a) Competitive antigen assay to detect the presence of human immunoglobulin (through a λ light chain epitope) in mosquito blood meal filter paper spots (produced by squashing trapped insects onto the paper). In this assay a monoclonal antibody specific to human Ig λ chain is used to coat ELISA wells. Enzyme-labelled standard antigen (IgGλ) binds fully to coating antibody, and a colour reaction develops to completion, in the absence of competing antigen in the eluted blood spot. The enzyme is HRP and the substrate is OPD. Standard competitor is purified human λ chain. **Rows A** and **B**, wells 2−11, are a doubling dilution series (in pairs along the rows) of standard λ chain inhibitor, from 25 μg/ml (row A, wells 2 and 3) to 40 ng/ml (row B, wells 10 and 11). **Row C**, wells 2−11 are a $\log_{10}$ dilution series of eluted normal human blood spots, starting at 3 × 10^{-2}, in pairs along the row. **Rows D** onwards, in pairs of wells, are 3 × 10^{-2} dilutions of eluted test blood meal spots used as competitor. D2+3 and H2+3 inhibit strongly and are human blood meal positive; D4+5, E2+3 and H4+5 are weakly inhibiting and come from older, partly digested human blood meals. The remaining test samples are negative in competition. **Column 12** is the 'positive' control reaction (nil competitor) and **column 1** is non-antibody mouse Ig-coated wells with standard antigen conjugate, as a zero binding control. (b) Competitive antigen assay inhibition curves for mosquito blood meal detection of human Ig. Standard curves are shown for human λ chain competitor dilutions and eluted normal human blood spots (sets 100% inhibition point). Two eluted mosquito blood meals (samples 1 and 2) give more than 50% inhibition and the amount of competing antigen can be determined from the 50% inhibiting dilution (ID50) by reference to the standard inhibition curve. Normal rabbit blood eluted spots are used as negative competitor controls (0% inhibition).

at 37°C for 1 h and then wash in saline–Tween in a Petri dish.

(vi) Develop the dot-ELISA by exposure of the strips in a solution of CNP substrate (for HRP-labelled antigen) (see *Tables 1* and *2*), in a Petri dish.

(vii) Wash the fully developed strips in PBS-T, dry and mount for visual analysis.

6.5.5 *Technical notes*

(i) The dot-ELISA has equivalent sensitivity to the plate assay but with the advantage that it can be performed under extremely simple laboratory conditions.

(ii) Dot-ELISA can be applied to other tests, for example those where solid phase antigens are used. A useful strategy for screening sera for antibodies to a range of infections, or to other panels of antigen, is to dot the appropriate antigens onto an ELISA plate-sized membrane and expose this to a single serum. Subsequent development with a labelled antiglobulin will reveal the pattern of specific antibodies.

6.6 **The antigen-capture two-site (sandwich) assay (assay 5)**

6.6.1 *Properties and advantages of antigen-capture assays*

An assay that captures and concentrates antigen onto an excess of solid phase antibody of defined specificity offers intrinsically high sensitivity and specificity. Such a system can potentially detect a single bound antigen molecule using a second labelled antibody to form a sandwich complex—the limits in practice being determined by features of the signal generated and the efficiency of its detection. Many commercial enzyme immunoassays now use this principle—the most sensitive allowing measurement of hormones and drugs previously only within the reach of radioimmunoassay. Use of high affinity monoclonal antibodies, one as capture and one as labelled reagent, has obvious advantages in standardization and sensitivity—the coating monoclonal offering exquisite specificity. The only major disadvantage of the double monoclonal system is that the antigen must present at least one target epitope on each side of the molecule. For most antigens a different monoclonal specificity will be required for initial capture and then labelled antibody binding. A second difficulty is that a signal-amplifying labelled antiglobulin cannot be used with two monoclonals in the system unless these are of different isotype or species. Partly for this reason methods for increasing substrate signal have tended to rely on use of an unlabelled polyclonal second antibody (of different species to the capture reagent), with a labelled species-specific antiglobulin, a co-enzyme system (e.g. avidin–biotin), enzyme cascades, or strategies such as enhanced chemiluminescence (see Section 5.2). The use of a polyclonal second antibody does not reduce the intrinsically high specificity of the assay provided by the capture monoclonal.

With antigen capture being the essential feature, the assay is amenable to modification to dip-stick technologies for antigen detection. In addition the replacement of the second antigen-specific antibody by a labelled antiglobulin converts the system into a specific immune complex test (assay 6) which, by use of anti-isotype-labelled antiglobulins, allows host antibody isotype profiles of complexes to be studied in chronic infections (52).

6.6.2 *Protocol*

Follow the instructions on reagent volumes, conditions for coating, washing steps, substrate reactions, stopping and reading plates detailed in Sections 4.3.3 and 6.5.1.

(i) *Steps involved.*

(1) Coat ELISA plates with capture antibody—monoclonal- or affinity-purified polyclonal (see Standardization 1).

(2) Apply dilutions of:

(a) standard antigen (see Standardization 2);
(b) reference positive samples;
(c) reference negative samples;
(d) test samples.

(3) Apply either:

(a) labelled second monoclonal antibody;
(b) labelled polyclonal antibody;
(c) unlabelled polyclonal antibody followed by
(d) labelled antiglobulin (to species different from that of coating antibody).

(4) Develop, stop and read reactions.

(5) Analyse results by reference to standard antigen binding curve.

(ii) *Standardization.*

(1) Antibody coating. Determine optimal antibody coating concentration as described in the antigen competition assay (Section 6.5.1) using either labelled antigen as the indicator or a pilot sandwich test. Coat a pattern of six pairs of wells with non-antibody immunoglobulin of same species for background antigen binding. *Figure 11a* illustrates a test for antibody coating.

(2) Standard antigen dilutions and controls. Use, as in other assays, initially an extended doubling (or $\log_{10}$) dilution series which can be later modified in the test itself, once the sensitivity is determined. Use OD values of antigen with non-antibody Ig control wells to check for low antigen background.

(3) Labelled second reagents. Titrate labelled antigen-specific second antibody to working dilution in pilot sandwich test. Check that labelled antibody does not bind to antigen-negative wells. Titrate labelled antiglobulin to working dilution as described in *Table 8*. Check that labelled antiglobulin does not bind in wells where second antibody is omitted.

(4) Prepare a standard antigen binding curve using reference positive sample to define 100% binding OD value, and non-antibody Ig-coated wells with antigen and labelled reagent to define the 0% binding OD value. A standard antigen curve is illustrated in *Figure 11b*.

(5) Quantitate test results at 50% binding dilution (or other point in linear part of dilution curve) against the standard antigen curve.

(6) In routine tests run a panel of eight or more negative samples through the assay to determine a mean negative value. Antigen-positive samples are defined as those with OD values greater than 2 SD above the mean of the negatives.

6.6.3 *Technical notes*

(i) The range of coating antibody is usually $1-5$ μg/ml.

(ii) Affinity purification of polyclonal antibodies, as can be used for coating, is described in Volume I, Chapter 5. It is difficult to purify high avidity polyclonal

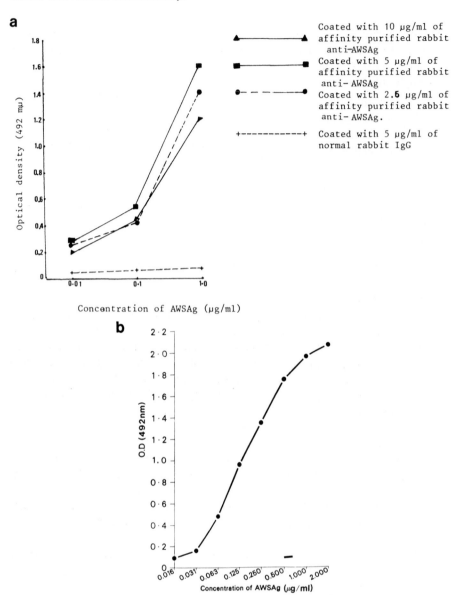

Figure 11. (**a**) Test for antibody coating concentration for an antigen-capture (sandwich) ELISA. The test system uses affinity-purified rabbit antibody to adult schistosome (worm) surface antigens (AWSAg), with coating at 10, 5 and 2.5 μg/ml. Normal rabbit IgG is used to determine background binding of antigen to non-antibody-coated wells; this gives minimal OD readings. Antibody coating is optimal at 5 μg/ml. Detection of adult parasite antigens is most sensitive in the 100 ng−1 μg/ml range in this standardization assay. The test can be used to detect antigen in schistosomiasis patients' serum before treatment in this sensitivity range, and to confirm loss of antigen after successful chemotherapy. (**b**) Standard antigen binding curve in antigen-capture ELISA for schistosome adult surface antigens. The assay shows near-linear quantitative binding of antigen in the range 30 ng−1 μg/ml. Test samples falling outside this range would need dilution adjustment. Greatest accuracy in determining test samples is achieved in readings falling between OD 0.5 and 1.8 (25−90% binding). 0% binding is set at OD 0.1 by non-antibody IgG-coated wells (see a). 100% binding is set for standard positive samples (not shown) which give, as with the standard antigen, an OD of 2.1.

antibodies with preserved binding activity, which is one reason why monoclonal antibodies have gained popularity in this assay and have allowed its development for many tests.

(iii) Tests based on antigen-capture by polyclonal antibodies are likely to be less specific. However, in some cases this can be turned to advantage in the search for putative antigens in test samples as a diagnostic aid. They can also be used successfully in measuring large molecular weight complex antigens such as serum proteins. The results of an assay for total serum IgE are illustrated as part of *Figure 8*. IgE is present in low concentrations in sera and cannot be easily measured by other means.

6.7 Modified antigen-capture assay to detect specific immune complexes and the isotypes of the bound antibody (assay 6)

6.7.1 *Protocol*

Protocol [as used to detect and measure specific complexes in schistosomiasis patients (52)].

(i) Coat ELISA plates with monoclonal antibody as ascitic fluid, using 5 μg/ml of specific antibody in coating buffer and 100 μl per well.

(ii) Titrate the plates overnight at 4°C in a humid box, wash five times in saline-T.

(iii) Dilute (on the previous day) human sera (reference positive and negative samples, test samples) in the range 1:20 to 1:100 in PBS-T and incubate the dilutions overnight at 4°C in wells of plates coated with 5 μg/ml of mixed purified normal rabbit and mouse Ig. This step removes any possible rheumatoid factors from patients' sera.

(iv) Dispense the absorbed serum dilutions in aliquots of 100 μl into the antibody-coated plates in duplicate.

(v) Incubate the coated plates at 37°C for 1 h, wash three times in saline-T.

(vi) Dispense 100 μl of HRP−antiglobulin reagent at its working dilution into the wells, incubate at 37°C for 1 h and wash the plates again in saline-T.

(vii) Dispense 100 μl of OPD solution in substrate buffer into each well and incubate in the dark at 37°C for 10−30 min until the standard positive reaction reaches an OD 492 nm value of 1.0 (after stopping).

(viii) Stop the reactions with 25 μl of 2 M H_2SO_4 or HCl and read using a 492 nm filter with a blank of substrate solution.

6.7.2 *Interpretation and technical notes*

(i) Positive reactions in the above test are taken as those that give readings 2 SD above the mean of a panel of negative control sera.

(ii) The test should include sera of non-infected patients with high levels of infection − non-specific immune complexes, used unabsorbed in the assay. Such samples can be obtained from rheumatoid and systemic lupus erythematosus patients. These sera demonstrate that rheumatoid factor and non-specific immune complexes do not give false positive reactions in this particular test.

(iii) The assay with the same test and control samples is repeated with each labelled antiglobulin specificity until a complete profile of antibodies in the samples has been accumulated. In such tests it is essential to standardize the dilutions of anti-isotype reagents so that each gives the same OD value for the same concentration of the respective immunoglobulin class. This is done in direct ELISA using purified isotypes as coating antigens (see Section 6.2.6). Once standardized, OD values can then be used directly to compare isotype levels in each sample.

7. STANDARDIZATION OF ELISA

7.1 Endpoint standardization

The signal provided by enzyme−substrate interaction is subject to many possible influences and its output is highly susceptible to variations in conditions. For a reproducible ELISA test it is essential therefore to standardize procedures and reagents with special attention being paid to reagent concentrations (including pipetting accuracy), temperature, pH and other buffer conditions. The aim is so to regulate the signal provided by the control (reference) positive serum wells, included in every assay, that the endpoint of the entire test, and of tests run on different days, becomes standardized. In practice this is attempted in one of two ways, either by stopping the reaction at a pre-set time, or when the reference positive serum has achieved a pre-determined absorbance value (e.g. OD 492 = 1.0). A modification of the more stringent but desirable second approach is to allow plates a set time for development but then to calculate and apply a correction factor based on comparison of actual and pre-set optimal reference positive serum values. The use of pre-set reference positive values is a major consideration in achieving reproducibility and a high standard of quality control within ELISA tests.

7.2 Reader (absorbance) and visual endpoints

A high degree of reproducibility cannot be achieved in tests based only on visual assessment of reactions. This is the basis of a common misunderstanding on the expected performance of ELISA when conducted under varying field conditions. It is true nevertheless that some assays can give perfectly acceptable results in qualitative work when read by eye alone, in the favourable circumstances that negative serum reactions give uniformly very low results whilst all positive sera give reactions that are reliably intense; that is when the test has a combination of optimal specificity and sensitivity. A visual interpretation of the results can then offer equivalent diagnostic precision to that obtained by absorbance measurement and use of a standardized endpoint. However, even when all ELISA systems can be developed to a robustness, specificity and sensitivity that offers good visual results, there remains a need to maintain exactly standardized protocols in the conduct of the test.

7.3 Precision of assay measurements

Precision and sensitivity of an ELISA test are important linked considerations. The measurement of precision is based upon comparing results of replicate tests of the same sample either within a single assay (i.e. replicate wells of one plate) or between assays (i.e. on different plates, perhaps on different days). The ratio of the standard deviation of these replicates to their mean value defines a correlation coefficient (CV) which is high when replicates vary greatly and low when replicates vary little. A CV of 10% or less is acceptable for within-plate or between-plate precision. It is clear that sensitivity of a test, that is the level of a signal—in ELISA the colour intensity or absorbance value—that can be reliably distinguished from negative or background (noise) values, is dependent upon precision. This is because with low precision a wider range of weakly positive reactions will be undetectable from background. The use of replicate wells to determine precision is an essential component of quality control. The absolute sensitivity of an indirect (antibody) ELISA test, that is the point at which a sample antibody reaction can be interpreted as positive as opposed to borderline, is influenced also by the reactions of the reference antibody-negative control sera of each test. This is in terms both of the size of the reactions and of the variation between samples and replicates. If the negative control values are close to zero and the variation is small, the test will be intrinsically of greater sensitivity because more borderline test samples will then fall above the upper limit of the negative range. It is evident that great importance can be attached to the use of reference panels of positive and negative control samples in each assay on each occasion, as a quality control of both precision and sensitivity in ELISA tests.

7.4 Recording the results—methods of data presentation

ELISA tests can be performed for qualitative or quantitative analysis of test samples.

7.4.1 *Qualitative assays*

The aim is to define positive from negative with the minimum proportion of borderline cases. There is no universally accepted formula for interpreting and presenting data but the following are some useful suggestions.

(i) *For visual readings.* Plate assays with low negative control reactions are needed. These are then scored as negative or ± reactions and positives can be placed on a scale of 4+ to 1+. Borderline samples can be reassessed at lower dilution with the negative controls also readjusted.

(ii) *For colorimetric readings.*
(1)   Threshold level approach. This depends on determining the range of a large group of control negative samples (ideally reference samples, of healthy individuals, from the endemic region). In simplest form positive results are all those that exceed the upper (threshold) limit of the negative range. The threshold is better defined as 2 SD units above the mean of the negative group.
(2)   Absorbance ratio or positivity index approach. The OD reading of each test sample is calculated as a value (ratio) related to the mean of the negative control group. A ratio value (positivity index) above a certain figure, say twice the negative

mean, is regarded as positive. Sera can be graded by degree of positivity in this approach.

7.4.2 *Quantitative assays*

The aim is to define the extent of positivity of samples, that is the relative amount of antibody or antigen, compared with either control negative or positive values. In quantitative assays, where titres are being compared one with another, a high degree of precision in the assay is demanded and the approach needs to take this into account. Thus assays based upon endpoint titre which give a variation of a two-fold dilution in the result actually have a reproducibility of $\pm 100\%$. The better approaches relate exact OD readings to single positive or negative values or to the points of a standard dilution curve of a control positive titration. In all these cases the reactions are read from a continuous scale which is more or less linear, by most readers, from values of $0.20-2.5$. This gives better reproducibility. It is essential to work within the linear limits of reader efficiency and for this reason all assays should be stopped whilst the included positive reference reaction lies on the linear part of the scale.

(i) *Absorbance value approach.* Reference positive samples are included in the test and form the basis of comparison with test samples. Thus a value of (e.g.) 1.0 would be given to a sample equivalent in antibody or antigen to the positive control; those greater than 1.0 would be of higher titre, and less than 1.0 would be lower titre down to the value of the negative control.

(ii) *Endpoint titre approach.* Samples are serially diluted in the assay down to negative values. The titre is the last dilution which gives a reaction above that of the negative controls run over the same dilution series.

(iii) *Standard curve approach.* Reference positive samples (or standard antigen) are titrated and a standard dilution (dose−response) curve prepared. The titre of the test sample is read from the standard curve. In this system it is best to use more than one dilution and to choose the result that falls closest to the centre of the linear part of the standard curve to calculate the titre. Test samples in this form of analysis can be assigned antibody or antigen units by comparison with the standard curve, or assigned a percentage of the standard value.

(iv) *Comparison with normal value approach.* A ratio of absorbance value of the test sample to the mean of the negative sample group is calculated, as in the simple positivity index approach above. However, the ratio value is then expressed as a 'multiple of normal activity' or MONA value, by relation to a dose−response curve of a reference positive sample (11).

8. NOTES ON QUALITY CONTROL OF ELISA

8.1 Sources of error in ELISA

8.1.1 *Factors affecting sensitivity, precision and specificity of tests*

The success of any immunoassay in its task of identifying or measuring antibody or antigen is achieved by combining satisfactory levels of sensitivity, precision and

Table 12. Sources of error in indirect ELISA.

	Source of error
Low assay sensitivity	1. Choice of solid phase.
	2. Antigen concentration (e.g. over-coating).
	3. Use of low-titre conjugates.
	4. Use of substrates with poor solubility.
	5. Presence of enzyme inhibitors in buffers (e.g. azide or phosphates, for peroxidase and phosphatase enzymes, respectively).
	6. Inadequate mixing of highly diluted samples (e.g. serum and conjugates).
Poor assay specificity (high background)	1. Quality of antigen.
	2. Choice of solid phase.
	3. Extended incubation periods.
	4. Use of unpurified conjugates containing free enzyme.
Low assay precision	1. Volumetric pipetting errors, especially critical in serum dilutions.
	2. Inadequate incubation periods (i.e. below equilibrium level).
	3. Poor endpoint standardization (i.e. effect of reaction rate variables).
	4. Operator errors; particularly important in routine laboratory tests.

Reprinted from ref. 48. Copyright 1981. The Institute of Medical Laboratory Sciences.

specificity within the test. These features are all subject to error and the continued high performance of an assay depends upon understanding the possible sources of error and how to avoid them. McLaren *et al.* (48) have discussed the major sources of error in the indirect ELISA, and *Table 12* is a list taken from their paper. Many of these points have been dealt with in previous sections of this chapter. Error is not exclusive to indirect ELISA; it has similar importance in all forms of enzyme immunoassay.

8.1.2 *Handling of collected samples*

This is a neglected area and concerns the collection, preparation, handling, storage and distribution of reference and test samples. The following are major points to consider.

(i)   Collect blood under sterile conditions and place in sterile containers to harvest the serum.

(ii)   Divide all reference samples into small aliquots, label adequately and store at −20°C (or lower if possible). Avoid adding preservatives that might interfere with enzyme activity (e.g. azide with peroxidase).

(iii)   Store test serum samples also at −20°C. If they are to be used for successive studies they should also be aliquoted. Avoid repeated freezing and thawing of the same sample.

(iv)   Do not allow reference or test samples to stand at room temperature when removed from cold storage before use—after thawing, store temporarily at 4°C or, preferably, stand them in an ice bucket.

(v)   Whole blood spots can be prepared on filter paper. These should be air-dried (and preferably placed in a desiccator to complete drying), then sealed in polythene envelopes each with a sachet of silica crystals. This is a useful way of transporting large numbers of test samples; however, although IgG antibody is stable under these conditions and can be eluted quantitatively, this may not be the case with all classes of immunoglobulin, all other serum proteins, contained antigens and immune complexes. Filter papers should be stored at −20°C. Elution of blood spots can be standardized by using a suitably sized paper disc punch. Discs can then be soaked in a suitable buffer (e.g. coating buffer, PBS-T, according to the use of the sample), overnight at 4°C. The volume of blood, and its dilution after elution, can be calculated from the size of the disc and the absorptive capacity of the filter paper. Whatman No.1 filter paper is a suitable format.

8.2 Quality control within and between laboratories

8.2.1 *Internal quality control*

The minimum requirement for daily quality control of an ELISA test is the use of internal positive and negative reference samples to act as internal controls. These will ensure a check on the uniformity of performance (precision) of the test from day to day in the one laboratory. The means and standard deviations of these internal standards may be plotted on specially designed quality control charts, for example the Shewart Chart (55).

8.2.2 *External quality control*

To ensure that uniformity of a test exists between laboratories it is necessary (where this applies) to use external positive and negative reference reagents which can act as external standards; these allow the accurate calibration of local standards for regular internal use. Some of these, listed by WHO (56), can be obtained from International Laboratories for Biological Standards, but many more have to be prepared. A mutual exchange of coded samples is another possibility for comparing the results of ELISA tests between laboratories.

9. ACKNOWLEDGEMENTS

Some parts of this chapter were prepared originally as a bench manual by ourselves and V.Houba which was issued by the World Health Organization (ref. 57). We are grateful to the WHO for allowing this information to be published. We have also drawn from data supplied by Dr G.Thorpe of the Wolfson Clinical Chemistry Unit, Queen Elizabeth Medical Centre, Birmingham, UK, and we thank him particularly for helping us with enhanced chemiluminescence (*Figure 6*). We have also used data from the work of Dr A.Jassim and Dr Z.Demerdash produced while working in our laboratory. *Figure 8* is from a recent paper (ref. 52) in *Parasite Immunology* and we thank the publishers (Blackwell Scientific Publications) for allowing us to reproduce it here. We thank the Institute of Medical Laboratory Sciences and Blackwell Scientific Publications for permission to reproduce *Table 12* from ref. 48. Finally we give our special thanks to Mrs F.O'Reilly for preparation of the manuscript.

10. REFERENCES

1. Engvall,E. and Perlmann,P. (1971) *Immunochemistry*, **8**, 871.
2. Van Weeman,B.K. and Schuurs,A.H.W.M. (1971) *FEBS Lett.*, **15**, 232.
3. World Health Organization (1976) *Bull. WHO*, **54**, 129.
4. Voller,A., Bartlett,A. and Bidwell,D.E. (1976) *Trans. R. Soc. Trop. Med. Hyg.*, **70**, 98.

5. Voller,A., Bartlett,A. and Bidwell,D.E. (1978) *Scand. J. Immunol.,* **8** (Suppl. 7), 125.
6. Voller,A., Bidwell,D.E. and Bartlett,A. (1979) Dynatech Europe, Guernsey, England.
7. Voller,A. and De Savigny,D. (1981) *J. Immunol. Methods,* **46**, 1.
8. Ambroise-Thomas,P., Desgeorges,P.T. and Monget,D. (1978) *Bull. WHO,* **56**, 797.
9. Bidwell,D.E. and Voller,A. (1981) *Br. Med. J.,* **282**, 1747.
10. Faubert,G.M. and Hartmann,D.P. (1979) *Can. J. Pub. Health,* **70**, 58.
11. Funke,M., Felgner,P. and Geister,R. (1981) *Zentralbl. Bakteriol. Mikrobiol. Hyg. (A),* **251**, 126.
12. Hillyer,G.V. and Gomez de Rios,I. (1979) *Am. J. Trop. Med. Hyg.,* **28**, 237.
13. McLaren,M., Draper,C.C., Teesdale,C.H., Amin,M.A., Omer,A.H.S., Bartlett,A. and Voller,A. (1978) *Ann. Trop. Med. Parasit.,* **72**, 243.
14. Nakane,P.K. and Kawaoi,A. (1974) *J. Histochem. Cytochem.,* **22**, 1084.
15. Wilson,M.B. and Nakane,P.K. (1978) In *Immunofluorescence and Related Staining Techniques.* Knapp,W., Holubar,K. and Wick,G. (eds), Elsevier/North Holland, Amsterdam, p. 215.
16. Pain,D. and Surolia,A. (1981) *J. Immunol. Methods,* **40**, 219.
17. Nilsson,P., Bergquist,N.R. and Grundy,M.S. (1981) *J. Immunol. Methods,* **41**, 81.
18. Yoshitake,S., Yamade,Y., Ishizaka,E. and Masseyef,R. (1979) *Eur. J. Biochem.,* **101**, 395.
19. Imagawa,M., Yoshitake,S., Ishikawa,E., Endo,Y., Ohtaki,S., Kano,E. and Tsunetoshi,Y. (1981) *Clin. Chim. Acta,* **117**, 199.
20. Lehtonen,O.O. and Viljanen,M.K. (1980) *J. Immunol. Methods,* **36**, 63.
21. Bos,E.S., van der Doelen,A.A., van Roox,N. and Schuurs,A.H.W.M. (1981) *J. Immunoassay,* **2**, 187.
22. Chandler,H.M. and Hurrell,G.R. (1982) *Clin. Chim. Acta,* **121**, 1144.
23. Ghosh,D. and Borkar,P.S. (1961) *Hind. Antibiot. Bull.,* **3**, 85.
24. Geetha,P.B., Ghosh,S.N., Gupta,N.P., Borkar,P.S. and Ramachandran,S. (1978) *Hind. Antibiot. Bull.,* **21**, 11.
25. Guesdon,J.I., Ternynck,T. and Avrameas,S. (1979) *J. Histochem. Cytochem.,* **27**, 1131.
26. Hofman,K., Finn,F.M., Fries,H.J., Diaconescu,C. and Zahn,H. (1977) *Proc. Natl. Acad. Sci. USA,* **74**, 2697.
27. Beastall,G.H. (1985) *Lab. Pract.,* **May**, 74.
28. Self,C.J. (1985) *J. Immunol. Methods,* **76**, 389.
29. Stanley,C.J., Johannsson,A. and Self,C.H. (1985) *J. Immunol. Methods,* **83**, 89.
30. Kricka,L.J. (1985) *Clin. Biochem. Anal.,* **17**.
31. Edwards,J.C., Martin,J.K., Davidson,G.P., Holion,J. and Mashiter,K. (1986) *J. Bioluminesc. Chemiluminesc.,* **1**, 96.
32. Carter,T.J.N., Groucutt,C.J., Stott,R.A.W., Thorpe,G.H.G. and Whitehead,T.P. (1982) UK Patent Application 8206263.
33. Whitehead,T.P., Thorpe,G.H.G., Carter,T.J.N., Groucutt,G. and Kricka,L.J. (1983) *Nature,* **305**, 158.
34. Thorpe,G.H.G., Haggart,R., Kricka,L.J. and Whitehead,T.P. (1984) *Biochem. Biophys. Res. Commun.,* **119**, 41.
35. Thorpe,G.H.G., Williams,L.A., Kricka,L.J., Whitehead,T.P., Evans,H. and Stanworth,D.R. (1985) *J. Immunol. Methods,* **79**, 57.
36. Thorpe,G.H.G., Whitehead,T.P., Penn,R. and Kricka,L.J. (1984) *Clin. Chem.,* **30**, 806.
37. Thorpe,G.H.G., Stott,R.A.W., Sankolli,G.M., Catty,D., Raykundalia,C., Roda,A. and Kricka,L.J. (1987) In *Bioluminescence and Chemiluminescence, New Perspectives.* Scholmerich,J., Andreesen,R., Kapp,A., Ernst,M. and Woods,W.G. (eds), John Wiley & Sons, Chichester, p. 209.
38. Valkirs,G.E. and Barton,R. (1985) *Clin. Chem.,* **31**, 1427.
39. Pappas,M.G., Hajkowski,R. and Hockmeyer,W.T. (1983) *J. Immunol. Methods,* **64**, 205.
40. Hawkes,R., Niday,E. and Gordon,J. (1982) *Anal. Biochem.,* **119**, 142.
41. Pappas,M.G., Hajkowski,R., Cannon,L.T. and Hockmeyer,W.T. (1984) *Vet. Parasitol.,* **14**, 239.
42. Pappas,M.G., Ballon,W.R., Gray,M.R., Takafuji,E.T., Mutter,R. and Hockmeyer,W.T. (1985) *Am. J. Trop. Med. Hyg.,* **34**, 346.
43. Kumar,S., Bond,A.H., Samantarey,J.T., Dang,W. and Talwar,G.P. (1985) *J. Immunol. Methods,* **83**, 125.
44. Weeks,I., Sturgess,M., Brown,R.C. and Woodhead,J.S. (1986) In *Methods in Enzymology.* Kolowick,S.P. and Kaplan,N.O. (eds), Volume 133, p. 366.
45. Zuk,R.F., Ginsberg,V.K., Houts,T., Rabbie,J., Merrick,H., Ullman,E.F., Fischer,M., Sizto,C.C., Stiso,S.N. and Litman,D.J. (1985) *Clin. Chem.,* **31**, 1144.
46. Gray,B.M. (1979) *J. Immunol. Methods,* **28**, 187.
47. Ito,J.I., Wunderlich,A.C., Lyons,J., Davis,C.E., Guiney,D.G. and Braude,A.I. (1980) *J. Infect. Dis.,* **142**, 532.
48. McLaren,M.L., Lilleywhite,J.E. and Au,A.C.S. (1981) *Med. Lab. Sci.,* **38**, 245.
49. Rotmans,J.P. and Delwel,H.R. (1983) *J. Immunol. Methods,* **57**, 87.

153

50. Pant,C.P., Houba,V. and Engers,H.D. (1987) *Parasitol. Today, 3*, 324.
51. Jassim,A., Catty,D. and Hassan,K. (1987) *Parasite Immunol., 9*, 627.
52. Jassim,A., Hassan,K. and Catty,D. (1987) *Parasite Immunol., 9*, 651.
53. Hewitt,J., Coates,A.R.M., Mitchison,D.A. and Ivanyi,J. (1982) *J. Immunol. Methods, 55*, 204.
54. Ivanyi,J., Krambovits,E. and Keen,M. (1983) *Clin. Exp. Immunol., 54*, 337.
55. Batty,I. (1977) In *Techniques in Clinical Immunology.* Thompson,R.A. (ed.), Blackwell Scientific Publications, Oxford, Chapter 11, p. 219.
56. World Health Organization (1984) *Biological Substances; International Standards, Reference Preparations and Reference Reagents.* WHO, Geneva.
57. Catty,D., Raykundalia,C. and Houba,V. (1983) WHO IMM/PIR.83.1.

CHAPTER 5

Immunoperoxidase methods

E.L.JONES and J.GREGORY

1. INTRODUCTION

Although the introduction of the immunofluorescent technique in 1950 (1) was a major advance in immunohistochemistry, it was subsequently found that these techniques had a number of limitations. Firstly a fluorescence microscope has to be used to observe the results, and secondly when viewing fixed tissue sections the orientation of tissue constituents and background details are very difficult to visualize. Thirdly the final preparations are not permanent, although there are now available techniques which inhibit the fading of the fluorochrome dyes (see Chapter 6, Section 4.8). However, because of the simplicity of the techniques and the ability of the fluorescent markers to be seen clearly at very low concentrations they remain popular, particularly when viewing individual structures such as renal glomeruli and when using unfixed frozen sections when the background detail is relatively unimportant. Methods for immunofluorescence are discussed in Chapter 6.

In the search for an alternative label to overcome the above disadvantages some enzymes were found to be an ideal substitute, particularly horseradish peroxidase (2). Other enzymes were subsequently introduced, namely alkaline phosphatase and more recently glucose oxidase. These enzymes are used histochemically to produce intensely coloured permanent precipitates which may be viewed using conventional light microscopy. Most of these precipitates are insoluble, thus enabling permanent preparations to be made. In addition they may be rendered electron dense by osmication, thus enabling suitably prepared material to be viewed in an electron microscope.

It is mainly a historical rather than a practical fact that immunofluorescence is used on cryostat sections and immunoperoxidase techniques on paraffin sections. Both procedures, however, can be used on material prepared by either technique (3).

The main disadvantages with the immunoenzyme techniques are firstly that some of the methods require more steps than the fluorescent techniques to increase the sensitivity. For comparison the unlabelled antibody – enzyme methods require three steps instead of two for the immunofluorescent sequence. Moreover by increasing the number of steps in the technique there is a risk of inducing an increase in non-specific staining and a decrease in the 'signal-to-noise ratio'. Therefore it follows that it is preferable to choose a tissue preparation method which renders the tissue as reactive and as sensitive as possible. Secondly, it is necessary to block endogenous peroxidase when using horseradish peroxidase as a label. Thirdly the substrate most popularly used in the histochemical visualization technique of peroxidase is the chemical diamino-benzidine (DAB) which was initially thought to be carcinogenic; however, recent reports suggest that this is no longer true. There are available several different alternatives to this particular chemical but they produce alcohol-labile precipitates which require the use of aqueous mountants which may not always give satisfactory preparations.

2. APPLICATIONS

In our laboratory the main uses of immunoenzyme techniques are for the differential diagnosis of lymphomas and tumours. The demonstration of surface and/or cytoplasmic immunoglobulin is an important step in the diagnosis of B cell lymphomas which make up the majority of non-Hodgkin's lymphomas. The application of T cell subset antisera to cryostat sections of lymphomas is also of value in the elucidation of T cell tumours. In routine histopathological diagnosis these techniques of immunostaining are being increasingly used to refine diagnosis of difficult tumours. This is especially useful in the differential diagnosis of anaplastic tumours, such as distinguishing between an anaplastic carcinoma and a high-grade lymphoma. Further examples of the use of these techniques are the typing of specific hormone secretion in various endocrine tumours, the investigation of glomerulonephritis and the demonstration of the different types of intermediate filaments in sarcomas and central nervous system tumours. These methods have also been extensively used in the investigation of the structure and normal immune functions of the cells of the lymphoreticular system.

3. FIXATION AND PROCESSING FOR PARAFFIN SECTIONS

All tissues that are required for histopathological examination should be fixed in as life-like a manner as soon as possible. This will decrease the effects of autolysis. Morphology is of prime importance in the practice of ordinary light microscopy; however, with immunocytochemistry several additional factors such as the immobilization of antigen, antigenicity and access of antibodies to reaction sites are all important. It is somewhat unrealistic to expect to find one particular technique that achieves all these ends, so in practice a compromise has to be reached between the various limitations.

It is, for instance, much better from a morphological point of view to fix and then process tissues through to paraffin wax. Unfortunately the antigenicity of some antigens will not survive the rigorous processing schedules that are necessary. Even when some antigens do survive paraffin wax processing, different fixatives may be required to preserve maximum antigenicity. Therefore, quenching and cryostat sectioning becomes first choice. Generally speaking, for demonstrating extracellular and surface antigens, fresh frozen cryostat sections post-fixed with acetone should be used. For the demonstration of intracellular antigens, however, tissue fixation followed by paraffin processing is generally preferred.

3.1 **Fixative solutions**

There are several different effective fixatives available and no particular one is entirely suitable for all purposes. Experimentation is often needed to determine the best fixative for the antibodies being used. At all times the tissues should be handled as gently as possible to avoid crushing and diffusion of antigens. Tissue slices not more than 2 mm in thickness are made using a sharp blade, preferably a de-greased razor blade. It is important to ensure that there is precise identification of the specimen by suitable labelling

Table 1. Formal − saline fixative.

1. Formalin	100 ml
2. Sodium chloride	8.5 g
3. Tap water	900 ml

Table 2. Formal − acetic fixative.

1. Formalin	100 ml
2. Tap water	900 ml
3. Acid sodium phosphate, monohydrate ($NaH_2PO_4.H_2O$)	4 g
4. Anhydrous disodium phosphate (Na_2HPO_4)	6.5 g
To the above solution add 5% glacial acetic acid.	

and that each piece of tissue is placed in at least 20 times its own volume of fixative.

3.1.1 *10% Formal − saline*

The composition of 10% formal − saline is given in *Table 1*.

Using formal − saline-fixed paraffin-processed sections, Taylor and Burns in 1974 (4) demonstrated immunoglobulin in plasma cells. This important discovery meant that retrospective studies could be carried out on blocks of tissue stored for many years. These earlier results, however, were fairly inconsistent and unpredictable. Various factors such as the consistency of the fixed tissue and whether the tissue had been left whole or sliced will affect the results obtained. Lymph nodes, for example, if left whole and then placed in fixative will show a marked fixation artefact, well-fixed tissue will be seen around the perimeter of the tissue with a poorly-fixed area centrally. When stained, the cells in the well-fixed area will be sharply demonstrated in a clear background while the cells in the poorly-fixed central areas will be poorly localized due to a marked degree of diffusion.

Positive staining of antigen may be effectively achieved with this fixative but the technique may have to be preceded by an unmasking process discussed later in Section 6. For example, immunoglobulins within plasma cells can be seen as a positively stained area next to the nucleus in only a relatively small number of cells. Following unmasking, many more positive cells are seen and the staining is observed throughout the cytoplasm. Formal − saline is a good general fixative and will immobilize and preserve the antigenicity of many antigens, some of which may require the unmasking procedure and some may not. The tissue is not rendered brittle if left in the fixative solution for a long period, adequate fixation occurring for thin blocks after 24 − 48 h.

3.1.2 *5% Formal − acetic*

The composition of 5% formal − acetic is given in *Table 2*.

5% formal − acetic is our fixative of choice in the demonstration of intracellular immunoglobulin (5). It is recommended that tissue slices should be fixed for a minimum of 48 h followed directly by dehydration. The main advantage with this fixative is that the masking of antigens that occurs by inter- and intra-molecular cross-linking in tissue fixed with aldehyde fixatives appears not to happen and therefore the unmasking technique is not required. The other advantage with this fixative is that the primary

Table 3. Formal – sublimate fixative.

1.	Saturated aqueous mercuric chloride	900 ml
2.	Formalin	100 ml

Table 4. Bouin's fluid fixative.

1.	Saturated aqueous picric acid	75 ml
2.	Formalin	25 ml
3.	Acetic acid	5 ml

antibodies can be diluted up to 10-fold compared with that required for formal – saline fixation.

3.1.3 *Formal – sublimate*

The composition of formal – sublimate is given in *Table 3*.

Formal – sublimate is another commonly used routine compound fixative. It is a combination of formalin and mercuric chloride, the latter being a powerful protein precipitant.

Its use was first suggested for the demonstration of immunoglobulin (Ig) in tissue sections in 1977 (6). Two significant disadvantages are, firstly, the formation of mercury pigment which needs to be removed before staining and secondly, mercuric chloride is so corrosive that containers with metal lids should be avoided. Its main advantage, however, over formal – saline, it is claimed, is that it does not create masking, although in our experience a certain amount of masking does occur (unpublished results).

The method that we recommend for the removal of the mercuric chloride crystals is as follows. This should be carried out immediately prior to the immunoperoxidase technique.

(i)   De-paraffinize the sample and wash in absolute alcohol.
(ii)   Treat sections with 0.5% iodine in 70% alcohol for 3 – 5 min.
(iii) Rinse in tap water.
(iv)   Treat with 2.5% sodium thiosulphate (hypo) until colourless, ~ 1 min.
(v)   Wash in tap water for 2 min.
(vi)   Proceed with immunoperoxidase staining.

3.1.4 *Bouin's fluid*

The composition of Bouin's fluid is given in *Table 4*.

This fixative contains formaldehyde, acetic acid and picric acid. The picric acid precipitates protein, forms picrates and produces intermolecular salt links. It is probably the inclusion of acetic acid in this fixative which preserves the antigenicity without masking. Our results show that the reaction product is sharply localized and background staining is minimal.

For a comprehensive review of the effects of fixation in tissue sections see Curran and Gregory (5).

Since fixation is probably the most important step in the preparation of tissues for

Table 5. Manual processing schedule.

1. Fixation
2. Incubation in 70% alcohol for 2 h
3. Incubation in 90% alcohol for 2 h
4. Incubation in absolute alcohol twice for 2 h
5. Incubation in chloroform overnight for 16 h
6. Incubation in paraffin wax twice for 3 h
7. Embed in fresh wax, and cool

immunohistochemistry, time and care must be taken in selecting the best one. Ideally the fixative chosen should allow for the highest dilution of primary antibody to be used, for the least number of stages required to give a good positive result and for the demonstration of antigen without unmasking.

3.2 Processing and sectioning

The tissue specimens may be processed through to paraffin wax either by hand in their individual containers or along with others in an automatic processing machine. This process involves dehydration and clearing, prior to embedding in paraffin wax.

3.2.1 *Dehydration*

Paraffin wax will not penetrate tissues in the presence of water so dehydration is an essential initial process. This is achieved by immersion of the tissues in ethyl alcohol. A 70% solution is optimum initially rather than using absolute alcohol, to try and reduce any distortion which might occur. Some distortion will inevitably occur, however, in all tissues subjected to paraffin processing. For details of tissue dehydration and manual processing schedules see *Table 5*.

3.2.2 *Clearing*

As alcohol is not miscible with wax, after dehydration it is necessary to treat tissue blocks with a reagent that mixes with both substances and which may in turn be eliminated in the process of wax impregnation. This step has traditionally come to be known as clearing because most of these reagents alter the refractive index of the tissues and render them almost transparent. As with fixation there are a number of alternatives. Xylene and chloroform are the most popular clearing agents used. It would seem from our experience that xylene is the most severe in action and will, after comparatively short exposures, further reduce the antigenicity of the tissue (unpublished results). Chloroform, however, even though it is considerably slower in its action than xylene, has little hardening effect on the tissue and better preserves antigenicity.

3.2.3 *Wax impregnation*

The hardness of the paraffin wax when set will be dependent on its melting point. Therefore the choice of wax will be dependent on the average temperature of the working area. It would prove very difficult for example to cut $3-5$ μm sections from wax with a 45°C melting point in a hot climate. In Great Britain wax with a melting point of $54-56$°C is suitable for most tissues. The wax should be melted by an electrically heated oven and not by a gas flame for safety reasons. The wax impregnation should remove the clearing agent and completely permeate the tissues. When cooled the wax will harden throughout to enable sections to be cut. Care should be taken not to heat the wax over 60°C, as this could cause polymerization of any plastic additives commonly found in paraffin wax which would then be difficult to remove from the section.

Good quality sections will only be produced by thoroughly impregnated tissues. Tissues that are under-impregnated will not cut easily and will almost certainly be washed off the glass slide during the immunoperoxidase techniques.

Although a certain amount of shrinkage and hardening will take place, the demonstration of intracellular and surface Ig can be achieved successfully after the tissues have been left in paraffin wax for a week at 56°C.

3.2.4 *Sectioning*

(i)   Cut sections at 3 μm (approximate thickness). They should be cut with a sharp knife as any pulling or ripping in the sections will produce a non-specific staining reaction. Disposable microtome blades are recommended.

(ii)   Mount the floating sections onto de-greased (by alcohol) glass slides from water heated to just below the melting point of the wax.

(iii) Heat the mounted sections to 60°C for 30−60 min to allow them to dry onto the glass.

If the tissue has been optimally processed and the glass slides are thoroughly cleaned there should be no problem with sections washing off. If this is found to be a problem there are several slide adhesive solutions commercially available. However, it should be noted that if these are used they can alter the concentration of primary antibody needed.

3.2.5 *De-paraffinization and rehydration procedure*

To ensure that all of the embedding medium is removed before staining, the slides should be heated to 60°C in the oven and then put straight into a bath of xylene. No longer than 60 sec should be required for this stage as overexposure to xylene will reduce antigenicity. In practise it is recommended that no more than 50 slides should be run through a 250 ml bath of xylene.

(i)   Place sections into a bath of xylene with intermittent agitation for 1−2 min.

(ii)   Remove from xylene and rinse with absolute alcohol from a wash bottle and place into a bath of absolute alcohol for 1 min with intermittent agitation.

(iii) Place into a bath of gently running water.

(iv)   Begin immunoperoxidase staining.

4. CRYOSTAT SECTIONS

It has been mentioned already that some cell surface antigens are destroyed by fixation and paraffin processing. To avoid this, the tissue can be rapidly frozen and sectioned in a cryostat, followed by brief fixation. Fixation is usually in acetone but other fixatives may be used; this depends on the nature of the antigen to be demonstrated.

4.1 **Quenching**

Specimens should be small in size, ideally about 1 cm square and 2−3 mm in thickness. The tissue should be wrapped in aluminium foil to enhance the cooling procedure and prevent desiccation, and then placed into liquid nitrogen or an ethanol/dry ice mixture. For speed and convenience in our laboratory the specimen is simply placed into a vacuum flask containing liquid nitrogen and held beneath the surface using forceps for around 20 sec or until the boiling has stopped. The specimen is then removed and may be stored in a small sealed plastic tube for long periods in a freezer at −70°C.

4.2 **Sectioning**

Frozen sections are cut in a cryostat usually set around −20°C. Modern cryostats have an independent setting for the chuck holder, which should be set lower than the temperature of the cryostat.

The frozen tissue is secured to a chuck in the cryostat by a commercially available freezing compound (e.g. Cryo-M-Bed, Bright Instrument Co. Ltd) and mounted on the chuck holder. Sections are cut at approximately 6 μm. The sections are picked up from the knife by placing a slide at room temperature close to the section. The slide should approach the tissue quite quickly so that the section 'jumps' across on to the slide and does not 'roll' across. If this procedure is not carried out as described it may affect the staining performance of the sections.

4.3 **Fixation**

The sections should be allowed to dry at room temperature for at least 30 min. At this stage sections may be put into acetone at room temperature for 5 sec and then wrapped in aluminium foil or cling film and stored in the freezer until ready for staining. For optimum results, however, cryo-sectioning should be done immediately before the staining procedure.

(i)   Allow the sections to dry at room temperature for 45 min.
(ii)   Place the sections in acetone at room temperature for 10 min.
(iii)   Remove the slides and allow them to stand at room temperature for 5 min.
(iv)   Continue with the first stage of the immunoperoxidase procedure.

Endogenous peroxidase activity is not blocked when using frozen sections because of the fixing effect that methanol would have on the sections. A negative control should be put through at the same time to demonstrate any endogenous peroxidase which may be present in the tissues.

5. SMEARS

Ideally it is best to make smears of one cell thickness, since problems may arise from reagents trapped between layers. Cyto-centrifuge preparations provide the best material. For the demonstration of cell surface antigens, fix with acetone for 10 min at room temperature, and for intracellular antigens use 10% formal−saline overnight. Blood smears should be placed straight into a mixture of methanol/H_2O_2 to fix at the same time as blocking the endogenous peroxidase. Fixed smears are stable at room temperature for a few days, or, if stored at −20°C, for several months.

6. EXPOSURE OF HIDDEN ANTIGEN

There are some tissue antigens that need to be unmasked by enzyme treatment before optimum immunoperoxidase staining can take place. The most common of the proteolytic enzymes used for unmasking antigens is trypsin (7). Trypsin is the least destructive to the tissue and its reaction can be easily controlled. Other enzymes commonly used are protease and pepsin.

6.1 Trypsin

The trypsin solution is prepared as follows.

(i)   Dissolve 0.1% trypsin and 0.1% calcium chloride in Tris−saline buffer at pH 7.8.

(ii)   Pre-heat the solution to 37°C and place it in a suitably sized beaker in a 37°C incubator on a magnetic stirrer (*Figure 1*).

(iii) Place the rehydrated sections vertically in a rack as shown, suspended in the solution for 30 min and gently stirred.

The time required for optimum digestion must be obtained by prior trial and error and 30 min seems to be optimal for tissues routinely fixed in our department. This incubation time, however, will vary according to the size of the tissue block being fixed, and the length of time that the tissues have been placed in the fixatives.

Over-digestion with proteolytic enzymes will damage the tissue morphology and even

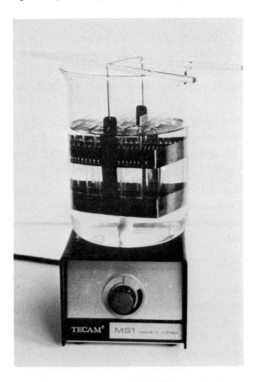

Figure 1. Mounted tissue sections suspended in trypsin solution.

cause loosening of the section from the slide. If an adhesive has to be used to attach the section to the glass slide a resistant one like chrome alum gelatin should be used.

In our experience the trypsin of choice is Difco 1:250. Some less pure trypsin preparations have failed to work effectively. To obtain the optimum incubation time a series of sections should be set up as follows.

(i)   No trypsin-buffer.
(ii)   10 min.
(iii)   20 min.
(iv)   30 min.
(v)   1 h.

If the digestion is not complete at 1 h then it is advisable to increase the strength of the trypsin probably to 1.0%, and repeat at the same times as before.

Trypsin digestion is not required for the demonstration of all antigens following aldehyde fixation. So the above test should be run not only for individual tissue specimens but also for each antigen that is to be demonstrated. Sometimes the denaturation and masking of the fixation process may be compensated for by increasing the concentration of the primary antibody or greatly increasing the incubation time. Sensitivity is also improved when using the peroxidase−anti-peroxidase (PAP) method instead of a direct or indirect immunoperoxidase technique. However, when these steps are taken they are likely to lead towards higher background staining.

6.2 Protease (Sigma: Type XXIV)

This is a more powerful enzyme than trypsin and is sometimes useful when trypsin has failed. It is best used as a 0.05% solution in Tris buffer, pH 7.4 for 30−60 min at 37°C. Once again experimentation is required to discover the optimum concentration and time. To demonstrate Ig in glomerular membranes (8) we use different concentrations of protease and exposure times depending on how the tissue is fixed. Following complete fixation in formal−saline it is usual to expose 2 μm paraffin sections of needle biopsies to 0.5% protease for 1 h at 37°C immediately preceding the immunoperoxidase technique. If, however, rapid fixation using heat has been employed then the concentration and exposure time of protease is decreased to 0.05−0.1% for 30 min at 37°C.

7. BLOCKING OF ENDOGENOUS PEROXIDASE

Before using horseradish peroxidase as the antibody label it is necessary first to inhibit or block any endogenous peroxidase present in the tissue sections because the substrate−chromagen reaction used to visualize peroxidase cannot distinguish between the extrinsic peroxidase label and the endogenous tissue peroxidase.

There are several ways of achieving irreversible blocking of endogenous peroxidase. The most popular method is to use a mixture of H_2O_2 and methanol.

(i)   Apply 1% of 100 vols of H_2O_2 in methanol for 10 min at room temperature.
(ii) Thoroughly wash the slide in water for 5 min.
(iii) Begin immunoperoxidase staining.

Other techniques that have proved useful include application of 2% HCl in methanol for 30 min. Absolute methanol with 1% sodium nitroferrocyanide and 0.2% acetic acid can also be used. Another effective technique is to incubate with 2.0% periodic acid for 10 min. This should be followed by a solution of 0.1 mg of sodium borohydride/1 ml of water for 10 min to reduce any aldehydes produced.

Alkaline phosphatase may also be used as a label and in this case endogenous peroxidase would not be a problem and blocking would not be required. There is however a small amount of endogenous alkaline phosphatase activity in some tissues which should be blocked using levamisole (9).

Another enzyme label now being used more often is glucose oxidase (10). This has the theoretical advantage over both of the previous labels that no known endogenous enzyme activity exists in mammalian tissues.

8. NON-SPECIFIC BACKGROUND STAINING

Non-specific background staining is seen as positive staining in tissue sections at sites other than where the specific antigen – antibody binding should have occurred. Usually it is paler than the specific reaction and the most common site is on highly charged collagen and connective tissues. It occurs when the molecules of the primary (antigen-specific) antibody non-specifically attach themselves to these highly-charged sites. When the labelled (antiglobulin) antibody is then added, binding takes place to primary antibody at all locations and non-specific staining occurs. It is possible however to reduce this background staining by the use of a combination of non-immune serum and determined optimally diluted antibodies. The non-immune serum should be from the same animal species that produced the second antibody. Thus, non-immune swine serum would be used with a three stage PAP sequence using rabbit anti-human antiserum (first stage), swine anti-rabbit antiserum (second stage) and rabbit PAP (third stage). The non-immune serum blocks background staining of the sections when added immediately prior to the primary antibody because the constituent proteins occupy all the highly charged non-specific sites, leaving available only the specific antigen sites for binding to the primary antibody. This serum is used at dilutions between 1:3 and 1:20. The optimum blocking dilution must be found because this determines the optimum dilution of the primary antibody. If the primary antibody is weak then non-immune serum should be omitted. Having incubated the non-immune serum on the tissue section for 10 min it should be carefully tipped off, leaving a film over the whole of the section. Care must be taken not to leave too much on the slide as this will cause dilution of the primary antibody, which is added to the sections by means of a Pasteur pipette, taking care not to drop directly onto the sections as this may cause them to wash off. The alternative to using a non-immune serum is to dilute all antibodies with buffer containing 2−5% bovine serum albumin (BSA).

Non-specific staining will also occur if the primary antibody used is too concentrated. This means that it is very important to test new antibodies with new tissues to achieve the optimum dilution.

When using monoclonal antibodies the use of non-immune serum is not required. If these antibodies are used at their optimal dilutions then there should be very little non-specific staining.

9. STAINING METHODS

There are several different staining methods available which may be discussed under the general heading of immunoenzyme techniques. These include the direct, indirect, unlabelled antibody – enzyme bridge techniques (single and double) and PAP techniques. All these techniques may be labelled with different enzymes such as peroxidase, alkaline phosphatase and glucose oxidase. In addition there are the avidin and biotin techniques.

9.1 Pre-treatment of sections

Unmasking and blocking procedure for paraffin sections.

(i)   De-wax 3 μm paraffin sections in xylene and rehydrate through alcohol to water.

(ii) Place the sections in trypsin solution at 37°C for required time (see Section 6.1).

(iii) Wash the sections in running water for 5 min.

(iv) Place the sections in endogenous peroxidase blocking solution of choice (see Section 7).

(v)   Wash the sections in running water.

(vi) Continue with the immunoperoxidase technique of choice.

9.2 Immunoperoxidase techniques

Peroxidase is the popular enzyme label of choice because it is easily and comparatively cheaply obtainable in a highly purified form. It is very stable during storage and application, and may be visualized with a wide choice of chromagens. It is also suitable for use with electron microscopy, being made electron dense following osmication.

An enzyme of similar value to peroxidase is alkaline phosphatase. This enzyme is generally employed in double enzyme techniques in conjunction with peroxidase. It is again inexpensive, and gives strong labelling with several different substrates. These two enzyme labels are still universally employed and there seems little reason at present for changing.

All incubations of antisera are carried out at room temperature in a wet chamber mounted on a rocking tray which ensures a movement of antiserum over the whole of the section, as in *Figure 2*.

9.2.1 Direct method

The sections are pre-treated as necessary followed by application of a labelled primary antibody which, when developed, identifies the antigen site. This technique is not often used in immunoenzyme techniques, the main disadvantage being that for each antigen to be localized a differently conjugated antibody is needed.

Proceed as follows.

(i)   Pre-treat the sections as described in Section 9.1.

(ii) Wash the sections in a buffer bath for 5 min.

(iii) Apply normal serum dilution 1:3 for 10 min (if required).

(iv) Tip off the excess serum and do not wash.

(v)   Apply enzyme-conjugated antibody, optimally diluted, for 45 min minimum.

(vi) Gently rinse with buffer from a wash bottle.

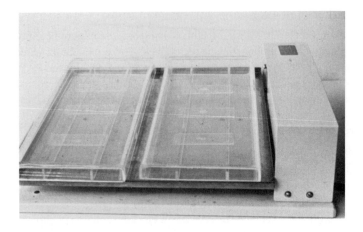

Figure 2. Mounted tissue sections incubating at room temperature on a rocking tray.

(vii)   Place the slide in the buffer bath for 10 min.
(viii) Carry out the visualization procedure.
(ix)   Counterstain and mount.

9.2.2 *Indirect technique*

After initial pre-treatment of sections, use unlabelled antibody to bind to the antigen in the section. After washing off excess antibody with buffer a second enzyme-conjugated antibody is applied from another species to bind to the first antibody to show specific antigenic sites in the section. The advantages over the direct technique are as follows.

(i)   Providing that all the primary antibodies are raised in the same species, one labelled antibody may be used as the second layer to locate any number of antigens without the need to label individually each primary antibody.
(ii)   The antigen will be more intensely labelled by this technique since the primary antibody will bind several molecules of the second antibody; therefore more molecules of peroxidase are available for the visualization of the antigenic site.
(iii)   Because of the increased sensitivity, higher dilutions of the primary antibody can be used.

There are two main disadvantages with this method.

(i)   It takes twice as long as the direct technique.
(ii)   It is liable to more non-specific reactions.

Proceed as follows.

(i)   Pre-treat the sections as described in Section 9.1.
(ii)   Wash in a buffer bath for 5 min.
(iii)   Apply normal serum dilution 1:5 for 10 min (if required).
(iv)   Tip off the excess serum and do not wash.
(v)   Apply the primary antibody, optimally diluted, for 45 min.
(vi)   Rinse gently with buffer from a wash bottle.

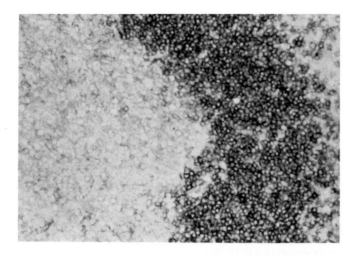

Figure 3. Indirect technique on an acetone-fixed cryostat section reacted for IgD, demonstrating surface immunoglobulin on lymphocytes of mantle zone of lymphoid follicle in a reactive node. ×173.

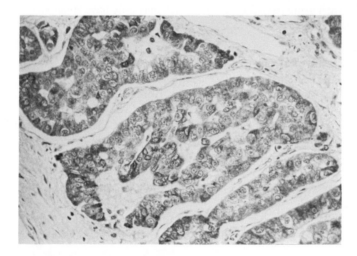

Figure 4. Indirect technique on a paraffin-processed section of an infiltrating ductal carcinoma of breast reacted for monoclonal epithelial membrane antigen. ×173.

(vii)   Wash in the buffer bath for 10 min.
(viii) Apply enzyme-conjugated second antibody, optimally diluted, for 45 min.
(ix)   Rinse gently with buffer from a wash bottle.
(x)   Wash in a buffer bath for 10 min.
(xi)   Carry out the visualization procedure.
(xii)   Counterstain and mount.

Examples of section staining by the indirect technique on an acetone-fixed cryostat section and on a paraffin-processed section are shown in *Figures 3* and *4*.

9.2.3 *Unlabelled antibody–enzyme bridge methods*

(i) *Single bridge*. This involves using a primary antibody followed by an unconjugated second antibody in excess, which is then followed by an antibody against peroxidase produced in the same species as the first antibody which binds to free combining sites of the second antibody (11). This is followed with peroxidase which is then visualized.

(ii) *Double bridge*. This technique is the same as above but the second and third layer sequence is repeated thus building up the number of available peroxidase reaction sites (12).

(iii) *Peroxidase–anti-peroxidase*. This modification of the bridge technique conjugates the peroxidase and anti-peroxidase together *in vitro* before reacting. After removal of excess peroxidase and antibody, a reagent containing stable cyclic formations of three peroxidase molecules to two antibody molecules is left. When this is substituted for the third layer in the bridge technique a much more sensitive technique is achieved and theoretically should minimize background staining.

With the introduction of a third stage antibody the technique again increases in length compared with the direct and indirect techniques and does in fact give rise to more background staining problems. The improved sensitivity, however, is advantageous, especially when using paraffin sections which may only have small amounts of antigen left after processing.

Proceed as follows.

(i)   Pre-treat the sections as described in Section 9.1.
(ii)   Wash the sections in a buffer bath for 5 min.
(iii)   Apply normal serum dilution 1:5 for 10 min (if required).
(iv)   Tip off the excess serum.
(v)   Apply primary antibody, optimally diluted, for 45 min (minimum).
(vi)   Gently rinse with buffer from a wash bottle.
(vii)   Wash the sections in a buffer bath for 10 min.

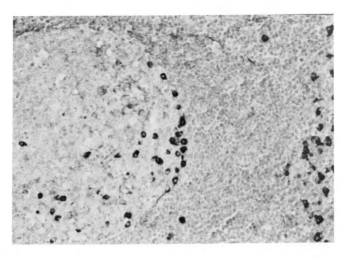

Figure 5. PAP technique on a paraffin-processed section reacted for *x* light chain, demonstrating cytoplasmic immunoglobulin in plasma cells in a reactive node. ×275.

(viii) Apply secondary antibody, optimally diluted, for 45 min.
(ix)   Gently rinse the sections.
(x)   Wash the sections in a buffer bath for 10 min.
(xi)   Apply PAP complex for 45 min.
(xii)   Gently rise the sections.
(xiii) Wash in a buffer bath for 10 min.
(xiv)   Carry out the visualization procedure.
(xv)   Counterstain and mount.

An example of a section stained by the PAP technique is shown in *Figure 5*.

9.3 Avidin—biotin techniques

When this technique was first introduced it was claimed to be superior to the PAP technique in sensitivity. The principle of the method is that the large glycoprotein molecule avidin, obtained from egg-white, binds with great affinity to molecules of the vitamin biotin. As with the PAP sequence, three stages are required. The first stage involves the specific primary antibody. This is followed by a second stage using a biotinylated antibody to react to the primary antibody. The third stage is the reaction of a complex of peroxidase-conjugated biotin and avidin, using the free sites on the avidin molecule to bind with the second antibody. These stages are followed by a visualization technique for the peroxidase to detect the antigenic sites in the tissue. Many molecules of peroxidase are able to bind to the second antibody molecule and hence to the tissue antigen.

One major disadvantage of the technique is the unwanted binding of avidin to endogenous biotin in the section. This is reduced by a technique of blocking the tissue sites by exposing them to unconjugated avidin and then unlabelled biotin (13).

Proceed as follows.

(i)   Pre-treat the sections as described in Section 9.1.
(ii)   Wash the sections in a buffer bath for 5 min.
(iii)   Apply primary antibody, optimally diluted, for 45 min.
(iv)   Rinse gently with buffer from a wash bottle.
(v)   Wash the sections in a buffer bath for 10 min.
(vi)   Apply biotinylated second antibody, optimally diluted, for 45 min.
(vii)   Gently rinse the sections.
(viii) Wash the sections in a buffer bath for 10 min.
(ix)   Apply peroxidase-conjugated biotin—avidin complex for 45 min.
(x)   Gently rinse the sections.
(xi)   Wash the sections in a buffer bath for 10 min.
(xii)   Apply substrate solution to give a coloured end-product.
(xiii) Counterstain and mount.

9.4 Alkaline phosphatase—anti-alkaline phosphatase technique (APAAP)

The APAAP technique has been introduced recently as a more sensitive technique when antigens have failed to be demonstrated by the indirect technique. APAAP consists of soluble complexes of alkaline phosphatase and mouse monoclonal anti-alkaline

phosphatase, thus delivering more molecules of label per molecule of antigen (14).
The APAAP technique is as follows.

(i)   Pre-treat the sections as described in Section 9.1.
(ii)   Wash the sections in a buffer bath for 5 min.
(iii)   Apply normal serum dilution 1:5 for 10 min (if required).
(iv)   Tip off the excess serum and do not wash.
(v)   Apply mouse primary antiserum, optimally diluted, for 45 min.
(vi)   Gently rinse with buffer from a wash bottle.
(vii)   Wash the sections in a buffer bath for 10 min.
(viii) Apply the second antiserum (rabbit anti-mouse Ig), optimally diluted, for 45 min.
(ix)   Gently rinse with buffer from a wash bottle.
(x)   Wash the sections in a buffer bath for 10 min.
(xi)   Apply mouse APAAP, optimally diluted, for 45 min.
(xii)   Gently rinse the sections.
(xiii) Wash the sections in a buffer bath for 10 min.
(xiv)   Carry out the visualization procedure for alkaline phosphatase.
(xv)   Counterstain and mount.

9.5 Buffers

During the staining procedures the buffer solution is used both to rinse and wash slides
and as the diluent for the antisera. The buffer generally used in our laboratory is Tris—
HCl/saline, pH 7.6. The addition of physiological saline to the buffer solution gives
it a higher salt concentration, thus effectively reducing non-specific background staining.
Another very commonly used buffer is phosphate-buffered saline (PBS, pH 7.2). This
has the advantage that it can be made up in large quantities and will remain at a constant
pH whereas the Tris buffer needs to be made up in smaller quantities for daily use.

Both of these buffers may be bought commercially. It is important to note, however,
that some manufacturers add sodium azide to the buffer formulation as an anti-bacterial
agent and this will inhibit the binding of peroxidase to the substrate in the visualization
procedure.

Ten-litre stock solutions of 0.2 M Tris, 0.1 M HCl and saline are stored in the
laboratory.

9.5.1 Stock solutions

(i)   0.2 M Tris. Dissolve 24.23 g of Tris in 1 litre of distilled water.
(ii)   0.1 M HCl. 8.5 ml of concentrated HCl in 1 litre of distilled water.
(iii)   Physiological saline. 8.5−9.0 g of NaCl in 1 litre of distilled water.

The stock solutions are mixed as follows.

Tris−HCl/saline buffer, pH 7.8, (for trypsinization) to make 600 ml.

(i)   150 ml of Tris.
(ii)   195 ml of HCl.
(iii)   255 ml of saline.

Tris−HCl/saline, pH 7.6, for use as diluent and for washing, to make 400 ml.

(i)   100 ml of Tris.
(ii)   150 ml of HCl.
(iii)   150 ml of saline.

  PBS 0.01 M, pH 7.2.

  Dissolve the following in 10 litres of distilled water.

(i)   Dibasic sodium phosphate, anhydrous (Na_2HPO_4)   14.8 g
(ii)   Monobasic potassium phosphate, anhydrous (KH_2PO_4)   4.3 g
(iii)   NaCl   72 g

This may be stored at room temperature.

9.6 Substrate solutions for peroxidase visualization

The coloured end product is formed at the site of enzyme activity and should not be soluble. This is achieved by the enzyme horseradish peroxidase (HRP) forming a complex with H_2O_2 together with an electron donor, forming an insoluble coloured end product, and water. The advantage of using this method is that the enzyme molecule is not depleted in the reaction and one molecule of enzyme may form many molecules of product.

$$HRP + H_2O_2 > HRP{\cdot}H_2O_2 > HRP{\cdot}H_2O_2 + \text{electron donor} >$$
$$\text{insoluble product} + H_2O + HRP$$

9.6.1 *3,3-Diaminobenzidine tetrahydrochloride* (11)

This electron donor is widely used and produces a dark-brown insoluble product. When used correctly it will give very clear and precise product formation. Its main disadvantage is that it could be a possible carcinogen.

  A stock solution may be made and aliquoted into 10 ml portions and stored at $-20°C$. Dissolve 60 mg of DAB in 100 ml of 0.05 M Tris buffer, pH 7.6.

  Proceed as follows.

(i)   Immediately before use thaw a portion of this solution and add 0.1 ml of 3% hydrogen peroxide.
(ii)   Cover the sections and incubate for 5–10 min at room temperature.
(iii)   Rinse off with running water.

  It is possible to microscopically observe and control the product formation but this is not recommended in view of the possible carcinogenicity. Always handle DAB with caution; any spills may be neutralized with bleach (sodium hypochlorite).

  There are a number of suggested alternatives to DAB.

9.6.2 *3-Amino-9-ethylcarbazole*

Stock solution (stable at room temperature): 0.4% 3-amino-9-ethylcarbazole (AEC) in dimethylformamide.

Working solution:

(i)   0.5 ml of stock solution;
(ii)   9.5 ml of 0.05 M acetate buffer pH 5.0;
(iii)   0.15 ml of 3% H_2O_2.

Filter on to the sections, and incubate at room temperature for 5−10 min. Mount the sections using an aqueous mounting medium.

9.6.3 *4-Chloro-1-naphthol*

(i)   Dissolve 3 mg of 4-chloro-1-naphthol in 0.1 ml of absolute ethanol.
(ii)   While stirring add this to 10 ml of 0.05 M Tris buffer, pH 7.6.
(iii)   Add 0.1 ml of 3% H_2O_2.
(iv)   Filter out the white precipitate before use.
(v)   Incubate the sections for 30 min at room temperature.
(vi)   Mount the sections using an aqueous mounting medium.

9.6.4 *p-Phenylenediamine dihydrochloride/pyrochatechol (Hanker−Yates)*

(i)   Mix 5 mg of *p*-phenylenediamine dihydrochloride with 10 mg of pyrochatechol.
(ii)   Dissolve the mixture in 10 ml of 0.05 M Tris buffer, pH 7.6.
(iii)   Add 1 ml of 3% H_2O_2.
(iv)   Incubate the sections at room temperature for approximately 15 min.
(v)   Sections may be mounted in DPX or Canada balsam.

In our experience these alternatives have proved to be less satisfactory in our laboratory than DAB since, with the exception of Hanker−Yates solution, they all produce alcohol-soluble end-products thus necessitating the use of water-based mounting media. Hanker−Yates solution, however, deteriorates on storage and is very capricious in its action.

9.7 Substrate solutions for alkaline phosphatase visualization

A coloured reaction product is formed by alkaline phosphatase as follows. The enzyme releases a 'coupler' from the substrate and this combines with a diazonium salt present in the incubating medium to form a coloured azo-dye.

There are two simple visualization techniques commonly used, one producing a blue colour which is useful in double labelling techniques as a contrast to the brown colour of the peroxidase−DAB reaction, and the other a red product which gives an excellent contrast with haematoxylin.

9.7.1 *Naphthol AS-MX and fast blue*

Dissolve 2 mg of naphthol AS-MX phosphate in 0.2 ml of dimethylformamide in a glass tube. Add 9.8 ml of 0.1 M Tris, pH 8.2.

This may be stored for several weeks at 4°C.

Proceed as follows.

(i)   Immediately before staining dissolve Fast Blue BB salt at 1 mg/ml in naphthol AS-MX phosphate buffer.

(ii)   Cover the sections with solution for 10−15 min.

(iii)   When the reaction is complete wash off with running water.

(iv)   Remember to mount the sections in a water-based mounting medium. To obtain a red reaction product simply alter the Fast Blue salt to Fast Red.

10. ANTIBODY DILUTIONS

It is essential to determine the optimal dilutions of all the antibodies used in the preceding techniques. Each antibody used will have its own optimum dilution. This will vary depending on a number of different factors. These are listed as follows.

(i)   Temperature of incubation.

(ii)   Length of time of incubation.

(iii)   The type of tissue section; frozen or fixed paraffin.

(iv)   Length of fixation.

(v)   Type of fixation.

(vi)   If an unmasking procedure has been used.

When using new antibodies it is often helpful to have some positive control tissue available. If excess antibody is present relative to the antigen in the section, reduced binding may occur with a poor result, a phenomenon that is similar to the prozone effect in agglutination reactions. When interpreting a result of immunostaining, a good positive result is where there is maximum contrast between the specific staining and the background.

10.1 Direct technique

The testing of an antibody for use in the direct technique is straightforward. There is only one antibody in use which is made up into 'doubling dilutions'. It is recommended to start with a dilution of 1:5, followed by 1:10, 1:20, 1:40, 1:80, 1:160, 1:320. To test these dilutions a minimum of seven sections would be required. If no positive staining has occurred the quality of the antibody must be checked and the visualization procedure should also be checked to confirm that it has been done correctly.

If there is all-over staining of the sections, increase the dilutions past the previous end point (1:320).

The correct dilution to use on the 'test' sections is selected from the section showing specific staining.

10.2 Indirect technique

Using the indirect technique the procedure becomes a little more complicated. Here we must set up a checkerboard titration. Using known positive controls we suggest that three or four dilutions are made for each antibody as set out in *Table 6*.

When the tests are complete all the slides are read and the optimal combination of dilutions will be the one that gives the maximum specific activity and the least amount of background staining.

10.3 The PAP technique

The PAP technique is more complicated because there are three stages in operation. In practise one stage is kept constant and the other two are varied.

Table 6. Checkerboard titration of antibody for the indirect technique.

		Primary antibody			
		1/50	*1/200*	*1/500*	*1/1000*
Secondary	1/50				
Antibody	1/100				
	1/200				

A minimum of 12 test sections are required.

Table 7. Checkerboard titration for the PAP technique.

		PAP		
		1/50	*1/100*	*1/200*
Secondary	1/50			
Antibody	1/100			
	1/200			

Initially the optimum working dilution for a primary antibody may be obtained either from the manufacturer's literature or from prior testing with the indirect technique. For example if we know it is in the region of 1:200 then keeping this constant a checkerboard for the secondary antibody and the PAP is set up as in *Table 7*.

The same conditions apply for determining the optimum dilution. In order to save costs select the highest working dilution of the PAP complex.

When the best combination between the secondary antibody and the PAP has been ascertained these then remain constant and the dilution of the first antibody is varied to discover its optimum titre.

In making the dilutions for these titrations it is recommended that high quality adjustable micro-pipettes are used. Using these pipettes there is a greater flexibility in the variety of dilutions prepared and the dilutions are more accurate and may be repeated.

Final volumes required will vary as to the size and number of sections to be covered. The absolute minimum amount required for small sections is 100 μl. It is easier to use 200 μl however but this is usually determined by the cost and availability of the antibody.

Dilution may be difficult to make for the inexperienced especially if a required volume is needed to be made from an already diluted antibody, e.g.

400 μl of 1:500 from a 1:100 dilution of antibody

so $\frac{500}{100}$ = 5 times original dilution.

$\frac{400 \, \mu l}{5}$ = 80 μl of original dilution.

so 80 μl original antibody with 320 μl of diluent = working dilution.

11. COUNTERSTAINING

The counterstaining and mounting technique used will be determined by which enzyme label and visualization techniques are used. With DAB the coloured end-products are alcohol fast, therefore alcoholic stains may be used followed by dehydration, clearing in xylene and mounting in Canada balsam or DPX.

The reaction products of AEC and chloronaphthol are soluble in alcohol and organic solvents, therefore the slides must be mounted directly from water in an aqueous mounting medium.

11.1 Insoluble end-product counterstaining

(i)   Stain the sections with Mayer's haemalum for 30 sec.
(ii)   Wash off with running water.
(iii)   'Blue up' in Scotts tap water substitute or running water for 15 min.
(iv)   Wash the sections in water after Scotts.
(v)   Dehydrate in alcohol.
(vi)   Clear in xylene and mount in Canada balsam.

11.2 Soluble end-product counterstaining

(i)   Stain the sections with an aqueous counterstain, for example neutral red or carmalum.
(ii)   Wash off with running water.
(iii)   Mount the sections from water in glycerol jelly.

12. CONTROLS

When staining for specific antigens in tissues, various controls should be employed to check the validity of the results. There are several different kinds of control in general use and some of them will be mentioned here.

The specific antibody in the primary antiserum may be absorbed with the purified antigen. This type of control, known as antigen absorption testing, is set up by making a series of dilutions of the relevant purified antigen using the working dilution of primary antibody as the diluent. When the specific antigen is present in sufficient concentration, then total absorption occurs and the reaction is blocked. As the antigen is diluted out then absorption is incomplete and positive staining occurs. With known positive controls the slides which have been reacted with the totally absorbed antiserum are negative, but as the antiserum becomes unabsorbed positive staining occurs.

This type of control may only be used if the purified antigen is readily available; this of course is not always the case and many purified antigens are very expensive.

In practice a very useful way to test antiserum specificity is to try and show that any staining present is not due to any non-specific antibodies in the serum. This may be done by substituting the primary antiserum with the serum of the animal used to raise the antiserum.

Certainly one of the best kind of controls is simply to stain a known positive section and a known negative section. Of course the tissue from which these sections are taken should be processed in an identical manner to the test tissue.

The second and third stage antisera should be controlled by substituting the primary antiserum with buffer only. Negative staining should occur and any staining which is observed is either due to non-specific staining by the antiserum or to endogenous peroxidase activity.

Each tissue examined also has its own 'intrinsic' control which occurs when a panel of specific antisera is being used. For example if reactive lymphoid tissue such as a tonsil is being examined and stained for γ, α, μ, δ, heavy chains, and $\varkappa$ and λ light chains, then each section will show different positive cell patterns. If, however, the same cells are being stained with each antiserum then some non-specific staining is occurring.

13. INTERPRETATION AND TROUBLE SHOOTING

When interpreting immunohistochemical results certain staining patterns will need to be identified, that is nuclear, intra- and intercytoplasmic, surface and non-specific.

As has been discussed earlier we are looking for distinct specific staining and a clear background. In practice, however, this may not be achieved very often and interpretation of results requires a careful examination of staining patterns and intensities and a knowledge of what to ignore on the sections.

If the required contrast has not been obtained then one or more of the following events may have happened during processing.

(i)   The tissue has been handled too roughly.
(ii)   The tissue has been left to dry before fixation.
(iii) The tissue has been put into fixative without slicing, leaving the central areas inadequately fixed.
(iv)   Excess tissue adhesive has been applied.
(v)   Paraffin-wax has not been completely removed from sections.
(vi)   There is omission of non-immune serum or haemolyzed non-immune serum has been used.
(vii) The primary antibody needs diluting (prozone effect).
(viii) The second and third antibodies are too strong.
(ix)   There is overdevelopment of the substrate reaction.

Negative staining may have occurred for the following reasons.

(i)   There is poor fixation and processing of tissues.
(ii)   Unmasking time was not long enough.
(iii) The antibody dilutions are incorrect.
(iv)   There is omission of an antibody incubation.
(v)   The antibody used is from an incorrect animal species.
(vi)   The substrate solution has been made up incorrectly.

14. ACKNOWLEDGEMENTS

We would like to thank Miss Jane Melhuish for typing the manuscript and Mr A.A. Cooper for photographic assistance.

15. REFERENCES

1. Coons,A.H. and Kaplan,M.H. (1950) *J. Exp. Med.*, **91**, 1.
2. Nakane,P.K. and Pierce,G.B.,Jr. (1966) *J. Histochem. Cytochem.*, **14**, 929.
3. Curran,R.C. and Gregory,J. (1978) *J. Clin. Pathol.*, **31**, 974.
4. Taylor,C.R. and Burns,J. (1974) *J. Clin. Pathol.*, **27**, 14.
5. Curran,R.C. and Gregory,J. (1980) *J. Clin. Pathol.*, **33**, 1047.
6. Bosman,F.T., Lindeman,J., Kuiper,G., van der Wal,A. and Kreunig,J. (1977) *Histochemistry*, **53**, 57.

7. Curran,R.C. and Gregory,J. (1977) *Experientia,* **33,** 1400.
8. Sinclair,R.A., Burns,J. and Dunnill,M.S. (1981) *J. Clin. Pathol.,* **34,** 859.
9. Ponder,B.A. and Wilkins,M.M. (1981) *J. Histochem. Cytochem.,* **29,** 981.
10. Rathlev,T., Hocks,J.M., Franks,G.F., Suffin,S.C., O'Donnell,C.M. and Porter,D.D. (1981) *Clin. Chem.,* **27,** 1513.
11. Graham,R.C. and Karnovsky,M.J. (1966) *J. Histochem. Cytochem.,* **14,** 291.
12. Ordronneau,P. and Petrusz,P. (1980) *Am. J. Anat.,* **158,** 491.
13. Wood,G.S. and Warnke,R. (1981) *J. Histochem. Cytochem.,* **29,** 1196.
14. Cordell,J.L., Falini,B., Erber,W.N., Ghosh,A.K., Abdulaziz,Z., Macdonald,S., Pulford,K.A.F., Stein,H. and Mason,D.Y. (1984) *J. Histochem. Cytochem.,* **32,** 219.

CHAPTER 6

Immunofluorescence

GERALD D.JOHNSON

1. INTRODUCTION

The possibility of covalently attaching fluorescent dyes to antibody molecules without significantly affecting their ability to react with antigen was demonstrated in 1950 by Coons and Kaplan (1). This provided a method which combines the sensitivity and specificity of immunological reactions with the topographical precision of microscopy. Fluorochromes emit light which is visible at very low concentration when viewed with appropriate equipment — staining of cell nuclei by antibody, for example, can be seen with as little as 10^{-15} g of fluorescein per nucleus. Efficient fluorescent conjugates are readily prepared in which the average molar labelling ratio is of the order 3:1; at this level the ability of antibody to bind specifically with antigen shows little impairment.

It is useful to compare immunofluorescence with the alternative immunohistochemical method which employs enzymes as labels and provides comparable sensitivity. Similar staining procedures are used in both techniques but the enzyme method requires an extra step to produce a coloured reaction product. This is visualized in a standard microscope whereas fluorescence microscopy requires a precisely tailored optical system. Double staining using two antibodies to give different colours at their respective sites of reaction is available by both techniques. However, due to the development of specific fluorescence filter systems which enable the individual contribution of each antibody to be separately assessed, immunofluorescence is the preferred method for studying *coincident* reactivity, especially when one reactant is predominant.

Previous shortcomings of the immunofluorescence procedure which encouraged the use of alternative labels have now been largely overcome as described below. Thus, fading of fluorescence during microscopy and storage can be considerably abated by the simple expedient of adding a retarding agent to the mountant; water-miscible media which solidify enable 'permanent' preparations to be made; the identification of reaction sites in complex tissues is facilitated by non-immunological fluorescent counter-staining.

Immunofluorescence has been exploited in all fields of biological science where appropriate antibody preparations are available. Recognition of the crucial importance of proper characterization of the reagents employed has resulted in considerable improvement in the quality of commercial conjugates available; in clinical immunology the introduction of the concepts of standardization and external quality control of tests for autoantibodies has drawn attention to the influence of variables in the procedure on the results obtained. Immunofluorescence provides a convenient method for screening large numbers of samples for specific antibody activity and is therefore widely employed in the development and characterization of monoclonal antibodies.

The following account describes the application of the immunofluorescent procedure and assessment by microscopy; the principles outlined are equally applicable to the preparation of samples for cytofluorimetric assay.

2. PREPARATION OF FLUORESCENT REAGENTS

High quality fluorescent reagents are essential for the successful application of immuno-fluorescence (IF). They must be prepared from suitably potent antibody preparations of the requisite specificity and conjugated with the optimal amount of fluorochrome. Recognition of the crucial importance of these parameters in determining the performance of the conjugate has resulted in a general improvement in the quality of commercial reagents and suitable preparations are now obtainable for most applications. Contrary to general belief, however, the conjugation procedure is very simple and, given a supply of suitable antiserum, conjugates can readily be prepared, very cheaply, that are at least as good as the best commercial reagents. The preparation of anti-species globulin conjugates (which have wide application) is described here. The principles apply equally to the production of conjugates with other specificities.

2.1 Selection of antisera

2.1.1 *Potency*

Conjugates prepared from potent antisera can be employed at high dilution thereby minimizing non-specific staining (NSS). Specific staining is generally correlated with the precipitating activity of the labelled antibody and for antiglobulin conjugates such as those used in the widely applicable indirect staining procedure a simple precipitin test therefore provides a convenient method of assessment. It should be noted that commercial unlabelled precipitating antisera may have already been identified by the manufacturer as being of inadequate potency for labelling although suitable for other applications. Methods for determining the antibody content of antisera are described in Volume I, Chapter 6. The reverse Marcini immunodiffusion procedure is recommended for evaluating materials for conjugation and in the analysis of conjugates. The anti-IgG content of suitable antisera is in the range of $0.4-2.0$ mg of antibody protein per ml.

A simple indication of precipitating activity can be obtained by the classical Ouchter-lony double diffusion method: a 1% solution of IgG is placed in the centre well and a series of doubling dilutions of antiserum in the outer wells. Suitably potent antisera show a precipitin line after overnight incubation at room temperature up to a dilution of 1:16 or more (diameter of wells 2.5 mm; distance from centre to centre 8 mm).

Table 1 details a useful practical procedure for screening preliminary bleeds for good responders following immunization.

2.1.2 *Specificity*

The specificity of antisera should be established by appropriate standard tests. In the case of antiglobulin reagents this is usually done by immunoelectrophoresis and double diffusion against purified immunoglobulin preparations. When available, a more sensitive indirect haemagglutination assay using antigen-coated cells as described in Volume I, Chapter 7 is recommended.

Table 1. Rapid screening test for potent antisera.

1.	Prepare a 4-step 10-fold series of dilutions of antigen from a solution containing 10 mg of IgG/ml in 0.15 M NaCl.
2.	Half-fill a vaccine capillary tube with *undiluted* antiserum, wipe dry the outside of the tube with absorbent tissue and complete filling the tube with antigen solution at each dilution.
3.	Stick the tubes vertically in plasticine with the antiserum on top.
4.	Leave at room temperature for about 10 min. Antisera suitably potent for labelling produce a copious precipitate throughout the length of the tube with at least one of the antigen dilutions corresponding to the equivalence zone.

Non-specific (i.e. unwanted) reactivity should be removed by immunoabsorption of the antiserum with insoluble antigen (see Chapter 1). It should be noted that neutralization of irrelevant antibody by adding an excess of soluble antigen is to be avoided since both the free antigen and soluble complexes may be subsequently conjugated with fluorochrome and lead to staining which could be interpreted as specific.

The sensitivity of the IF procedure is such that staining is produced by conjugates in high dilution at concentrations which do not give positive precipitin reactions. Unwanted reactivity capable of producing irrelevant (albeit specific) staining cannot therefore be excluded on the basis of negative precipitin results; for example, the failure of an anti-IgG serum to precipitate with IgM does not exclude its reactivity with IgM by IF when the antiserum is conjugated with fluorochrome.

2.2 Preparation of globulin fraction for conjugation

Conjugates must be prepared from antibody-rich fractions of antisera since other proteins — particularly albumin — have a higher affinity for the fluorochrome than γ-globulin and therefore label preferentially. Furthermore the process of conjugating proteins with isothiocyanates results in an increased negative charge so that proteins that are themselves negatively charged acquire potent NSS potential for basic sites in tissues by electrostatic binding. The removal of albumin from the antibody preparation before labelling is therefore paramount.

The following types of preparation are used for the production of fluorescent conjugates.

(i)   An immunoglobulin-rich fraction prepared by simple salting-out procedures.
(ii)   A chromatographically pure immunoglobulin fraction obtained by ion-exchange chromatography.
(iii)   Specific antibody prepared by immunoadsorption.
(iv)   Divalent $F(ab')_2$ obtained by proteolytic cleavage.

The methods of carrying out these fractionation procedures are described in Chapters 4 and 5 of this book. Satisfactory conjugates for general use can be conveniently prepared by the user from the fraction obtained by salting-out, and a method which the author has found useful is described below. On a commercial scale, conjugates should be prepared from chromatographically pure fractions. Labelled $F(ab')_2$ fragments are useful where Fc binding may be a problem and also in double-staining in order to avoid interspecies cross-reactivity between the reagents. Conjugates prepared from specific antibody may be desirable in particular research applications, especially in direct staining systems.

Table 2. Preparation of globulin-rich fraction by salting-out.

1.	Add 0.4 ml of antiserum to a centrifuge tube containing 9.6 ml of a solution containing 193 g ammonium sulphate and 40 g NaCl per litre in distilled water.
2.	Mix for 2 min at room temperature.
3.	Centrifuge for 1 h at 300 g at 4°C.
4.	Remove the supernatant and re-suspend the precipitate in the precipitating mixture.
5.	Centrifuge as before.
6.	Remove the supernatant and take up the precipitate in the minimum amount of 0.15 M NaCl to enable it to be transferred to a dialysis bag with minimum dilution.
7.	Dialyse overnight at 4°C against 0.15 M NaCl.
8.	Remove the small amount of insoluble protein by brief centrifugation.

An important consideration arises from the use of sheep antiserum for the preparation of anti-species conjugates for use in indirect staining (2). Such conjugates are widely employed for studying surface membrane-associated antigens of human lymphocytes since the cells do not possess receptors for sheep Fc. Two IgG components are obtained by ion-exchange chromatography, both of which show specific antibody activity demonstrable by passive haemagglutination; however only the 'faster' gamma 1 fraction shows precipitating activity and produces satisfactory fluorescent conjugates. On the other hand, the precipitating activity of horse and rabbit antisera is mainly associated with 'slow' IgG and this fraction produces satisfactory conjugates.

The simple method outlined in *Table 2* is suitable for preparing fractions for labelling from small amounts of antiserum with very little contamination with non-immunoglobulin protein (3).

For most applications steps 4 and 5 of *Table 2* may be omitted as, with care, the level of contaminating protein is insignificant. It is clearly good practice to confirm the activity of the fraction to be conjugated, however it is produced. The rapid capillary tube method described in *Table 1* is convenient for this purpose.

Unlabelled antibody-containing fractions (and fluorescent conjugates) are often preserved by the addition of sodium azide up to a concentration of 0.1%. It should be noted, however, that conjugation with isothiocyanate derivatives is inhibited by azide and it is therefore essential to remove the preservative, for example by dialysis against 0.15 M NaCl, before conjugation is attempted.

2.3 Choice of fluorochrome

The original definitive description of the IF method (1) was based on the use of fluorescein-labelled conjugate. Fluorescein continues to be the primary fluorochrome of choice on account of its superior performance when compared with alternative compounds that have been proposed over the last 35 years. Fluorescein conjugates show an absorption maximum of 495 nm and have a strong fluorescence emission which is apple-green, a colour rarely encountered in mammalian tissues as autofluorescence and which also corresponds to a region of high retinal sensitivity. The Isomer 1 form of the isothiocyanate derivative is generally used. This is easily coupled to protein to produce stable conjugates having predictable labelling ratios. Amorphous dye is much cheaper than the crystalline form and is generally satisfactory. Commercial preparations certified by the Biological Stain Commission (USA) contain at least 70% of the pure material. When conjugating small amounts of protein it is convenient to use a 10% dispersion of the dye on an inert carrier, Celite, which is easily removed after conjugation by centrifugation; satisfactory material is obtainable from British Drug Houses (Poole, Dorset, UK).

The principal alternative to fluorescein is rhodamine. Conjugates of this dye show an absorption maximum of 555 nm and an orange fluorescence giving good contrast with fluorescein. It is therefore widely employed in dual-fluorescence studies. The tetramethyl isothiocyanate is generally used; it is obtainable from Cambridge Research Biochemicals (Cambridge, UK).

An alternative orange/red-emitting fluorochrome, Texas Red, has been proposed (4). The absorption maximum of this dye (596 nm) is further removed from that of fluorescein compared with rhodamine. In a dual laser system incorporating a tunable dye laser it can therefore provide more efficient spectral separation from fluorescein excitation.

Phycoerythrin (5) has recently been introduced to provide an alternative fluorescent colour to fluorescein for use in single laser fluorescence-activated analysis. Unlike rhodamine this dye shows orange fluorescence on excitation by light of similar wavelength to that used to excite fluorescein. However, since the fluorescence spectrum of fluorescein extends into the red region, the use of phycoerythrin in discriminatory double fluorescence analysis should be approached with caution.

A recent study (6) has drawn attention to a previously unrecognized additional hazard when phycoerythrin (RPE) is employed in dual fluorescence with fluorescein staining. This arises due to the spectral overlap between the absorbance curve of RPE and the emission curve of fluorescein which can result in an appreciable loss of the fluorescein signal in the presence of high intensity RPE staining. Control tests in which RPE is omitted are therefore essential in order to avoid misinterpretation of results—especially of subpopulation analysis by single laser FACS. See Section 5.3 for a fuller consideration of the rationalization of filter systems in relation to the dyes employed.

2.4 Analysis of fluorochrome by thin layer chromatography

As indicated above, reliable preparations of fluorochromes are commercially available. Confirmation of their relative purity can be easily demonstrated by thin layer chromatography performed on silica-gel plates (Merck). The dye is dissolved in acetone and the plate is developed in the ascending manner using a solvent system containing, for example, 1 part methanol in 30 parts of diethyl ether. After about 2 h the plate is dried and inspected under a UV scanner. Pure crystalline fluorescein isothiocyanate (FITC) which gives a single spot may be run for comparison. Use of this procedure in the author's laboratory revealed the presence of a green-emitting contaminant in a commercial preparation of rhodamine which was therefore clearly unsuitable for use in double fluorescence staining.

2.5 Conjugation procedures

2.5.1 *General method*

Isothiocyanate compounds bind to protein readily at pH $9.0-9.5$ in aqueous solution with minimum loss of antibody activity. The basic procedure given in *Table 3* has been

Table 3. Fluorescein conjugation.

1.	Prepare the protein fraction of the antiserum as described in Section 2.2.
2.	Prepare the conjugation buffer (0.5 M carbonate/bicarbonate, pH 9.5) by adding 5.8 ml of 5.3% Na_2CO_3 to 10 ml of 4.2% $NaHCO_3$. Check the pH and adjust if necessary.
3.	Prepare the reaction mixture containing 10 mg/ml of the protein fraction in 0.15 M NaCl and 10% by volume of the alkaline buffer.
4.	Add 30 μg of FITC/mg of protein. This ratio is satisfactory for the BDH Isomer 1 product; the optimum amount for materials of different purity should be determined by trial conjugation. As mentioned in Section 2.3, the 10% dispersion on Celite may be more easily weighed when conjugating small amounts of protein.
5.	Rotate the mixture gently (e.g. on a Matburn type mixer) for 1.5 h at room temperature.
6.	Remove unreacted dye as described in Section 2.7.

employed by the author to prepare conjugates from a wide range of antisera produced in various species. It is rapid, economical in materials and yields conjugates with predictable labelling ratios.

2.5.2 *Rhodamine conjugation*

Rhodamine conjugates are prepared in a similar way with the following modifications. The amorphous form of the tetramethyl rhodamine isothiocyanate (TRITC) isomer R is satisfactory and the labelling ratio for the Cambridge Research Biochemicals product is 30 μg/mg of protein. It has been shown (7) that better conjugates are obtained with a lower protein concentration (4 mg/ml) than is used with FITC. The dye is less readily soluble and conjugation is therefore allowed to proceed overnight at 4°C. An alternative procedure (8) is to dissolve the dye in dimethyl sulphoxide (DMSO) (1 mg/ml) and add the solution drop-wise to the buffered protein solution in the ratio 25 μg TRITC per mg of IgG. Conjugation is accomplished in 2 h at room temperature.

2.5.3 *The biotin−avidin system*

An alternative to the use of fluorochrome-labelled antibodies is provided by the biotin−avidin system (9). In the procedure the water-soluble vitamin biotin is conjugated to the antibody protein, and the fluorochrome attached to the egg white protein avidin, which has a high affinity for biotin. Commercial reagents based on this system are now available.

The procedure for biotinylation of antibody protein as described by Goding (10) is as follows.

(i)   Adjust the protein concentration to 1 mg/ml and dialyse against 0.1 M $NaHCO_3$.

(ii)   Dissolve biotin succinimide ester (Calbiochem, Sigma) in DMSO (1 mg/ml) immediately before use and add to the protein with mixing.

(iii) Keep at room temperature for 4 h then dialyse against phosphate-buffered saline (PBS) containing 0.1% NaN_3. The optimum labelling ratio is in the range 50−250 μg of the ester per mg of protein and is determined by trial conjugation.

2.6 **Detection of free dye**

A substantial proportion of the fluorochrome added to the conjugation mixture remains unbound to protein. Such free dye is a potent source of NSS and produces high levels

Table 4. Test for free fluorochrome.

1.	Prepare a suspension of Sephadex G25 or G50 (medium grade) in PBS.
2.	Allow to settle, remove the supernatant and pour the slurry onto a microscope slide.
3.	Remove the surplus fluid by holding paper tissue against the edge of the slide. Do not allow the Sephadex to dry out completely.
4.	Arrange the slide between two Petri dishes at an angle of $10-20°$ and attach filter paper wicks at each end.
5.	Fill the dish at the upper end with PBS and allow the fluid to flow for a few minutes.
6.	Apply a few microlitres of the conjugate about 1 cm from the upper end.
7.	After $15-20$ min examine the slide under a UV scanning lamp. [Alternatively arrange the slide on the stage of a fluorescence microscope equipped for incident illumination but without the objective lens installed, and view through an appropriate (Section 5.3) barrier filter held to the eye.] Labelled protein will be seen as a discrete spot several centimetres from the origin whereas free dye will remain trapped in the Sephadex at the point of application.

of background fluorescence in concentrations as low as 5 μg of FITC/ml. Furthermore, after storage for long periods, conjugates begin to dissociate and liberate free dye with consequent increase in NSS. This is particularly a feature of rhodamine conjugates. When this is suspected it is useful to test the solution for free dye by the chromatographic procedure described in *Table 4*.

2.7 **Removal of free dye**

Removal of unconjugated fluorochrome is best accomplished by passing the conjugate through a 'molecular sieve' comprising Sephadex G25 or G50 medium grade. The sample volume should not exceed 30% of the bed volume which should be contained in a long narrow column. The conjugated protein is present in the exclusion peak; by carefully observing the fluorescence of the outflow it is possible to recover the conjugate in a similar volume to that of the sample applied, i.e. without significant dilution. Rhodamine conjugates often produce a long 'tail', probably due to insolubilization of some of the free dye in the column. This can be avoided by preliminary dialysis against PBS for 1 or 2 h followed by centrifugation. Simple dialysis was employed originally for removal of free dye but this takes several days with frequent changes of dialysing solution and the more definitive separation procedure as described is recommended.

2.8 **Fractionation by ion-exchange chromatography**

Conjugates as prepared contain a heterogeneous mixture of protein molecules having different labelling ratios. If the reaction mixture is satisfactorily constituted most of the protein will be optimally labelled. However, the random distribution of dye inevitably results in the presence of a population of antibody molecules with low levels of labelling, the presence of which may inhibit binding of optimally-labelled antibody; the population of over-labelled molecules on the other hand may produce high background staining due to the increased net negative charge resulting from the attachment of the isothiocyanate derivative via the thiourea linkage. Conjugates prepared from potent antisera are generally employed at such high dilution that the effects of the minor populations of under- and over-labelled antibody molecules are minimized and for most applications the whole conjugate may therefore be successfully employed. When less potent antisera, however, are only available and in more critical applications the opti-

Table 5. Fractionation by chromatography.

1.	Equilibrate the conjugate against starting buffer (0.0175 M phosphate pH 6.3).
2.	Prepare a DEAE−cellulose (DE 52-Whatman) column containing 5 g of cellulose/100 mg of protein.
3.	Elute with starting buffer — this fraction contains the under-labelled fraction.
4.	Elute with starting buffer containing 0.125 M NaCl — this provides the optimally-labelled fraction.
5.	Conjugate remaining in the column has a high labelling ratio and may be recovered by elution with starting buffer containing 0.25 M NaCl.

Table 6. Preparation of tissue homogenate.

1.	Obtain fresh tissue, e.g. liver, spleen from an appropriate species—e.g. absorption with human tissue would improve the performance of sheep anti-mouse Ig conjugate used for testing the reactivity of mouse monoclonal antibodies with human tissues.
2.	Homogenize in an equal volume of 0.15 M NaCl in a blender.
3.	Transfer to a large cylinder and add 5 vols of acetone.
4.	Allow the particles to sediment, remove the supernatant by suction and wash three times with 0.15 M NaCl, filling the cylinder each time with washing fluid.
5.	Remove any remaining lipids by further washing with acetone.
6.	Transfer to a filter funnel and wash through with acetone.
7.	Dry the material overnight at 37°C spread on filter paper.
8.	Grind to a fine powder in a mortar and remove fibrous particles by passage through a fine sieve.
9.	Slake in PBS, distribute in tubes, centrifuge and discard the supernatant. A volume of ~0.5 ml of packed material in a 3 ml tube is convenient.
10.	The stoppered tubes can be stored indefinitely at −20°C.

Table 7. Absorption procedure.

1.	Add 2 vols of conjugate to 1 vol. of packed homogenate and mix thoroughly.
2.	Gently rotate the tube for 20−30 min at room temperature.
3.	Centrifuge for 10 min (3000 r.p.m. in a bench centrifuge), remove the supernatant and re-centrifuge in order to eliminate highly fluorescent particles from the solution.
4.	Add preservative (0.1% NaN$_3$); this is essential because conjugates otherwise rapidly become infected after absorption with tissue.

mally-labelled fraction may be separated by ion-exchange chromatography based on the altered charge on the protein produced by conjugation described above. The step-wise elution procedure (9) given in *Table 5* is satisfactory.

2.9 **Purification by absorption with tissue homogenate**

This empirical method of improving the performance of fluorescent conjugates was originally described in 1950 (1) and is still a useful procedure. Optimal recognition of specific fluorescent staining is determined by two factors related to the performance of the conjugate; the intensity of specific staining and its contrast with the level of background 'noise'. It is important to recognize that unwanted (background) fluorescence may be associated with (i) true NSS, mainly due to electrostatic binding and (ii) irrelevant but *specific* staining due to immunological cross-reactivity with the substrate tissue. Selective removal of both factors with minimal reduction of significant staining is generally accomplished by absorption with appropriate tissue homogenate (*Tables 6* and *7*). This enables conjugates to be employed at higher concentrations [for example as required in direct staining (Section 4.2)] which would otherwise give unacceptable levels of background staining, and also in double immunofluorescence.

2.10 Determination of dye labelling ratio by spectrophotometry

The simplest method of obtaining an assessment of the degree of labelling is by comparison of the optical densities of a solution of the conjugate at the wavelength corresponding to peak absorption by the fluorochrome and at 280 nm — the tyrosine absorption peak. The conjugate is diluted 1:20−1:40, FITC is measured at 495 nm and TRITC at 555 nm. Optimally-labelled fluorescein conjugates have an absorbance ratio F:P approaching unity; values below 0.5 indicate low labelling and conjugates giving a value greater than 1.0 would be expected to show unacceptable NSS on tissue sections. In the case of rhodamine conjugates the optimal ratio is in the range 0.2−0.5:1.

2.11 Determination of labelled antibody specificity

The precipitating activity of labelled antibodies with isolated antigens can usually be demonstrated by standard techniques, as described elsewhere in this volume. In the case of antiglobulin conjugates, for example, immunoelectrophoresis against whole serum should confirm the reactivity of the conjugate with particular immunoglobulin components. Since immunofluorescent procedures show a higher sensitivty than precipitin reactions (of the order of 16-fold) however, the *absence* of a precipitin line does not exclude the presence of unwanted labelled antibody which would be manifest in an immunofluorescent test. For this reason the specificity of fluorescent reagents is best identified by 'performance testing' on known material. Immunoglobulin class specificity of anti-human Ig conjugates may be determined by staining preparations of bone marrow obtained from patients with myelomatosis in which the tumour cells contain the characteristic 'para-protein'. A satisfactory method (12) of preparing the marrow cells is given in *Table 8*.

An alternative method to the direct staining procedure for characterizing antiglobulin conjugates is the indirect procedure employing middle-layer antibodies of known isotype specificity. For example IgG anti-nuclear antibody obtained by ion-exchange chromatography from the serum of a case of active systemic lupus erythematosus is an appropriate reference preparation for evaluating IgG-specific conjugates used in autoantibody

Table 8. Preparation of bone marrow for immunofluorescence.

1.	Collect the marrow in 1 ml of 5% EDTA.
2.	Centrifuge at 900 *g* for 5 min at 4°C.
3.	Discard the supernatant, transfer the cell deposit to a microhaematocrit tube, centrifuge at 700 *g* for 5 min at 4°C.
4.	Remove the buffy coat layer and wash the cells in 30 ml of a solution containing 60 ml PBS, 8 ml 5% EDTA and 20 ml of 20% bovine serum albumin (BSA) solution.
5.	Centrifuge at 175 *g* for 10−15 min at 4°C.
6.	Resuspend the cell pellet in 0.5 ml of washing solution and prepare cytocentrifuge slides.
7.	Store the slides in sealed packets at −20°C.
8.	Before staining, fix the slides in 5% acetic acid in 96% ethanol at −20°C for 15 min.
9.	Wash in PBS for 1 h at 4°C.

Table 9. Block titration of antiglobulin conjugates.

1.	Prepare a 2- to 4-fold dilution series of an appropriate middle-layer serum (e.g. a serum known to contain anti-nuclear antibody).
2.	Apply the series of dilutions to tissue sections and test them in chessboard fashion against a 4-fold series of the antiglobulin conjugate using the indirect staining procedure described in Section 4.3.
3.	Determine the maximum obtainable 'titre' for the middle-layer antibody.
4.	Determine the maximum dilution of the conjugate with which the maximum titre for the middle-layer antibody is obtained.

testing; similarly, the heterophile antibody occurring in infectious mononucleosis which is demonstrable on sections of bovine tissue by immunofluorescence (13) provides an exclusively IgM reagent which can be used without serum fractionation. Isotype-specific anti-mouse immunoglobulin conjugates are characterized by testing their reactivity with a range of monoclonal antibodies of known isotypes.

2.12 Determination of the potency of conjugates

The potency of fluorescent reagents relates to the combined effects of the antibody concentration and its relative avidity. This determines the amount by which a conjugate may be diluted without losing demonstrable reactivity and is important not only from the point of view of economy in the use of the reagent but also because optimal staining efficiency is achieved by using conjugates at high dilution in order to increase the signal-to-noise ratio. The *precipitating* antibody activity of conjugates may be measured by standard immunological techniques. For example a reversed Mancini procedure has been described (14) in which the diameter of the precipitation zone produced in agar containing appropriate antigen is compared with that obtained with a reference standard whose specific antibody-N is known. A similar procedure may be employed using agar containing specific antibody to quantify *antigen* in conjugated antigen preparations. It must be emphasized, however, that the most meaningful assessment of conjugate potency is obtained by testing the performance of a conjugate in the application for which it is intended to be used. For direct staining this is effected by simple titration on the substrate preparation. Antiglobulin conjugates employed for indirect staining should be evaluated by block titration as described in *Table 9*.

This single test provides all the information needed to characterize the conjugate in terms of potency. Most preparations show a plateau for the titre of the middle-layer antibody which extends over a range of dilutions of the conjugate. The plateau height is determined by the antibody content of the first antibody and also by the labelling ratio of the conjugate; at high conjugate concentration the extent of NSS is demonstrated; the length of the plateau is related to the amount of antibody in the conjugate. At dilutions of conjugate beyond the plateau the observed titre for the first antibody falls rapidly. Conjugates prepared from potent antisera show a plateau titre for the first antibody at conjugate dilutions well beyond the range showing NSS. The working dilution of such a conjugate *for applications requiring a similar level of sensitivity to that employed in the evaluation test* should contain twice the concentration of conjugated antibody at the plateau endpoint. Simple titration of the conjugate against a single dilution of a potent middle-layer serum at high concentration is not recommended since this will give a higher observed titre for the conjugate resulting in false-negative tests when over-diluted conjugate is employed with weakly-positive sera.

2.13 Characterization of conjugates by use of defined antigen substrate spheres

An alternative to the use of biological materials such as cells and tissue sections for immunostaining is the defined antigen substrate sphere (DASS) system (15). This is based on the use of purified proteins coupled to an inert support — Sepharose beads. The method has potential where a standardized substrate is required and pure antigen available, and in quantitative fluorescence assays. The use of labelled beads has been proposed as a fluorescence standard for microscopy (16). Methods of attaching proteins to activated Sepharose are described elsewhere in this volume. Application of the DASS system to immunofluorescence assays follows the general procedures outlined in this chapter and requires a rigid experimental protocol.

3. PREPARATION OF TISSUES AND CELLS FOR IF

3.1 Cryostat sections

Tissues must be obtained as fresh as possible and care taken to avoid excessive handling which would disrupt the architecture. The process of rapid freezing may be accomplished in several ways as described below. It should be noted that simply allowing tissue to freeze by placing it in a deep-freeze cabinet or dropping it directly into liquid nitrogen is not satisfactory.

(i) *Use of solid CO_2.*
(1)   Add small pieces of solid CO_2 to industrial methylated spirit (74 O.P.) in a wide-mouthed Ewer flask until the mixture ceases to 'boil' i.e. at a temperature of $-70°C$.
(2)   Place the tissue to be frozen (up to 0.5 cm thick) on the inner wall of a hard glass tube, about 30 mm in diameter, and immerse the tube in the freezing mixture to bring the tissue below the level of the fluid.
(3)   After the tissue is completely frozen, prise it off the glass, transfer to a small polythene bag and place it in the freezing cabinet at $-20°C$, preferably $-70°C$. It is imperative that the tissue does not come in contact with the alcohol as this prevents proper freezing. This method is recommended for handling large specimens.

(ii) *Freezing with gaseous CO_2.* This is the method of choice for assembling composite tissue blocks and enables four or five different tissues to be cut simultaneously in a single section. Equipment for this procedure is available from SLEE Ltd, South London Electrical Equipment Co. Ltd, Lanier Works, Hither Green Lane, London, UK. The tissues are suitably orientated and placed as closely as possible on the face of a hollow microtome chuck. Rapid freezing is effected by passing CO_2 through the chuck from a 'snow-making' cylinder.

(iii) *Liquid nitrogen.* Blocks of tissue, preferably attached to metal foil, may be frozen by repeatedly dipping the foil into the liquid so that the tissue is gradually frozen. If this is done too quickly the tissue is liable to crack.

A more satisfactory method of employing liquid nitrogen is to use the coolant to chill iso-pentane which is then used to freeze the tissue directly by repeated immersion. This procedure is recommended for freezing very small pieces of tissue, especially where correct orientation is essential, e.g. small punch biopsies of skin and gut. A small capsule is formed of metal foil and filled with OCT Compound (Miles Laboratories, Inc.); the tissue is orientated as necessary near the surface of the viscous liquid and the capsule repeatedly immersed in iso-pentane which has been cooled in liquid nitrogen; when the block is entirely frozen the foil is removed, excess OCT Compound trimmed and the block attached to a cold chuck with a small amount of water.

(iv) *Preparation of cryostat sections.* The following points should be followed in order to obtain sections of the requisite quality.

(1)   Frozen tissues must not be allowed to thaw.

(2)   Cut sections 4−6 μm thick.

(3)   Minute adjustment of the anti-roll plate is vital with respect to angle and height in relation to the cutting surface of the knife, and distance from the knife.

(4)   The knife edge should be of very high quality and should be kept grease-free by occasionally cleaning with acetone.

(5)   The leading edge of the anti-roll plate must be undamaged and it should also be grease-free.

(6)   Sections taken onto glass slides at room temperature must be immediately dried by placing under a fan. The time required for complete drying varies with the tissue from 10 to 30 min.

(7)   The optimal temperature for cutting most tissues is −20°C. In practice the cabinet is usually maintained at −30°C so that the inevitable rise in temperature associated with making the initial adjustments produces the desired temperature for cutting.

(8)   Properly dried sections can be stored for long periods in a freezer at −20°C, preferably −70°C. They should be placed in sealed polythene bags. Before use the slides are allowed to reach room temperature before opening the bags in order to avoid the disastrous effects of water from condensation.

(9)   The use of Multispot Slides (17) is recommended when large numbers of tests are required. These enable as many as 12 separate tests to be processed on a single microscope slide (25 × 75 mm) and mounted under one coverslip. This effects considerable economy in labour and materials. Pre-coated slides in a wide range of formats are obtainable from C.A.Hendley (Essex) Ltd, Oakwood Hill Industrial Estate, Loughton, Essex, UK. A Teflon spray useful for making coated slides is supplied by Marshall Howlett, PO Box 39, Betsham Road, Gravesend, Kent, UK under the name Klingerflon. The test area is covered with an obdurator of suitable size before spraying.

3.2 **Imprints**

This simple alternative to tissue sections has been used by some authors where architectural detail is not required. Substrate slides are prepared by lightly touching the cut surface of the fresh tissue on the glass and immediately drying. The method may be useful for certain applications. In the author's laboratory imprints of rat liver were found to give a higher incidence of positive anti-nuclear antibody tests than cryostat sections of the same tissue.

3.3 Cytocentrifuge preparations

High-quality preparations of cells suitable for intracellular staining can be consistently prepared in the cytocentrifuge. The suspension should contain about 10^6 cells/ml and a suitable volume is 50 μl per spot. After spinning, the slides should be thoroughly air-dried; the use of Teflon to define the test areas as described in Section 3.1 is strongly recommended.

3.4 Cell spreads

This is an alternative to the cytocentrifuge procedure where large numbers of tests on a cell preparation are required. The method requires careful attention to technical detail to achieve consistent results. The final cell suspension is made in 0.04 M NaCl (hypotonic) and applied to the slides as rapidly as possible. One drop containing 10^6 cells per ml is placed onto 3 mm test areas; after 1 min the supernatant fluid is removed by suction and the slide rapidly dried under a fan.

3.5 Cells for surface staining

Specific techniques for preparing live cells in suspension are described elsewhere in this volume. The final suspension should contain $2-5 \times 10^5$ cells per test, preferably in glass tubes and maintained on ice.

3.6. Fixation

Originally immunofluorescence procedures were devised for studying immunological reactions involving tissues in their native state and for this reason the use of frozen unfixed tissue was developed in order to maintain maximum reactivity. However, there is now an extensive literature on the use of fixatives in immunolabelling and it is generally appreciated that the visual quality of (for example) frozen sections can be improved by mild fixation without detriment to antigenic reactivity. Since antigens vary in their sensitivity to different chemicals used as fixatives it is not possible to make general rules covering all systems but the following considerations apply.

(i) Cross-linking reagents such as formaldehyde have a considerable inhibiting effect on many antigens and this may be partially neutralized by enzymes such as trypsin and pepsin.

(ii) Many antigens are resistant to organic solvents such as ethanol, methanol and acetone which nevertheless may enhance the appearance of the tissue.

(iii) In the author's laboratory all cryostat sections and dried preparations of cells are fixed for 5 min in acetone at room temperature.

The procedure detailed in *Table 10* based on fixation in ethanol was devised (18) to provide tissue sections for immunofluorescence by a modification of the normal histological tissue processing by paraffin embedding. It is strongly recommended when high quality sections are essential or the use of cryostat sections of frozen fresh tissue is not feasible, provided the relevant antigen is alcohol stable.

Table 10. Cold alcohol fixation.

1.	Place a block of tissue not more than 5 mm thick in 95% ethanol pre-cooled to 4°C. Leave for 1 h at 4°C.
2.	Trim into slices 2−4 mm thick and leave for a further 15−24 h at 4°C.
3.	Dehydrate in four changes of pre-cooled absolute alcohol, 1−2 h each.
4.	Clear in three changes of xylene 1−2 h each at 4°C.
5.	Embed in paraffin, four consecutive baths, 1−2 h each at 56°C.
6.	The blocks may be stored at 4°C for several months.
7.	Sections are cut in the normal way but flotation on water at 40°C should be as brief as possible.
8.	Dry the sections at 37°C for 30 min, de-paraffinize in two baths of cold xylene for 10−15 sec each.
9.	Remove the xylene in three baths of cold 95% ethanol (10−15 sec each) and remove the alcohol by gentle agitation in three baths of cold PBS, each lasting about 1 min.
10.	Carry out immunofluorescent staining immediately.

4. STAINING PROCEDURES

4.1 General considerations

Slides should be treated with antibodies and conjugates in a damp chamber to minimize evaporation. The time of application is normally 30 min at room temperature. Washing is best accomplished in three steps in order to remove unreacted material efficiently:

(i)   an initial rinse with PBS from a wash bottle (avoid directing the jet onto the test area itself);

(ii) brief immersion in a jar of PBS;

(iii) the slides are finally transferred to a carrier suspended over a stirring bar in a bath of PBS on a magnetic stirrer.

Unless this procedure is adopted it is possible for very potent antibody preparations to produce false-positive tests by contamination in batches of slides. Conjugates should be employed at their optimal concentration as described in Section 2.12. Sections and cell preparations on slides should be mounted in 90% glycerol in PBS. Since the fluorescence of fluorescein is pH dependent it is essential that the mounting solution is buffered in the range pH 8.0−9.0 (optimum 8.6). It should be noted that, on storage, glycerol may have a considerably lower pH than the range indicated. An alternative mountant which is water-miscible and which sets to give permanent preparations has recently been described (19). This contains 20 g of polyvinyl alcohol dissolved in 80 ml of PBS to which is added 40 ml of glycerol. This has been found especially suitable for mounting cells stained in suspension. The use of chemical incorporated in the mountant to retard fading during microscopy (Section 4.8) is now becoming standard practice.

An important source of artefacts occurring during the staining procedure should be emphasized. It is imperative that the test area on the slide does not become dry at any stage because of the effects of local high salt concentration. For this reason when large batches of slides are processed one slide at a time should be taken from the washing bath, surplus moisture removed *and the next reagent applied* before removing the next slide from the bath.

Table 11. Direct staining method.

1.	Pre-wet slides in PBS.	
2.	Apply diluted conjugate for 30 min.	
3.	Wash sections for 60 min and cell preparations for 30 min.	
4.	Mount.	
	Controls:	(a) Stain irrelevant material lacking the appropriate antigen.
		(b) Pre-treat the slide with unlabelled antibody in order to inhibit specific staining.
		(c) Dilute the conjugate in unconjugated antiserum — this should markedly reduce specific staining.
		(d) Absorb the conjugate with purified antigen, preferably in insoluble form.
		(e) Use a conjugate which is not directed against the antigen in question.

Table 12. Indirect staining method.

1.	Apply diluted antibody preparation for 30 min. (Stored sections should be pre-wetted in PBS.)	
2.	Wash in PBS for 10 min.	
3.	Stain with diluted conjugate for 30 min.	
4.	Wash sections for 60 min and cell preparations for 30 min.	
5.	Mount.	
	Controls:	Since the conjugate is directed against globulin of the first antibody this system is easier to control than the direct method. It is usually adequate to include known positive and negative sera at the first stage.

4.2 Direct method

This is the least sensitive immunofluorescent staining procedure and requires up to 10 times the concentration of conjugated antibody compared with the indirect method. For this reason it is usually advisable to absorb the conjugate with tissue homogenate in order to reduce background staining. The procedure is described in *Table 11*.

4.3 Indirect method

This is based on the use of conjugated antiglobulin antibody to demonstrate the site of reaction of previously applied unlabelled antibody (*Table 12*). In general, the conjugate should be specific for the species in which the first antibody was derived; however antiglobulin reagents often show cross-reactivity with various species. In order to avoid direct staining of the tissue by the antiglobulin conjugate it is often useful to make up the conjugate solution in PBS containing 10% serum from the same species as the tissue.

4.4 Anti-complement method

The presence of *in vivo* bound complement in tissues is demonstrated by the direct method using appropriate anti-complement conjugates. A modification of the indirect method can be employed to determine whether a particular antibody has complement-fixing activity (*Table 13*).

4.5 Double staining

4.5.1 *General method*

As discussed above, the ability to identify two different antigens — particularly when

Table 13. Test for complement-fixing activity.

The following procedure is used to determine whether a mouse monoclonal antibody to a human tissue component is complement-fixing.

1. Treat the section with the diluted antibody to which has been added an equal volume of fresh human serum to act as a source of complement.
2. Wash for 5 − 10 min.
3. Stain with diluted anti-human C3 conjugate.
4. Wash for 30 − 60 min.
5. Mount.
    Controls: This is very precisely controlled by including a test in which the added fresh human serum is previously de-complemented by heating at 56°C for 30 min. The complement system can also be validated by using a known complement-fixing antibody. When the test with unheated serum is negative it is useful to confirm the reactivity of the primary antibody by staining with antiglobulin conjugate in parallel.

Table 14. Sequential double-staining procedure.

In the following procedure the proportion of cells reactive with mouse antibodies to x and y are determined with fluorescein and rhodamine, sheep anti-mouse Ig conjugates.

Sequence 1

1. Apply mouse anti-x
2. Stain with rhodamine anti-mouse Ig
3. Apply mouse anti-y
4. Stain with fluorescein anti-mouse Ig

Sequence 2

1. Apply mouse anti-y
2. Stain with rhodamine anti-mouse Ig
3. Apply mouse anti-x
4. Stain with fluorescein anti-mouse Ig

Interpretation.

In Sequence 1 cells that are *only* stained by the fluorescein conjugate are $x^- y^+$ and in Sequence 2 cells that are exclusively fluorescein stained are $x^+ y^-$. By simple computation it is possible to determine the proportion of cells that are respectively $x^+ y^-$, $x^- y^+$, $x^+ y^+$, $x^- y^-$. It should be noted that cells reactive with the first antibody are inevitably stained by both conjugates because: (i) the second conjugate can become attached to antibody notwithstanding the presence of the first conjugate and (ii) the second (unlabelled) antibody can be bound to free antibody sites on the first conjugate. Notwithstanding this reservation, however, the discriminatory potential of this method as described above is valid provided that the second antibody and conjugate are applied in excess.

they occur at the same site — is one of the most important attributes of the immunofluorescent procedure. The simplest application is by direct staining using conjugates specific for each antigen labelled with fluorescein or rhodamine. The conjugates should be prepared from antibodies produced in the same species and they should show no interaction. The direct procedure is performed with a mixture of the two conjugates as indicated in *Table 11*.

The advantages of the indirect method may also be exploited in double staining as follows.

(i) Primary antibodies produced in different species are applied (usually as a mixture) followed by a mixture of the species-specific conjugates, preferably produced in one species.

(ii) Primary antibodies produced in one species, but having different isotypes, are applied as a mixture followed by a mixture of isotype-specific conjugates produced in one species. This is a powerful method of identifying a sub-population of cells, for example, with monoclonal antibodies.

Table 15. Combined surface and intracellular staining procedure.

1.	Stain cells in suspension (Section 4.6) either by the direct method using rhodamine-labelled conjugate, or by the indirect method.
2	Make cytocentrifuge preparations of the stained cells.
3.	Re-stain the dried cells by the direct method with identical conjugate but labelled with fluorescein (or by the indirect method using the same antibody preparation as before and conjugate with the alternative label).

Interpretation.
Intracellular antigen is stained only by the second conjugate, whereas membrane-bound antigen is stained by both conjugates as discussed above.

Table 16. Cell surface staining procedure.

1.	In a *glass* tube place $2-5 \times 10^5$ cells, lightly centrifuge and discard the supernatant.
2.	Re-suspend the pellet in 200 μl of diluted antibody in PBS containing $5-10\%$ foetal calf serum and 0.1% NaN_3.
3.	Incubate on ice for $30-60$ min with gentle shaking.
4.	Fill the tube with PBS, centrifuge and wash again with PBS.
5.	Discard the supernatant and re-suspend the pellet in fluorescent conjugate diluted in the same mixture as in step 2.
6.	Incubate again on ice for $30-60$ min with gentle shaking.
7.	Wash twice with PBS as in step 4.
8.	Re-suspend the pellet in one drop of PBS followed by one drop of mountant.
9.	Transfer to a microscope slide.

(iii)   When the primary antibodies have the same isotype the sequential double-staining procedure (*Table 14*) is employed to identify cells stained with either or both antibodies (20).

4.5.2 *Differentiation between cell surface and internal staining*

A special application of the double-staining methodology is in the demonstration of the same antigen on the cell membrane and simultaneously within the cell. The procedure outlined in *Table 15* was originally devised for studying the cellular location of immunoglobulin (21) and subsequently (22) for discriminating between surface-bound and phagocytosed IgG in studies on polymorphonuclear cells. The essential requirement is paired conjugates having identical specificity for the antigen in question.

In this protocol (*Table 15*) the method is used to demonstrate Ig on and within lymphocytes.

4.6 Surface staining

The basic indirect method of staining cell membrane-asociated antigens has been found to give reproducible results (*Table 16*).

4.7 Counterstaining

A serious criticism of the immunofluorescence procedure as originally practised was the difficulty in visualizing unstained areas. With the development of fluorescent counterstains however it is possible to identify with confidence the sites of reaction (and non-reaction) in the most complex tissue. An early approach was the use of rhodamine-labelled BSA; this has a high propensity for NSS due to its negative charge without interfering with the specific reactivity of a fluorescein-labelled conjugate. The reagent is still usefully employed for identifying NSS, for example, of mast cells and eosinophils which bind the specific conjugate.

A more recent development is the use of fluorescent nuclear counterstains. Ethidium bromide and propidium iodide intercalate with nuclear DNA to form a highly fluorescent compound which has a bright orange fluorescence. This can readily be detected in the fluorescence microscope with the filter system employed with fluorescein conjugates and thus gives a clear definition of the topography of a complex tissue section which contrasts with the green of specific staining. The staining is accomplished by merely immersing the slides immediately before mounting in a solution of the halide in PBS containing 1 μg/ml. After 2 or 3 min the solution is rinsed off with PBS and the slides mounted in the usual way. This procedure is employed in all applications of immunofluorescence involving sections and fixed cell preparations in the author's laboratory. It has proved useful not only in localizing specific staining in complex tissue sections such as tonsil and kidney but also in identifying cell types in preparations of mixed cells. Since the fluorescence excitation and emission of the halides is indistinguishable by microscopy from that of rhodamine it is necessary to use an alternative nuclear counterstain in dual fluorescence staining. Bisbenzimide (Hoechst 33258 or 33342) is satisfactory and produces blue nuclear fluorescence when excited with UV light (360 nm). The dye is used at a concentration of 20 μg/ml or less (23). Unlike the halides used for nuclear counterstaining, bisbenzimide can enter live cells and it therefore provides a useful morphological marker in the analysis of cell populations by surface fluorescence staining.

4.8 Retardation of fading

For three decades the inevitable fading of fluorescence during microscopy was accepted as an inherent and intractable problem, and this no doubt played a large part in the quest for alternative non-fluorescent immunolabelling systems. In 1981 the use of para-phenylene diamine was reported (20). This has a very potent effect in retarding fading and is employed at a concentration of 10^{-2} M in the mountant. However, this material undergoes rapid photo-oxidation and furthermore is a recognized skin sensitizer. A more convenient compound was reported in 1982 (21) which although not as potent as para-phenylene diamine in retarding fading nevertheless has a marked effect. This was 1,4-diazabicyclooctane (DABCO) which is extremely stable, non-ionizing and cheap and can be stored without special precautions to avoid skin contact and exposure to light. It is used at a concentration of 2.5 g% in the mountant and can be confidently recommended for all applications of immunofluorescence.

5. FLUORESCENCE MICROSCOPY

The essential requirements for successful fluorescence microscopy are:

(i)   a potent light source with high emission of light corresponding to the excitation wavelength of the fluorochrome used;

(ii) an efficient illumination system for transferring the light energy to the specimen;

(iii)   an appropriate set of filters.

It should be noted that these components can usually be incorporated in a standard microscope to provide a highly efficient but relatively inexpensive instrument.

5.1 **Light source**

Most fluorescence microscopes are equipped with a high-pressure mercury vapour burner. These have a high output of visible as well as UV light although (contrary to earlier belief) the fluorochromes in use require *visible* light for maximum excitation. These light sources have a limited life, e.g. 100 h for the HBO 50 (Wotan) lamp. After this time the quartz capsule becomes increasingly blackened with considerable loss of excitation efficiency and there is, furthermore, increasing risk of explosion. It is therefore essential to monitor the duration of usage, preferably by means of a built-in hour counter.

An alternative light source is the quartz−halogen bulb. This is relatively cheap to instal, requiring only a simple rheostat; it does not lose efficiency with use and eventually the filament fails without risk of explosion. UV output is minimal and although it does not show the mercury lines in the visible region which enhance the excitation of rhodamine (Section 5.3) it provides very satisfactory excitation for fluorescein, especially for immunohistological applications.

5.2 **Illumination systems**

Transmitted light systems based on the use of high performance dark-ground condensers were successfully employed during the development of the immunofluorescence procedure. These have now been superseded by the incident system in which the specimen is illuminated through the objective lens so that the actual surface viewed is exposed directly to the fluorescence-exciting radiation. This system depends on the use of beam-splitting, dichroic mirrors which *reflect* the excitation light onto the specimen and *transmit* back to the ocular the light of wavelength corresponding to the fluorescence emission. The special merit of this system is particularly seen with high magnification objective lenses since all the illuminating light is concentrated on the area that is in view.

The apparent intensity of fluorescence, in addition to the factors dicussed above, is determined by the effective magnification and lens performance. Thus, since brightness is a function of unit area the effect of *doubling* the eye-piece magnification, e.g. from $5\times$ to $10\times$ is to reduce the apparent brightness by a factor of *four*! Similarly an objective lens having a numerical aperture of, for example, 0.9 gives twice the intensity shown by a lens of the same magnification with a numerical aperture of 0.65.

5.3 **Filters**

Two filters are required for fluorescence microscopy; they are complementary and their specification is determined by the spectral characteristics of the dyes employed. The *primary* filter should transmit light of wavelength corresponding to the absorption/excitation peak of the fluorochrome (fluorescein 495 nm, rhodamine 555 nm); light of longer wavelength, in particular corresponding to the fluorescence emission wavelength maximum (fluorescein 525 nm, rhodamine 575 nm) must not be transmitted. This requirement calls for a near-vertical cut-off and is met by the use of interference filters. In the case of the fluorescein filter *broad band* excitation is usually employed, maximum transmission ranging over the visible blue region. *Narrow band* excitation of rhodamine by taking advantage of the high energy peak transmission of the mercury burner in the green region avoids the possibility of incidental excitation of fluorescein with the primary filter used for rhodamine excitation. This is of crucial importance for discrimination between the fluorochromes since the fluorescence emission of fluorescein, which is generally considered to be apple-green, includes an orange/red component. This is easily demonstrated by viewing bright FITC fluorescence through an orange/red coloured glass.

The requirements of the secondary filter are generally met by the use of simple inexpensive glass filters which act as a barrier to the light employed for excitation but give high transmission of the fluorescence emission. A complete filter set for a particular fluorochrome can be assembled in a single unit comprising the primary and secondary filters between which is incorporated the appropriate dichroic mirror; sets of filters for different fluorochromes should be mounted in a simple changeover device so that individual cells (say) may be easily studied for their content of each fluorochrome in turn.

5.4 Photography

Successful photographic recording of the results obtained by immunofluorescence, especially in applications that involve differential staining by two fluorochromes, should be regarded as standard procedure. This can be regularly achieved by attention to the following points.

(i)   Do not attempt to photograph staining that does not appear bright by eye (prolonged exposure merely reduces the contrast with the background).

(ii)   Automatic camera systems rarely give results as good as those obtained by manual control. With experience, the assessment by eye of the relative intensity of specific fluorescence in the context of the total light in the field gives a better indication of the optimum exposure than automated control by full field or 'spot' measurement.

(iii) The camera attachment to the microscope should incorporate a beam-splitter for pre-viewing the field *which can be removed* from the light path before exposure, so that 100% of the light reaches the film.

(iv)   Very high speed emulsions are not necessary. In the author's laboratory immunofluorescence photography is made on standard colour film 64-100 ASA with standard processing (exposure time 10 sec to 1 or 2 min).

(v)   When recording two-colour immunofluorescence it is usually better to take separate exposures for each fluorochrome and subsequently to display the photographs side by side, rather than make double-exposures on a single frame.

(vi)   The use of DABCO to retard fading as recommended in Section 4.7 is a considerable advantage especially for prolonged exposures.

5.5 Confocal microscopy

The recent development of a fluorescence microscope imaging system in which both illumination and detection are confined to a single point in the specimen has eliminated the problem of out-of-focus interference (26). This enables structures to be sectioned optically and has the potential to reveal features that are completely obscured by conventional fluorescence microscopy. It is likely that this new technique will have a considerable impact on studies of cellular structure and organization.

6. STANDARDIZATION

Methods of applying the immunofluorescence procedure cannot be rigidly standardized, and there are many variables in the technique which determine sensitivity. These include, *inter alia*, the choice of substrate, potency of reagents, level of background staining, efficiency of the microscope and observer experience.

In order to monitor sensitivity and thus enable meaningful comparisons of results between laboratories it is necessary to use *internal* standards which have been calibrated against *external* reference preparations. The WHO/IUIS Standardization Committee has made considerable progress in providing such preparations in the field of human autoantibody detection. International Standard Conjugates of FITC-labelled anti-human Ig, IgG and IgM are available from the WHO Immunology Unit, Geneva. These provide yardsticks for assessing the potency *and specificity* of commercial (and other) conjugates in use. Similarly, International Reference Preparations are provided for homogeneous and speckled anti-nuclear antibodies, anti-actin and, most recently, antibodies to double-stranded DNA. It is therefore possible to quantify specific reactions in tests for these antibodies in uniform terms throughout the world.

National External Quality Assessment Schemes for autoimmune serology have now been established. Their function is to monitor the performance of routine clinical laboratories by regular distribution of samples for analysis. The number of participating laboratories in the UK has already reached 192.

In other fields of application no reference preparations are currently available and the only possibility of standardization therefore is by exchange of materials. Progress — at least in terms of specificity — is dependent on the outcome of collaborative Workshops designed to provide a consensus on the reactivity of antibodies with putative specificity.

7. REFERENCES

1. Coons,A.H. and Kaplan,M.H. (1950) *J. Exp. Med.*, **91**, 1.
2. The,T.H. and Feltkamp,T.E.W. (1970) *Immunology*, **18**, 865.
3. Wolfson,W.Q., Cohn,C., Calvary,E. and Ichiba,F. (1948) *Am. J. Clin. Pathol.*, **18**, 723.
4. Titus,J.A., Haughland,R., Sharrow,S.O. and Segal,D.M. (1982) *J. Immunol. Methods*, **50**, 193.
5. Oi,V.T., Glazer,A.N. and Stryer,L. (1982) *J. Cell Biol.*, **93**, 98.
6. Chapple,M.R., Johnson,G.D. and Davidson,R.S. (1988) *J. Immunol. Methods*, **111**, 209.
7. Amante,L., Ancona,A. and Forni,L. (1972) *J. Immunol. Methods*, **1**, 289.
8. Goding,J.W. (1976) *J. Immunol. Methods*, **13**, 215.
9. Bayer,E.A. and Wilchek,M. (1980) *Methods Biochem. Anal.*, **26**, 2.
10. Goding,J.W. (1980) *J. Immunol. Methods*, **39**, 285.
11. Goldman,M. (1968) In *Fluorescent Antibody Methods.* Academic Press, New York, p. 105.
12. Hijmans,W., Schuit,H.R.E. and Klein,F. (1969) *Clin. Exp. Immunol.*, **4**, 457.
13. Johnson,G.D. and Holborow,E.J. (1963) *Nature*, **198**, 1316.
14. Beutner,E.H., Wick,G., Sepulveda,M. and Monin,K. (1970) In *Standardization in Immunofluorescence.* Holborow,E.J. (ed.), Blackwell, Oxford, p. 165.
15. van Dalen,J.P.R., Knapp,W. and Ploem,J.S. (1973) *J. Immunol. Methods*, **5**, 49.
16. Haajman,J.J. and van Dalen,J.P.R. (1974) *J. Immunol. Methods*, **5**, 35.

17. O'Neill,P. and Johnson,G.D. (1970) *J. Clin. Pathol.*, **23**, 185.
18. Sainte-Marie,G. (1962) *J. Histochem. Cytochem.*, **10**, 250.
19. Freer,S.M. (1984) *J. Immunol. Methods*, **66**, 187.
20. Johnson,G.D. and Walker,L. (1986) *J. Immunol. Methods*, **95**, 149.
21. Owen,J.J.T., Wright,D.E., Habu,S., Raff,M.C. and Cooper,M.D. (1977) *J. Immunol.*, **118**, 2067.
22. Johnson,G.D., Goddard,D.H. and Holborow,E.J. (1982) *J. Immunol. Methods*, **50**, 277.
23. Bainbridge,D.R. and Macey,M.M. (1983) *J. Immunol. Methods*, **62**, 193.
24. Johnson,G.D. and Nogueira Araujo,G.M.de C. (1981) *J. Immunol. Methods*, **43**, 349.
25. Johnson,G.D., Davidson,R.S., McNamee,K.C., Russell,G., Goodwin,D. and Holborow,E.J. (1982) *J. Immunol. Methods*, **55**, 231.
26. White,J., Amos,W.B. and Fordham,M. (1987) *J. Cell Biol.*, **105**, 41.

CHAPTER 7

Fluorescence activated cell sorting

ANDREW VAUGHAN and ANNE MILNER

1. INTRODUCTION

Flow cytometry developed as a technique for quantifying the visual picture obtained by microscopic examination of cells or tissues stained with specific antibodies (1). The technique of cytometry allows certain questions to be asked about the antigen distribution on cells that are either impossible to determine microscopically or can be done much faster and inherently more accurately using cytometry. Since its development the applications of flow cytometry have expanded to include quantitation of cellular DNA, both for use in determining cell cycle phases and in the analysis of chromosomes. Other more specialized applications are being continually developed. This chapter will concentrate on the practicalities of getting started in flow cytometry by describing actual studies undertaken with cytometry equipment. Most of the applications discussed here may be carried out on all currently available machines, though some devices are not sold with a cell sorting capability. The particular studies described below were undertaken primarily with a Becton Dickinson (BD) fluorescence activated cell sorter (FACS) 440, though some data was taken from an Ortho Cytofluorograph IIs.

Examples of the studies made possible by cytometry can be contrasted with microscopy.

(i) Antigen expression through a population of cells. Cells stained with a specific fluorescent antiserum and examined with a microscope may appear brighter or duller than the average. Though an attempt may be made at quantitation of this effect by a skilled microscopist, a more accurate method is the automatic recording of the fluorescent content of each cell using cytometry.

(ii) Small populations of antibody reactive cells. It is a very time-consuming task to examine slides of stained material in the search for antigen expression at very low frequency. Using cytometry, large numbers of single cells, typically 1000/sec, may be examined and the percentage of the target population recorded.

(iii) Cells stained with two or more antisera. Both the above applications could be carried out using only a microscope. Some studies, however, cannot realistically be attempted without the speed and recording ability of a flow cytometry system. Here the ability to record the fluorescent content of single cells using two or more fluorochromes attached to different antibodies allows a picture of the expression of antibody reactive molecules in that population. Such pictures can, with appropriate controls, be stored for comparison with repeat experiments or with data from other centres.

The above list provides only a very brief illustration of the potential applications of flow cytometry. Before considering specific applications we will review the technology that makes cytometry possible.

2. BACKGROUND TECHNOLOGY

To those who are unfamiliar with the theory and practice of cytometry the hardware can seem initially very complex. Though, to their credit, the major manufacturers have marketed increasingly 'user friendly' devices, there is still an aura of mystique that surrounds cytometry. In fact the underlying theory of cytometry is very simple. There are many extensive and excellent reviews on the subject (2−8) and so here we will concentrate only on the basic principles of cytometry operation.

A strong light source, usually a laser but not necessarily so, illuminates single cells passed through it in a thin stream of fluid. If a cell passing through the light contains a fluorochrome this will be stimulated to emit light of a different colour which may be detected by a photomultiplier tube (PMT). In addition, the original light beam will be deflected by the cells' presence. This deflected beam may also be detected by a PMT and gives crude information on the cell size. The PMT is similar in concept to television but running in reverse, the PMT taking in light signals and turning them into electricity, the amount of which is recorded by an appropriate medium, such as a floppy disc.

There are therefore three principle stages in cytometry as shown in *Figure 1*. Here we will consider the salient parts of each stage in turn.

2.1 **Light source**

This is usually either a laser or a mercury arc lamp. The latter sources are to be found in small bench top devices used primarily for simple repetitive analyses. The laser power source is able to generate a more intense light spot on the cell and therefore offers a more sensitive system.

2.2 **Optics**

To work effectively the light beam, sample stream and collection optics all have to be correctly aligned. The adjustment of these parameters is very important and each manufacturer has their own recommended procedure. All, however, are quite straight-forward in that they depend on adjusting for optimum signal output into each PMT. It is important that these adjustments are regularly checked as the device will work with incorrect settings but the data recorded cannot then be compared with repeat studies. After the light signal has been generated it is passed through appropriate lenses and mirrors to reach the PMT detector. Within this process optical filters are used to isolate the appropriate colour so that each detector is exposed only to the desired light signal such as green, red or scattered light.

2.3 **Data accumulation**

After light has interacted with the cell the PMT detectors will record all the light of each particular colour associated with each cell. This information is transmitted by the PMT as a specific voltage to the data collection device. Put simply, weakly fluorescent

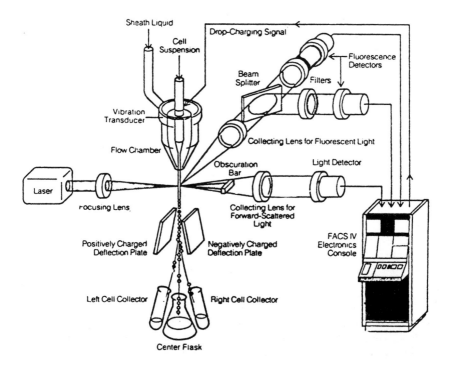

Figure 1. Diagrammatical representation of a Becton Dickinson FACS IV flow cytometer, demonstrating the light source, optics, data collection and sorting capability.

cells give rise to a low voltage signal and strongly fluorescent cells give rise to a high voltage signal. The data is then recorded as a digital code reflecting the magnitude of the original light output.

The data is usually represented in one of two ways; either a frequency histogram or a two-dimensional correlated plot as in *Figures 2* and *3*, respectively. The histogram is constructed by setting a scale from low to high voltage (equivalent to each cell's light output) and a unique position is assigned to each cell within the scale. The accumulation of individual data gives a profile of the measured parameter through the population. The correlated plot does the same thing but records two parameters for each event, thus a two-dimensional representation of the data is obtained. A third option of three parameter representation is available where another parameter is correlated to the first two. This requires some computer processing to give the appearance of three dimensions on a flat screen. Our individual experience of this form of data is that it looks very impressive but is difficult to interpret routinely or explain to a third party; far better to draw a series of one- or two-dimensional plots.

Operation of cytometers can generate large volumes of data very rapidly; thus it is important to have sufficient room for storage on either hard or floppy disc systems. The manipulation of data after recording is handled almost entirely by the in-house computer programmers of the major manufacturers. This makes subsequent utilization of data a relatively simple task and is dependent on the manufacturer's expertise. The

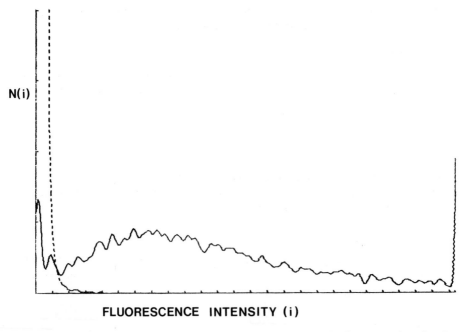

Figure 2. Single colour quantitation of a determinant on the cell surface. The fluorescence intensity of a specific monoclonal antibody (solid line) was compared with that of an irrelevant antibody (dotted line).

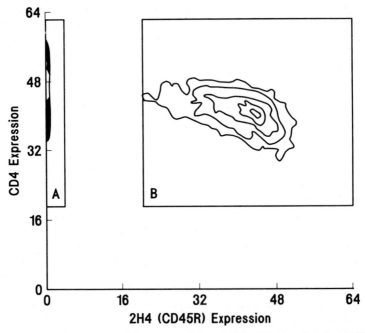

Figure 3. Two colour analysis of the expression of CD4 and 2H4 (CD45R) on the cell surface. Red fluorescence (2H4−PE) was plotted versus green fluorescence (CD4−FITC). Cells expressing both antigens appeared in the upper right-hand quadrant (**B**). Cells expressing only CD4 appeared in the upper left-hand quadrant (**A**).

competitive nature of the market-place has made the data processing software in general very good, and responsive to changing demands from users.

3. GETTING STARTED

The decision to purchase a cytometer is constrained by many factors, not the least being financial. In terms of equipment the two major manufacturers, Becton Dickinson and Coulter, offer a similar range of machines in terms of applications; these cover a three tier system aimed at different application areas.

3.1 **Level 1 equipment**

The least expensive are bench top analyser machines with a relatively low power light source. These are primarily aimed at repetitive routine studies as might be found in a hospital-based diagnostic laboratory.

3.2 **Level 2 equipment**

The second level of equipment consists of fully automated, laser-beam cytometers with the option of a cell-sorting capability. These machines are now largely automated and make a suitable 'entry level' purchase for research-based applications.

3.3 **Level 3 equipment**

The most expensive devices retain a substantial degree of manual control over all operational settings and are thus both more adaptable to novel research needs and more complex in terms of routine operation. It is clear that the purchase of a suitable machine requires some care in order that current and any future applications can be met with the chosen equipment. The larger machines may have specific requirements such as three-phase power supplies and water cooling that require the machine location to be carefully considered in terms of service access. If at all possible any cytometer should have a specific sole-use room assigned to it.

Most of the applications listed below can be carried out on all cytometers. In those cases where there is a restriction on a technique this is noted as being suitable for level 1, 2 or 3 equipment, level 1 being the simplest machines and 3 the most complex, according to the grading system above.

After the selection of appropriate equipment the next most important step is to ensure that the equipment is supported by an active users' group. These organizations are usually benevolently sponsored by the major manufacturers and are a vital link between the manufacturer's support of the hardware and the day-to-day operations of the equipment in order to generate data. These organizations offer an invaluable resource as a forum for the exchange of techniques and applications; for the newcomer to cytometry their importance cannot be over-emphasized. Finally the journal *Cytometry* contains many articles dedicated to theory, practice and research with this type of equipment.

4. CYTOMETRY OPERATION

4.1 **Calibration**

For any application in cytometry it is essential that the machine is optimally adjusted. In practice this means that the optical system is so arranged that it intersects the cell stream at the correct point for optimal generation of fluorescence or scatter data. To enable this to be done accurately standard particles are offered which possess carefully controlled scatter and fluorescence properties. The two most widely used are:

(i)   Fixed chicken red blood cells. These cells are of quite uniform size and fluoresce in the green wave band when exposed to blue laser light.

(ii)   Stained latex beads. These particles have the advantage of being available in a range of sizes attached to a variety of fluorochromes and are accurately controlled in the amount of fluorochrome and intrinsic size.

  A typical calibration procedure would be as follows.

(i)   Attach the calibration particle sample to the machine and start the flow of sample through the system, using between 100 to 500 mW if laser-based. It is easiest to calibrate the machine by accumulating dual parameter data, that is displaying each particle event on a TV screen in terms of both its light scatter and fluorescence properties.

(ii)   The machine optics and sample stream controls are then adjusted to generate maximal signals on the TV screen. The adjustments themselves differ for each machine; for this refer to the manufacturer or appropriate users' group.

(iii)   When the signals are optimized the effectiveness of the calibration may be quantified by reference to the coefficient of variation (CV) of both the scatter and fluorescence signal according to the formulae below.

$$CV = 100 \times SD/X$$

More simply, for a display that approximates to a Gaussian distribution the mean channel is equal to the peak channel number and the CV can be taken from the width of the distribution at half the maximum peak height:

$$CV(hm) = 0.424 \times W(hm)/100X$$

where X is the mean channel number of the distribution, SD is the standard deviation and $W(hm)$ is the width of the distribution at half the peak height.

  As is clear from the formulae, the derived CV is dependent on the channel number of distribution; it is therefore important to accumulate data in the same region for each analysis. *Figure 4a* and *b* shows histograms of results for both correctly and incorrectly set up fluorescent latex beads. In the case shown the poor resolution was produced from an incorrect alignment of the optics. Poor resolution may be due to any or all of the problems mentioned in Section 4.2.

4.2 Factors highlighted by calibration procedure

4.2.1 *Incorrect optical or cell stream adjustment*

(i)   Correctly align the optics starting closest to the laser entry to the optical system and end at the relevant PMT. Inspection of the data histograms will show the location of problems.

(ii)   If both forward scatter and 90° fluorescence and scatter are poor, the basic

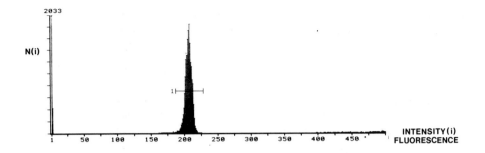

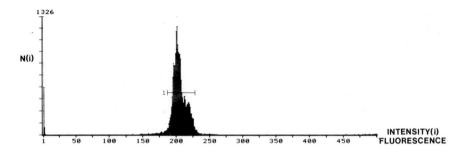

Figure 4. Fluorescence histogram of 1.9 μm fluorescence-stained polystyrene beads recorded on an ortho cytofluorograph IIs. (**a**) Optics aligned; CV = 2.4; (**b**) slightly defocused; CV = 4.4.

alignment of the laser/stream interaction should be looked at. An adequate fluorescence signal but poor forward scatter indicates that adjustment is probably required beyond the laser/stream intersection point on the forward scatter side. However, this is unfortunately not a foolproof rule as most adjustments will perturb both axial and 90° light impulses. This finding is significant in machine operation and occurs with some level 2 and all level 3 machines. Level 1 machines are much simpler to adjust.

4.2.2 *Dirty optics*

The cleaning procedures are important and must be done carefully. A golden rule here is never to rub the lenses with anything. In the sample stream area, lenses may become contaminated with salt and cellular debris. Most lenses in this area are vertical.

(i)   Apply a small amount of distilled water to a folded lens tissue and place it on the lens; it should adhere. Wait a few seconds for the deposits to dissolve and gently slide off the tissue. Repeat as necessary.

(ii)   For stubborn deposits, perhaps burnt on by laser heat, use either ethanol or acetone.

4.2.3 *Particle blockage*

This may be only slight but sufficient to disturb the CV.

(i)   Flush sample collector through with water or 5% sodium hypochlorite.
(ii) Less likely is a degradation of the laser signal due to incorrect lasing conditions. See the laser manual for the appropriate check list.

5. APPLICATIONS OF CYTOMETRY

5.1 **Measurement of cell cycle**

5.1.1 *Theory*

The division of mammalian cells is classically separated into 'G$_1$', a gap phase, followed by 'S', where DNA synthesis occurs leading to 'G$_2$', a further gap followed by 'M', mitosis. From G$_1$ to G$_2$/M the amount of DNA essentially doubles; a DNA-specific dye will therefore give cells in G$_2$M twice the fluorescence of those in G$_1$. Cytometry detects these fluorescence increases and from that it is possible to estimate the proportion of cells in each part of the cell cycle (*Figure 5*).

5.1.2 *Equipment*

Bench centrifuge
Cytometer level 1−3
37°C water bath

5.1.3 *Method 1, using dispersed living single cells*

(i) *Reagents.*

Fixing buffer; 0.07% paraformaldehyde, 0.1% Triton X-100 in saline
DNA stain (see below). Stock solution of 2 mg/ml propidium iodide (PI) in water
PI-stained beads

(ii) *Protocol.* Wash cells twice with appropriate ice-cold medium, and resuspend in fixing buffer at a concentration of one million/ml. Add the DNA stain to give a final concentration of 50 μg/ml and leave for 15 min prior to analysis.

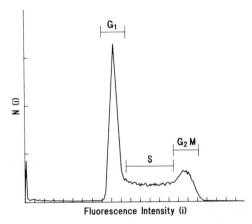

Figure 5. Cell cycle analysis of the CHO cell line. Cells were stained with PI and analysed for fluorescence intensity.

5.1.4 *Method 2, from paraffin-wax-embedded material*

This method may be used with any conventionally fixed and paraffin-wax-embedded material. It allows the retrospective determination of the cell cycle in historical samples of fixed tissue.

(i) *Reagents.*

(1)   Ethanol−water solutions; 100, 90, 70 and 50% with respect to ethanol.
(2)   1% Pepsin solution of activity 2500−3500 U/mg in 0.9% saline made to pH 1.5 with 2 M HCl (Sigma).
(3)   0.01 M Tris buffer containing 5 μM $MgCl_2$, pH 7.0.
(4)   PI stain; 1 mg/ml in Tris buffer (Sigma).
(5)   Ribonuclease Type 1-AS; 2 mg/ml, 50−75 U/mg, in Tris buffer (Sigma).
(6)   35 μm nylon mesh (R.Cadish, Finchley, London, UK).

(ii) *Protocol.*

(1)   Cut two 30 μm thick sections from the fixed tissue and place in xylene for 10 min to remove the wax.
(2)   Rehydrate the specimen by placing in 100, 90, 70, 50% ethanol for 10 min each, ending up in distilled water.
(3)   At this stage incubate in the pepsin solution for 1 h with frequent shaking, preferably by vortex mixing.
(4)   Count the number of cells recovered; greater than 100 000 is preferred, otherwise reprocess a further section(s).
(5)   Centrifuge them for 10 min at 2500 r.p.m. and resuspend in 1 ml of the Tris buffer.
(6)   Filter through 100 μm nylon gauze and store at 4°C.
(7)   Prior to analysis, incubate the cells with 0.5 ml of PI stain, and an equal volume of the ribonuclease solution for 15 min at 37°C to remove double-stranded DNA.
(8)   Run the sample as shown below. If cell clumping is still a problem pass the cells through a 25-G needle and filter through 35 μm nylon mesh.

5.1.5 *Method 3, from fresh tissue (tumour etc.)*

This method is generally applicable to a range of tumour types. Other, more complex, recipes have been used containing enzyme mixtures such as trypsin and collagenase and these should be investigated in cases of difficulty.

(i) *Reagents.*

(1)   0.5% Pepsin solution at 2500−3500 U/mg in 0.9% saline, made to pH 1.5 with 2 M HCl.
(2)   Fixing buffer; 0.07% paraformaldehyde and 0.1% Triton X-100 in phosphate-buffered saline (PBS).
(3)   Staining buffer; made by adding 45 ml of 0.1% sodium citrate to 45 ml of fixing buffer and 10 ml of PI solution (20 μg/ml in water).
(4)   Ribonuclease Type 1-AS (Sigma).

(iii) *Protocol.*

(1) Cut samples of tumour into approximately 3 mm cubed pieces. Chop pieces as small as possible using two crossed scalpel blades working against each other. It is easier if no medium is present at this stage to restrict the movement of tissue.

(2) Place the pieces in a 10 ml Pyrex centrifuge tube with 3 ml of the pepsin buffer. Incubate for 30 min at 37°C whilst drawing sample up and down a hypodermic syringe using a 19-G needle.

(3) Filter the suspension through the nylon gauze and centrifuge the result at 500 *g* for 10 min.

(4) Resuspend the pellet in 2 ml of staining solution and add 0.1 g of RNase and incubate for 15 min at 37°C.

5.1.6 *General method of analysis*

(i) Prepare the machine by setting an appropriate light path to a PMT for the collection of red fluorescence and calibrate with PI beads, record all machine settings, PMT voltages, gains, etc.

(ii) The most usual activating light source will be the 488 nm line from an Argon laser. This will require a filter system such as a 620 nm long pass, in front of the PMT collecting the red fluorescence. This filter will only transmit light of longer wavelength than 620 nm (red) and will thus not respond to the activating 488 nm (blue) laser line. The exact filter set will depend on the light source and fluorochrome used (see *Table 1*, p. 221).

5.1.7 *Data acquisition*

(i) Run the sample and collect data from at least 20 000 cells as red fluorescence from the PI in the DNA.

(ii) Show the data in histogram format and spread this out such that the G_1 can be discriminated from the S and G_2/M stages (if present).

(iii) Store data on computer for subsequent analysis.

5.1.8 *Analysis*

Almost without exception cytometers are supplied with some programme or method for quantitating the relative proportion of cells in G_1, S and G_2/M. With cell cycles derived from material in normal growth such patterns are easily interpreted to discriminate each component of the cell cycle. Cells from tumour material that contain variable amounts of DNA per cell are not suitable for an automated analysis system and will require individual inspection to determine the best analytical approach. The approach used will depend on both the cell type and the information required (9 – 11).

5.1.9 *Points to note*

There are a range of fluorochromes that will bind to DNA and can be used to analyse the cell cycle, these may be useful for particular light sources in individual machines (see *Table 1*, p. 221 for listing).

The Hoechst dyes have the advantage of being able to penetrate living cells and bind to DNA. This gives the potential for sorting viable cells based on cell cycle phase.

However, the intimate association of the dye with DNA may affect the subsequent viability and biological activity of such labelled cells. In addition the dye requires activation in the UV region, a considerable disadvantage for most equipment (13−16).

5.2 Single colour analysis for the quantitation of a single determinant on human cells (HLA class II)

5.2.1 *Theory*

Monoclonal antibodies recognize a single unique determinant and will bind to this on the surface of or within cells. The tagging of antibodies with a fluorochrome allows for the quantitation of the determinants through a population of cells (*Figure 2*).

5.2.2 *Equipment*

Bench centrifuge
Cytometer level 1−3

5.2.3 *Method*

(i) *Reagents*

(1)   Specific antibody.
(2)   Irrelevant antibody of same species and subclass.
(3)   Second antibody recognizing the first antiglobulin linked to fluorescein isothiocyanate (FITC), this may be a F(ab)$_2$ fragment.
(4)   Diluent medium; 10% fetal calf serum and 1% human serum in PBS.
(5)   Human lymphocytes.

(ii) *Protocol.*

(1)   Set up an appropriate light path to a PMT. If using laser 488 nm excitation place a 530 nm long pass filter in front of the PMT to accept the green FITC light and exclude the blue 488 nm.
(2)   Calibrate the machine with FITC-labelled beads.
(3)   Wash one million cells twice with diluent medium and resuspend cell pellet.
(4)   Incubate 200 μl of specific antibody, at a concentration of approximately 1:20 (if bought commercially), or irrelevant control antibody with the cells held on ice for 30 min. Certain antibodies can be used at a lower concentration; this must be found by experiment.
(5)   Wash twice with ice-cold medium and incubate cells with labelled second antibody for 30 min on ice.
(6)   Wash twice with ice-cold medium and analyse within 1 h.

5.2.4 *Data acquisition*

Run sample with the suspected highest fluorescence first and ensure that the brightest cells are collected on the data screen. For antibody-stained cells it is possible to collect data on a log scale; this is particularly useful for cells expressing a wide range of fluorescent intensities or for detecting small populations with low antigen expression. In this case it may also be beneficial to increase the laser power to 500 mW. Collect

20 000 events and store the histograms.

The median channel number is the most appropriate way to quantitate fluorescence distributions. This is more accurate than a mean figure as it takes into account the shape of the distribution. The median of the control sample may be subtracted from the test data to give an index of the specific fluorescence in each population. More use may be made of the data by quantitating the number of cells expressing a particular degree of brightness and using this to compare different populations. If using a log scale the peak fluorescent channel is used to represent the distribution (17−20).

5.2.5 *Points to note*

There are a range of fluorochromes that can be used for single colour analysis. These may be bought commercially attached to a variety of antibodies (see *Table 1*, p. 221).

5.3 **Two colour analysis for the quantitation of two human lymphocyte populations (CD4 and a subgroup CD45R) in human peripheral blood: introduction to gating**

5.3.1 *Theory*

The use of two colour fluorescence supplied by different specificities of antibody allows for the quantitation of two determinants on the same cells, and analysis of cell populations expressing one, or both antigens, or neither.

5.3.2 *Equipment*

Bench centrifuge
Cytometer level 1−3

5.3.3 *Method*

(i) *Reagents.*

(1)   CD4 monoclonal antibody (BD) coupled to FITC and 2H4 (Coulter) monoclonal antibody (anti-CD45R) coupled to phycoerythrin (PE).
(2)   Irrelevant antibody of same species and subclass as control.
(3)   Washing and diluent buffer; 2% BSA and RPMI 1640.

(ii) *Protocol.*

(1)   Prepare a human monoclonal cell suspension by Ficoll centrifugation using standard techniques. Wash three times in buffer to remove traces of Ficoll which otherwise can cause non-specific absorption of antibodies.
(2)   Add anti-CD4 at a dilution of 1:40 in buffer and anti-CD45R at a dilution of 1:50.
(3)   Incubate both antibodies together with the cells, on ice to prevent capping. The use of directly labelled antibodies is required for dual label studies because a second layer antiglobulin (e.g. goat anti-mouse immunoglobulins) would not discriminate between the two mouse monoclonal antibodies of different specificity, unless they were antibody isotype-specific, which is unnecessarily complex.

(4) Wash three times in buffer at approximately 300 g for 10 min and resuspend at one million/ml. Set appropriate light paths to the PMT tube using selective filters as described in *Table 1* (p. 221).

5.3.4 *Data acquisition*

(i) Most equipment will require adjustment for spill-over of fluorescence from the green to red channels and vice versa. Set the equipment to acquire data on two parameters, green in the x direction and red in y. For BD FACS 440 equipment the green (FITC) sample is run first and examined for signal contamination in the red channel; this is removed by altering the signal compensation. The green signal is further adjusted to place the events in the upper (x) half of the screen. Similarly run the red sample (PE) only and adjust the compensation and gain to place these events on the right (y) half of the screen. Double-positive cells should now fall in the upper right screen quadrant, double-negative in the lower left and cells expressing single colours will occupy their own specific quadrants (*Figure 3*).

(ii) Collect 20 000 events for each sample and run calibration beads of both green and red fluorescence to standardize the machine settings (21−25).

5.3.5 *Points to note*

(i) Logarithmic scales are preferable to linear for dual colour work as this emphasizes the distinction between positive and negative cells. In this case the peak channel is the appropriate parameter for quantifying the data.

(ii) The number of channels per decade will vary for each machine and this should be determined for each machine, especially if cross-comparisons between machines are envisaged.

(iii) A useful control for direct dual label experiments is a cell line that does not express either determinant.

(iv) Though an indirect labelling assay could be devised using appropriate antibody specificities, a problem may be encountered using PE in that the large size of the molecule may sterically inhibit the binding of other antibodies, especially in a multi-layer system.

(v) For a single laser cytometer the combination of FITC and PE are the most effective in monitoring two determinants. A single laser can also be used to monitor the cell cycle in combination with an FITC antibody, though in some cases the PI can quench the FITC signal; an FITC sample alone would be needed to check this. Dual laser machines may use a greater number of alternative fluorochromes, which increases the possible number of determinants that can be measured in the same cell population.

5.3.6 *Gating*

With the data acquired by dual fluorescence analysis many questions can be asked concerning the expression of each target determinant through the population of cells. It is possible with most equipment to pre-select a particular population of cells for acquisition. For example it may be that only cells with both markers are of interest.

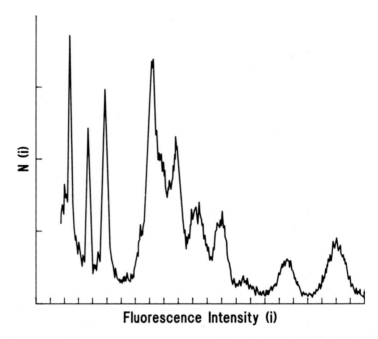

Figure 6. Fluorescence histogram of chromosomes prepared from the CHO cell line. Individual pairs of chromsomes bind varying amounts of PI and appear as discrete peaks with varying fluorescence intensity.

In this case an electronic 'gate' can be set around these cells, in the upper right quadrant in this example. The machine will then only accumulate data that arrives through this gate. There is not much point in doing this in the example quoted but the technique is a powerful one in that gates may be set around parameters other than those being accumulated on-screen. In the example used a gate might be set around a particular light scatter property of the cell that is associated with larger proliferating lymphocytes (see Section 6). Thus the distribution of the determinants analysed is restricted to these larger cells. In this way more data is gained about the distribution of the target determinants in relation to the physiology of the cell. Specifically this technique compresses more information into the dual or single parameter plot.

5.4 Analysis of the individual chromosomal content of cell populations using the Chinese hamster ovarian (CHO) cell line as a model

5.4.1 *Theory*

Individual chromosomes vary according to the amount of DNA they possess; their physical size is one of the principal parameters used to identify them unambiguously. A direct DNA stain such as PI will quantitatively bind to the DNA such that the largest chromosomes have the most stain. A histogram of PI fluorescence should show peaks of light intensity corresponding to the relative DNA content of chromosomes of varying size (*Figure 6*).

5.4.2 *Equipment*

Cytometer level 2 or 3

5.4.3 *Method*

(i) *Reagents.*

Hypotonic buffer; 50 mM KCl, 10 mM $MgSO_4$, 5 mM Hepes salts
0.15 mg/ml RNase A, pH 8.0, in the buffer
Colcemid (Gibco)
CHO cells
PI stain 20 μg/ml in water
Triton X-100
PI-stained calibration beads (1−5 μm)
Balanced salt solution

(ii) *Protocol.*

(1) Grow cells in a monolayer culture in 250 ml culture flasks and use when in log phase growth.
(2) Block cells in metaphase by the addition of 10 ml of a balanced salt solution containing 0.05 μg/ml Colcemid for 2 h prior to harvesting.
(3) Shake off mitotic cells and centrifuge for 8 min at 100 g.
(4) Resuspend cells in the hypotonic buffer. Centrifuge and resuspend in same buffer pre-warmed to 37°C and leave for 10 min at that temperature.
(5) Adjust the cell concentration to 100 000/ml and cool on ice for 10 min.
(6) Add 10% of total volume of 2.5% Triton X-100 and incubate for 10 min on ice; release chromosomes by passaging 4−5 times through a 22-G needle.
(7) Stain with PI to a final concentration of 50 μg/ml, leave on ice for 15 min, then analyse.

5.4.4 *Data acquisition*

(i) Run the PI beads with an appropriate filter (*Table 1*) and set up the machine to give the smallest CV for both forward scatter and fluorescence. This set up is most important for chromosome analysis in that multiple peaks are expected; their individual resolution will directly depend on the accuracy of the setting of the optical system.
(ii) Run the sample at a flow rate of less than 500/sec and inspect the fluorescence histogram. Adjust the gain settings such that the histogram fits into the screen and collect 50 000−100 000 events. The large chromosomes will be displayed on the right and the small on the screen left (25−29).

5.4.5 *Points to note*

(i) This technique is one of the more difficult to accomplish successfully. The reasons for this are not entirely clear but the majority opinion is that it can be attributed to the cells and their processing. It may be that certain cells, in particular the chemical or physical makeup of the nuclear chromatin, are not suitable for this type of analysis. Some workers have suggested that the buffers used to release the DNA are critical. Digitonin has been used to prepare the chromosomes in place of the hypotonic buffer plus Triton X-100, though with considerable batch-to-batch variability. It remains a matter of experiment to design the most appropriate conditions for the cells used.

(ii)   Alternative DNA dyes such as Hoechst 33342 and 33258 have been used and these give good resolution when at least 100 mW of UV laser power is available. Ethidium bromide can also be used but this may give more cross-talk if used in conjunction with an FITC probe.

(iii)   Further processing of the data may usefully be done to improve the resolution by examining a dual parameter plot of forward scatter against fluorescence. This displays the chromosomes as discrete islands according to scatter and fluorescence. Setting individual gates around each island and accumulating fluorescence data through them can give improved resolution on a subsequent fluorescent histogram.

(iv)   There has been much interest in using this technique to construct libraries of human genetic material. This depends on isolating individual chromosomes by making use of the sorting capability of some cytometers (see Section 5). This task is perfectly possible but is restricted by the numbers of chromosomes that can be isolated. If 1000 chromosomes may be sorted per second (a considerable feat with most commercial equipment) then a 1 h sort would generate approximately 3.6 million chromosomes, or about 1 μg of DNA. In practice considerably less would be expected. Depending on the application this may severely limit construction of DNA libraries containing worthwhile amounts of genomic material.

5.5 Cell and particle sorting: isolation of G_1 and G_2/M cell populations

5.5.1 *Theory*

Particles passing through a cytometer system are analysed extremely quickly, the process is complete within a few millimetres of particle transit time after laser interaction. Sorting exploits this rapid analysis by causing an oscillation of the sample stream such that the stream breaks up into droplets after the analysis process has taken place. Prior charging of the sample stream with a negative or positive charge makes the droplets containing the cells move in response to an external electric field set up by two high voltage plates either side of the sample stream. Rapid switching of the polarity of these plates causes particular particles to move either left or right according to parameters that have been pre-programmed into the particle analysis. Luckily, the practice of sorting is rather simpler than the theory surrounding it! Although most systems differ in the way they are set up, all require that the analytical step is meshed with the final sorting process such that the correct particle is selected. The following protocol specifically describes the FACS 440 system.

5.5.2 *Equipment*

Cytometer level 2 or 3
Cells stained for cell cycle (see Section 5.1)

5.5.3 *Method*

(i) *Droplet formation.* Set the machine for sample stream flow but no sample throughput. Switch on the head drive unit (this is a piezioelectric transducer incorporated within the stream nozzle). This will vibrate the nozzle such that droplet formation occurs. Droplet formation is visualized by a stroboscopic lamp triggered by the transducer frequency. This 'freezes' the droplet production process for inspection. The formation of droplets can be checked by microscope, if no droplets are seen, adjust the head drive frequency and amplitude.

(ii) *Side stream selection.* Check that right and left side stream controls are at 8 o'clock and the centre control at 12 o'clock. Switch on the 'calibrate' signal, 'test sort' and 'high tension' to the plates. This will send a test signal to the sorter processor such that equal proportions of drops are sorted left and right. This should enable the side streams to be visualized. Some care in the lighting of the sample chamber, dimming the room lights for example, may help in identifying them. Adjust the central and side streams with the controls to deposit the streams into the central and side containers. At this stage adjust the stream controls to hit the sample tube obliquely to slow the cells down before coming to rest. This avoids the stream impacting with high velocity at the base of the tube. Final side stream adjustment is carried out with the phase control to produce a clean wisp-free jet.

(iii) *Meshing drop selection with analysis step.* Switch off 'calibrate' and 'test sort'. Start the sample running and measure the drop delay from the laser intersection to the first drop constriction. The measurement will be shown on the micrometer gauge attached to the microscope. Input this measurement via the 'drop delay' switch. Set number of deflected drops to three. Inspect the two-dimensional display of scatter versus DNA fluorescence and set windows around the required G_1 and G_2M regions.

The machine should now be sorting the cells into the required populations $(30-34)$ (*Figure 7*).

5.5.4 *Points to note*

(i)   Sterile sorting can be achieved by flushing the system with 70% ethanol for 30 min prior to sorting. Take the usual steps to sterilize all other equipment in contact with the cells.

(ii)   The jet diameter is important in determining the drop break-off point. For each nozzle this point will have to be determined separately. If no droplets can be seen try a smaller nozzle size.

(iii)   Determine the drop delay when the sample is running, as the sample's presence can affect the cut-off point.

(iv)   Partial blockages will change the break-off point so it is important:

    (a)   to watch the sample streams;

    (b)   to make sure the sample is as free as possible from debris and clumps of cells.

(v)   The droplet selection of three is the slack in the analysis system. If the particle

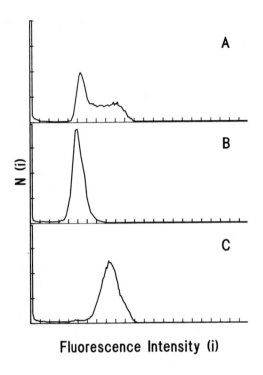

Fluorescence Intensity (i)

Figure 7. Cell cycle sort gates were placed around the G_0/G_1 and G_2M phases of the cell cycle which were then sorted. (**A**) Represents the original cell cycle; (**B**) the resulting G_0/G_1 sort and (**C**) the resulting G_2M sort.

is actually in the droplet behind or in front then this will be collected as all three droplets go the same way. Further accuracy can be achieved by:

(a)   reducing the cell concentration in the sample below one million/ml;

(b)   reducing the droplet selection below three.

(vi)   It is useful to cross-check the performance of the machine by examining the sample microscopically and comparing the yield of cells sorted with the electronic report the machine generates.

(vii)   A high flow rate will generate more aborted sorts as the selection criteria cannot be met; this will not affect purity, however. With slow flow rates evaporation may be a problem unless the collection tubes are pre-filled with medium. This latter point is worthwhile whatever the flow rate as media may be placed in the tubes which both cushions the cells arrival and offers a more appropriate medium for cell survival than the PBS used in the flow system.

(viii)   Glass tubes are preferred for the collection of sample as they do not readily become charged, unlike plastic, which would deflect the sample streams. Siliconized glass is the best of all.

5.6 **Identification of leukocyte contamination in lymphocyte preparations using correlated light scatter**

5.6.1 *Theory*

Narrow angle light scattering from a perfect, spherical particle has been described mathematically and, in general, larger particles scatter more light. However, even for perfect spheres, the mathematics are very complex. Thus for approximations of spheres, such as cells, it is empirically a reasonable first assumption that larger cells will scatter more light. However, it must be remembered that the relationship between cell size and light scatter is only a rough approximation, unlike Coulter sizing which measures volume directly. Therefore the relationship between light scatter and cell size must always be used cautiously. In addition to narrow angle light scatter most machines can also accumulate light scatter at 90°, or side scatter. This is presumed to indicate scattering events that occur within cells such that multiple reflective events generate the high angle of reflection. For cells this can be used to give information on the internal structure of the cell.

The cells of the blood offer a unique system in terms of light scatter analysis in that they possess a wide range of cell sizes. These range from the small lymphocytes to large granulocytes and in the latter cell type they express a structurally unique cell constitution in terms of the many cytoplasmic granules. It is therefore possible to discriminate between the white cells of the blood based on only dual light scatter measurements.

5.6.2 *Equipment*

Bench centrifuge
Cytometer levels 2 and 3 (some level 1)

5.6.3 *Method*

(i) *Reagents*.

Fresh whole blood
Buffered salt solution
Lymphoprep (Flow Labs)

(ii) *Protocol*.

(1)   Separate a lymphocyte-rich population from whole blood using an appropriate separation medium such as Lymphoprep. Remove the lymphocyte-rich layer at the blood/Lymphoprep boundary by pipette aspiration.
(2)   Wash the result three times in medium to remove debris and Lymphoprep.
(3)   Resuspend cells in PBS at one million/ml and run on the machine using 488 nm laser light and collecting forward and 90° scatter in a correlated plot. The various components of the blood will appear as shown in *Figure 8* (35,36).

5.6.4 *Points to note*

(i)   It is possible to get a better illustration of the total leukocyte content of blood using other separation methods. In almost all cases conventional, automated

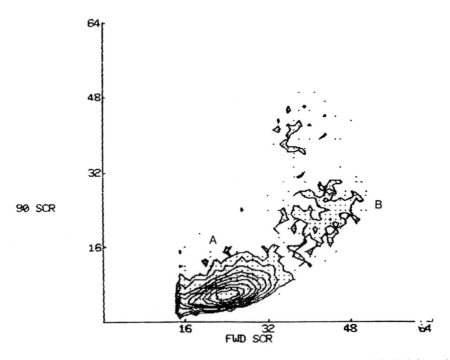

Figure 8. Light scatter analysis of leukocyte sub-populations. Leukocytes were analysed for both forward and 90° scattered light. Lymphocytes could be seen as a distinct population (**A**). Monocytes (**B**) scattered more light in the forward and 90° direction.

       techniques of routine cytology give a more rapid and preferable method of total leukocyte counts. Light scatter analysis is primarily useful as a method of checking that antibody binding occurs within a defined population of cells.

(ii)   The complexity of light scattering mathematics means that other laser wavelengths will give unique distributions of cell populations.

6. OTHER APPLICATIONS

Described above are the basic operations carried out with flow cytometers. There are a large number of more specialized applications that have made use of flow cytometry analysis, some of which are briefly discussed below. For further information consult the references given. In almost all cases the advantage to be gained from using a flow system is the generation of data from single cells rather than entire populations.

6.1 Fluorescence polarization measurements

Certain chemicals such as 1,6-diphenyl-1,3,5-hexatriene (DPH) exhibit changes in the plane of polarization of the emitted light dependent on the local environment. For example free fluorescein is almost completely depolarized but when attached to albumin it becomes polarized. DPH when incorporated into cell membranes can give information on the 'fluidity' of the membrane environment (37).

Table 1. Principal excitation and emission lines of fluorochromes used in flow cytometry.

	Exciting wavelength (nm)	Emission wavelength (nm)
Fluorochromes that bind to DNA		
Ethidium bromide	518	610
Propidium iodide	540	625
Mithramycin	421	575
Hoechst 33342, 33258	352	460
Fluorochromes suitable as antibody labels		
Fluorescein isothiocyanate (FITC)	494	517
Texas red isothiocyanate	545	575
Phycoerythrin (PE)	488	600

6.2 Bioreductive reactions leading to fluorescent compounds

Many human and animal tumours contain a significant number of hypoxic cells that are relatively resistant to radiotherapy. Certain compounds such as Nitroakridin 3582 are capable of being nitroreductively metabolized into a fluorescent product within the oxygen-deficient environment of hypoxic cells. This technique could therefore be used to detect the presence of hypoxic cells *in vivo* by the rapid extraction and analysis of tumour material (38).

6.3 DNA damage

Nuclei extracted from irradiated cells have been analysed by laser scatter and used to indicate DNA damage. Here the damage within the nucleus results in a relaxation of the supercoiled arrangement of nuclear DNA, causing a physical expansion of the extracted nucleus as the supercoils unwind (39).

6.4 Calcium ionophores

Certain compounds have the ability to fluoresce specifically when bound to particular metals. Indo 1 has been used to follow the rapid time course of calcium mobilization in platelets, a change that takes place over a $10-15$ sec period (40).

7. REFERENCES

1. Herzenberg,L.A., Sweet,R.G. and Herzenberg,L.A. (1976) *Sci. Am.*, **234**, 108.
2. Fulwyler,M.J. (1980) *Blood Cells*, **6**, 173.
3. Kruth,H.S. (1982) *Anal. Biochem.*, **125**, 225.
4. Norman,A. (1980) *Med. Phys.*, **7**, 609.
5. Miller,R.G., Walande,M.E., Mccutcheon,M.I., Stewart,S.S. and Price,G.B. (1981) *J. Immunol. Methods*, **47**, 13.
6. Horan,P.K. and Wheeless,L.L. (1977) *Science*, **198**, 149.
7. Van Dilla,M.A., Dean,P.N., Waerum,O.D. and Melamed,M.R. (1985) In *Flow Cytometry: Instrumentation and Data Analysis*, Van Dilla,M.A. (ed.), Academic Press, New York.
8. Melamer,M.R., Mullaney,P.F. and Mendelsohn,M.L. (1979) *Flow Cytometry and Sorting*.
9. Fried,J. (1976) *Comput. Biomed. Res.*, **9**, 263.
10. Dean,P.N. (1980) *Cell Tissue Kinet.*, **13**, 299.
11. Gray,J.W. (1976) *Cell Tissue Kinet.*, **9**, 499.
12. Lyndon,M.J., Keeler,K.D. and Thomas,D.G. (1980) *J. Cell. Physiol.*, **102**, 175.
13. Crissman,H.A. and Tobey,R.A. (1974) *Science*, **184**, 1298.
14. Krishan,A. (1975) *J. Cell Biol.*, **66**, 188.
15. Fallon,R.J. and Cox,R.P. (1979) *J. Cell. Physiol.*, **100**, 251.

16. Walker,L., Guy,G., Brown,G., Rowe,M., Milner,A.E. and Gordon,J. (1986) *J. Immunol.*, **58**, 583.
17. Abo,T. and Balch,C.M. (1981) *J. Immunol.*, **127**, 1024.
18. Balch,C.M., Ades,E.W., Loken,M.R. and Shore,S.L. (1980) *J. Immunol.*, **124**, 1845.
19. Lowe,J., Ling,N.R., Forrester,J.A. and Cumber,A.J. (1986) *Immunol. Lett.*, **12**, 263.
20. Gordon,J., Walker,L., Guy,G., Brown,G., Rowe,M. and Rickinson,A. (1986) *Immunology*, **58**, 591.
21. Scollay,R. (1982) *Adv. Exp. Med. Biol.*, **145**, 157.
22. Parks,D.R., Hardy,R.R. and Herzenberg,L.A. (1983) *Immunol. Today*, **4**, 145.
23. Rudd,C.E., Morimoto,C., Wong,L.L. and Schlossman,S.F. (1987) *J. Exp. Med.*, **166**, 1758.
24. Salmon,M., Kitas,G., Gaston,J.S.H. and Bacon,P.A. (1988) *Immunology*, in press.
25. Watson,J.V., Sikora,K. and Evan,G.I. (1985) *J. Immunol. Methods*, **83**, 179.
26. Turner,B.M. and Keohane,A. (1987) *Chromosoma*, **95**, 263.
27. Young,B.D., Ferguson-Smith,M.A., Sillar,R. and Boyd,E. (1981) *Proc. Natl. Acad. Sci. USA*, **78**, 7727.
28. Gray,J.W., Carrano,A.V., Steinmetz,L.L., Van Dilla,M.A., Moore,D.H., Mayall,B.H. and Mendelsohn,M.L. (1975) *Proc. Natl. Acad. Sci. USA*, **72**, 1231.
29. Stubblefield,E., Cram,S. and Deavan,L. (1978) *Exp. Cell Res.*, **94**, 464.
30. Gregory,C.D., Edwards,C.F., Milner,A.E., Wiels,I., Lipinski,M., Rowe,M., Tursz,T. and Rickinson,A.B. (1988) in press.
31. Mekada,E., Yamaizumi,M. and Okada,Y. (1978) *J. Histochem. Cytochem.*, **26**, 62.
32. Hulett,H.R., Bonner,W.A., Barrett,J. and Herzenberg,L.A. (1969) *Science*, **166**, 747.
33. Schaap,G.H., Van Der Kamp,A.W.M., Ory,F.G. and Iongkind,J.E. (1979) *Exp. Cell Res.*, **122**, 422.
34. Stovel,R.T. and Sweet,R.G. (1979) *J. Histochem. Cytochem.*, **27**, 284.
35. Salzman,G.C., Cromwell,J.M., Martin,J.C., Trutillo,T.T., Romero,A., Mullaney,P.F. and Labauve, P.M. (1975) *Acta Cytologica*, **19**, 374.
36. Loken,M.R. and Houck,D.W. (1981) *J. Histochem. Cytochem.*, **29**, 609.
37. Schrepp,G.H., Josselin de Joy,J.E. and Jonkind,J.F. (1984) *Cytometry*, **5**, 188.
38. Begg,A.C., Hodgkiss,R.J., McNally,N., Middleton,R.W., Stratford,M.R.L. and Terry,N.H.A. (1985) *Br. J. Radiol.*, **58**, 645.
39. Milner,A.E., Vaughan,A.T.M. and Clarke,I.P. (1987) *Radiation Res.*, **110**, 10.
40. Davis,T.A., Dratts,D., Weil,G.J. and Simons,R. (1988) *Cytometry*, **9**, 138.

CHAPTER 8

Antibodies for tumour immunodetection and methods for antibody radiolabelling

GILLIAN D.THOMAS, PETER W.DYKES and ARTHUR R.BRADWELL

1. INTRODUCTION: HISTORICAL PERSPECTIVE

This chapter describes the sequence of techniques involved in the production of an antibody scan for *in vivo* radioimmunodetection (RAID) of a tumour expressing a given antigen. Where relevant methods have been detailed elsewhere in this book the reader is referred to the appropriate chapter.

Administration of antibodies for diagnostic or therapeutic purposes is not a new concept. Passive immunotherapy was introduced to clinical practice in 1891 when Emil von Behring developed the first diphtheria anti-toxin. This was followed by an attempt to raise antisera against a human osteogenic sarcoma in two dogs and an ass in 1895 (1). Injection of antibody was followed by a reduction in the size of a tumour on the chest wall. Subsequently, 50 cases were treated in this way and successful results claimed (2). Other workers were unable to substantiate these results at that time and even in recent years there has been an almost complete failure to show more than minimal and transient anti-tumour effects in occasional patients.

Proof of specific *in vivo* antibody localization in tumours awaited the development of techniques for isotopic protein labelling. Radioiodinated rabbit anti-kidney antibodies were shown to localize in rat kidney (3), and subsequently anti-tumour antibodies injected i.v. in mice showed similar localization to the antigenic site (4). Convincing evidence for specific antibody localization was provided in 1957 by a paired-labelling technique (5) in which a specific tumour antiserum and non-immune serum, each labelled with a different radioisotope, were injected into tumour-bearing animals. Specific antibody localization was confirmed by counting both isotopes in tissue samples. This group further demonstrated that tumours in animals could be shown by external scintigraphy after radioactive antibody localization (6). These results suggested the possibility of similar studies in humans but there was, at this time, little knowledge of human tumour antigens. The first successful imaging of human tumours was described in 1967 when fibrinogen in tumours was targeted using radioiodinated rabbit anti-fibrinogen and uptake was convincingly demonstrated. The first clinical radioimmunotherapy study followed (7).

The discovery of tumour-associated antigens (TAAs) provided the next impetus. Carcinoembryonic antigen (CEA) was the first of such antigens and radiolabelled anti-CEA localization in patients with a variety of cancers was elegantly demonstrated in 1978 (8). Other localization studies followed rapidly (9,10) and included other targets such as human chorionic gonadotrophin and α-fetoprotein (AFP) (11,12). The advent

Table 1. Clinical studies with radiolabelled antibodies.

Antibody type	Tumour type	Uptake ratio (U)	% Injected activity/g tumour	Reference[a]
AP	mixed	2.5	–	1
Pab	germ cell	40[b]	–	2
Mab	kidney	2.3	–	3
Pab	colon	2.5	–	4
AP	colon	3.6	0.0033	5
Mab	mixed	4	0.0026	6
Mab	colon	2.3	0.005	7
AP	hepatoma	5	–	8
Mab	colon	2–5	–	9
Mab	melanoma	4.3	0.0057–0.01	10
Mab	breast	4	–	11
Mab	colon	2.5	–	12
Mab	colon	3	–	13
Mab	breast	>2	–	14
Mab	melanoma	2.3	0.0036	15
Fab$_2$	melanoma	2.4	0.0017	15
Mab	ovary	2.2	–	16
Mab	various	1.22–35.8[c]	0.015	17
Mab	bone	2.8[b]	–	18

Pab, Polyclonal antibody; AP, Affinity purified polyclonal; U, Tumour to normal tissue ratio in surgically resected samples.
[a]For full citation of table references see Appendix in Section 9 of this chapter.
[b]One sample only.
[c]Sample taken 12 days post-injection.

of monoclonal antibodies (Mabs) allowed many novel TAAs to be discovered. This accelerated research and there are now many publications indicating the use of antibodies for localization and therapy (see *Table 1*). Nevertheless, therapeutic and diagnostic success has been limited and many problems remain.

The term 'uptake ratio' has been used to describe the ratio of radioactivity within the target tissue relative to that in control normal tissue. It is difficult (or perhaps impossible) to prepare an antibody absolutely specific for a tumour, and non-specific uptake of macromolecules by tumours and other tissues masks the accumulation from the specific antibody–antigen interaction. In the majority of studies uptake ratios of below five have been obtained and it must be stressed that RAID is still an experimental and not a routine procedure.

2. CHOICE OF ANTIBODY
Antibody properties which may affect the uptake ratio are considered in this section.

2.1 Monoclonal versus polyclonal
The advent of Mabs seemed theoretically to offer the ideal answer to many difficulties. They could be prepared exclusively to tumour-specific antigens with no cross-reacting antibodies, and there would be no need for affinity purification. Indeed, there is some *in vitro* and animal work to show that some have superior tumour uptake in comparison

with polyclonal antisera, but this has not yet provided important clinical benefits. There are several reasons for this.

(i) No human tumour-specific antigen has been discovered; indeed CEA is as specifically tumour-related as many of the more recently described antigens.

(ii) An apparently specific Mab may bind unexpectedly to similar determinants on other antigens.

(iii) The affinity of the antibody may have to be high, which has not been easy to achieve.

(iv) Mabs also have idiosyncratic properties which create difficulties in purification, radiolabelling and *in vivo* stability.

2.1.1 *Specificity*

Polyclonal antisera contain both specific and irrelevant antibodies. The proportion of the former should be as high as possible for RAID. Affinity chromatography has been used to isolate the antibody fraction which reacts with the target antigen from the irrelevent fraction. Problems which may arise from the use of this technique, however, include antibody damage resulting from harsh disruptive elution conditions (13) or loss of high affinity antibody if less severe elution conditions are applied. The results obtained in RAID studies with crude polyclonal antibodies and affinity purified antibodies have been similar. In general, Mabs tend to be of lower affinity and it has proved difficult to improve on high-grade polyclonal antisera.

Screening of antibody interaction with a range of normal tissues is required even for affinity purified or monoclonal antibodies as unexpected cross-reaction may occur; for example a Mab against a peptide sequence in a tumour-associated protein may recognize a similar sequence in a completely different antigen. The extreme specificity of Mabs may reduce tumour accumulation if the quantity of antigen is limited, especially if the antibodies can only recognize one binding site (epitope) per antigen molecule. In contrast, several antibody molecules may attach to each antigen when a polyclonal antiserum is used.

As regards the relevance of the antigen location, it is logical to aim the antibody at a cell surface antigen, although successful scans have been performed with antibodies directed against antigens that are not primarily cell surface components, for example AFP (12) and thyroglobulin (14). By this means the observed 'capping' and loss of cell-surface-bound antibody (modulation) that occurs with (divalent) antibodies is avoided. Overall, the antibody localization results were similar to those obtained with surface antigens, perhaps reflecting the multiple factors that determine scanning success in patients. Monoclonal antibodies may not induce modulation, but this needs to be investigated. Alternatively, use may be made of modulation by labelling the antibody with an isotope which is subsequently retained intracellularly (see Section 3).

2.1.2 *Affinity and avidity*

It has been assumed that a high affinity antibody is required for RAID, with a suggested affinity constant of at least 10^{10} M^{-1} (15) but supporting experimental data is not available. The avidity of an antibody may be defined as the net combining strength of an antibody with antigen and is determined by both affinity and valency. IgM antibodies have the highest avidity despite their low affinity and for this reason might be expected to perform well as imaging agents; however, the relatively slower release of this much larger molecule from the circulation has to be taken into consideration. Successful imaging of xenografts in animals has been achieved using both intact monoclonal IgM and its pepsin-derived antigen-binding fragment F(ab')$_2$ (16) but clinical reports are lacking.

2.1.3 *Species and subclasses*

Radiolabelled sheep or goat IgGs have been used predominantly as the scanning agents in RAID studies involving polyclonal antisera. The main consideration in the choice of an appropriate species has been the requirement for low uptake of immunoglobulin by Fc receptor-bearing cells in the recipient. High Fc interaction results in rapid clearance from the circulation, allowing insufficient time for antibody uptake by tumour and resulting in accumulation of labelled antibody in the liver, spleen and bone-marrow. This results in poor tumour localization and false positive areas on the scans, but can, by contrast, be advantageous for a second antibody given to clear background radiation once the first has bound to its target (see Section 2.3). The affinity of heterologous immunoglobulin for human Fc receptors shows differences both between species and between different immunoglobulin classes and subclasses (17). Rabbit IgG is bound strongly by human Fc receptors while sheep IgG$_1$, for example has particularly low Fc interaction. Murine IgG$_{2a}$ has high Fc interaction whilst murine IgG$_1$ has intermediate characteristics. Idiosyncratic results may occur in the case of individual Mabs and each subclass varies in its stability during purification, labelling and storage. Careful selection of Mabs is therefore essential. Reticulo-endothelial uptake of murine Mabs has presented difficulties *in vivo* in RAID studies (18). This problem may be circumvented by selection of a polyclonal antibody from a species with low Fc interaction, for example sheep, or by selection of a murine Mab with low Fc uptake from a panel of antibodies. An alternative approach is to prepare Fab fragments of an antibody in which Fc uptake has proved a problem (see Section 2.2).

2.2 **Fab fragments**

One approach to improving uptake ratios has been the use of antigen-binding antibody fragments. Diffusion of these fragments into tumours occurs more rapidly than with whole immunoglobulin (15) but excretion is also faster. Higher uptake ratios have been achieved with both Fab' and F(ab')$_2$ fragments of four anti-CEA Mabs than with the intact antibodies in xenograft models (19). However, the absolute concentration of fragments in the tumours was lower than that of intact antibodies due either to their more rapid elimination or lower affinity. The advantage of an improved uptake ratio is therefore counterbalanced by a loss in absolute counts. Clinical RAID studies (20) suggested that better results were obtained with a F(ab')$_2$ fragment than with the intact murine Mab, but the percentage of positive scans which was achieved with intact antibody was lower than usual. Studies using either intact affinity purified goat polyclonal antibody or its Fab' fragments or murine Mabs for anti-CEA imaging in humans showed no difference in the results (21).

Removal of the Fc portion of the immunoglobulin molecule does offer advantages when Fc uptake of the intact immunoglobulin has presented a problem. $F(ab')_2$ fragments of a monoclonal anti-melanoma antibody have been shown to be superior to whole immunoglobulin for RAID due to a marked reduction in antibody uptake by bone-marrow, liver and spleen resulting from the Fc interaction which occurred with a murine Mab (18).

2.3 Second antibody

A further approach to improved uptake ratios has involved the administration of a clearing second antibody directed against the first (22). The resultant immune complex is cleared by the reticulo-endothelial system, which recognizes Fc regions, and then degraded with elimination of the label. The second antibody technique is most effective at removing circulating antibody, but extravascular sites are poorly cleared. The probable mechanism of second antibody clearance is combination with first antibody followed by reticulo-endothelial uptake (liver, spleen and bone-marrow) via Fc receptors. The second antibody must have a strong affinity for human Fc receptors, and rabbit IgG seems ideal. It should preferably be affinity purified and needs to be given in a specific antibody dose at least 5-fold greater than that of the first antibody. The optimal time of injection appears to be at 24 h, but repeated doses may be preferable, and there is little detailed data on the best regimen.

The second antibody removes little unbound first antibody from the extravascular space, and since this contains at least 50% of the injected dose the effect is inevitably limited. The redistribution of radioactivity to other organs achieved by the second antibody is a disadvantage in terms of scan interpretation because false positive hot spots may arise in the liver, spleen and marrow. However, a substantial increase in clearance of unbound labelled first antibody has been achieved in animals by using a second antibody and in patients given second antibody, counts of radioactivity in the blood have fallen more than twice as quickly as in control subjects, yet tumour counts have been maintained (23).

This second antibody technique can be applied to whatever antibody system is being used provided it does not generate spurious uptake in reticulo-endothelial sites. The optimal system has yet to be evaluated.

3. CHOICE OF RADIOISOTOPE

Selection of a suitable antibody radiolabel requires consideration of a number of factors. These include the physical and biological half-lives, γ energies emitted, decay products, particle radiation, availability, expense and the ease of antibody radiolabelling. Ideally, radionuclides which are particularly suited for imaging should have a physical half-life of $2-4$ days with a similar biological half-life, a γ energy range of $150-200$ keV, small abundance and low energy particulate radiation and good radiolabelling chemical properties and stability. The biological half-life is dependent upon the antibody biochemistry and the isotope chemistry. If the isotope forms a stable bond with the antibody and there is no antibody damage, then the biological handling (rate of removal) is similar to that of the native antibody. This will have a half-life of days to weeks (25 days for normal human IgG), depending upon the species of origin, immune status of the patient, size of the tumour, etc. Release of isotope usually occurs during antibody catabolism but it may be stripped off before the protein is broken down. Once released, the isotope chemistry determines its subsequent fate. Thus one of the problems associated with use of iodinated antibodies is dehalogenation *in vivo*. This has been suggested as a major factor in the low tissue uptakes observed, and in the elution of radioactivity from tumours. Some isotopes, notably metals including Indium-111 (^{111}In) (Section 3.2.1), are retained intracellularly so this rapid loss of free label is avoided.

There are relatively few isotopes which have the required properties for antibody imaging and none which is completely ideal. ^{111}In and three isotopes of iodine have been shown to be suitable: ^{99m}Tc is being evaluated for labelling fragments.

3.1 Radioiodine

Iodination is a safe, reliable method for radiolabelling proteins, and antibodies in particular seem tolerant of it. Nearly all studies of radiolabelled antibodies have used iodine isotopes.

3.1.1 Iodine-131

Iodine-131 has been used as the radiolabel in most RAID studies. The physical properties of this isotope include a 360 keV γ emission, β particulate radiation and an 8 day half-life which is compatible with the peak tumour accumulation of antibody 24−48 h after administration. The biological half-life of free iodine is approximately 2 days. The whole body dose received from 74 MBq (2 mCi) of ^{131}I-labelled antibody is 1 rem (24) which is acceptable if not ideal, and radioiodination procedures are straightforward. The disadvantages of this isotope are that the emission of β particles increases the tissue dose about 5-fold without adding externally detectable radiation, and that the high energy γ emission is relatively poorly detected by present γ cameras; the count density of the resultant scan is therefore low. When all factors are considered, however, there is no clearly superior alternative.

3.1.2 Iodine-123

Iodine-123 has an ideal decay energy for γ camera detection (159 keV) but its short half-life (13 h) requires early localization. This isotope has been used successfully for RAID studies (25) but the availability of this isotope is limited, the labelling efficiency is lower than ^{131}I and the isotope is costly. In addition the 159 keV photopeak overlaps with that of technetium (140 keV) which cannot therefore be used for background subtraction (Section 3.2.2).

3.1.3 Iodine-124

Iodine-124 has a half-life of 4 days and emits positrons which produce characteristic 'annihilation radiation' of 511 keV on interaction with electrons. Positron emission tomography requires a very sophisticated camera (of limited availability) which detects the source of this radiation with good spatial resolution and high sensitivity. However, the isotope is not generally commercially available, is expensive, and conjugation to antibody has proved difficult.

3.2 **Radiometal chelates**

The binding of antibody to cell surface antigens may result in rapid movements of the membrane and either shedding of the antibody – antigen complex, or internalization and degradation. In the case of iodine-labelled antibodies, rapid de-iodination and excretion occurs. In contrast, a stable cellular label leads to trapping and intracellular concentration. Indium and other metals are retained in this way but, unlike the iodine isotopes, cannot be induced to form covalent bonds with proteins. Labelling is by covalent attachment of a strong chelating group to the antibody and this then binds the metal.

3.2.1 *Indium-111*

The potential advantages of this radiolabel include an optimal physical half-life of 68 h and twin photopeaks of 171 and 245 keV. The major disadvantage is that significant hepatic accumulation of radioactivity occurs and the long biological half-life results in an absorbed dose equal to that from [131]I. Count rates achieved with ^{111}In are high but it is only suitable for use in scanning organs distant from the liver.

3.2.2 *Technetium 99m*

(i) *Labelling.* This is the most widely used isotope for tracer studies in nuclear medicine, with a half-life of 6 h giving a high count rate over the period of investigation and a wide margin of safety for out-patient use. It decays with a peak γ emission energy of 140 keV and is conveniently prepared locally by elution of a column of [99]Mo, its parent compound, which has a half-life of 67 h. Technetium decays rapidly, its chemistry is poorly understood, and the method of production results in a very impure preparation. Despite this it has been used to label proteins but its short half-life makes it unsuitable for RAID in which accumulation of antibody occurs at the tumour site over a period of days unless fragments are used, in which case labelling with ^{99m}Tc may be optimal.

(ii) *Subtraction.* A useful technique is to use the longer-lived ^{131}I or ^{111}In as the antibody label and to give ^{99m}Tc alone just before scanning when the antibody has had time to accumulate. The distribution of ^{99m}Tc should be the same as that of the antibody except where there is specific antibody – antigen binding and so, in theory, subtraction of the technetium from the iodine or indium scan yields an image of the tumour only (26).

3.3 **Indium-111 versus iodine-131 scans**

Because half of a given amount of ^{111}In has decayed after 68 h, while for ^{131}I the same process takes 8 days, there must be proportionately more disintegrations per second (Becquerels) detectable from the ^{111}In source, mole for mole. Hence ^{111}In as an antibody label gives higher count rates and hence better resolution on the scan for a given number of antibodies bound to tumour than does [131]I (*Figure 2*), but with the disadvantage of being concentrated in the liver (*Figure 1*). This means that a large area of the abdomen and a common site of metastatic spread cannot be assessed for positivity. Iodine is concentrated by the thyroid gland in the neck (and to a lesser extent by the gastric mucosa), but this can be prevented by the prior administration of thyroid-blocking

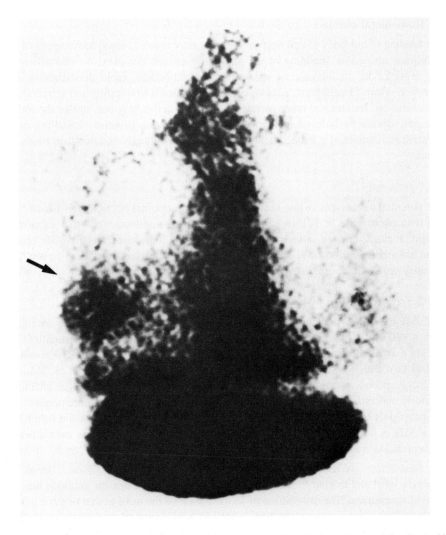

Figure 1. Anterior view of the chest showing a 5 cm carcinoma in the right breast (arrowed) localized with an ^{111}In-labelled sheep antibody against epithelial membrane antigen. The tumour to normal tissue uptake ratio was 7:1 3 days after injection. (Reproduced from ref. 42 with permission.)

drugs. Once the antibody is metabolized, free iodine is rapidly excreted allowing repeat scans to be performed and minimizing the whole body dose, while indium scans remain positive for a very long time and result in larger whole body doses since the source of radiation is trapped intracellularly.

4. PREPARATION OF LABELLED ANTIBODY FOR INTRAVENOUS INJECTION

Antibodies to the chosen TAA are prepared from immunized animals in the form of polyclonal antisera or Mabs as described in Volume I, Chapters 2 and 3, respectively.

An IgG-rich fraction can be prepared from polyclonal antisera by precipitation followed by ion-exchange chromatography (Volume I, Chapter 2) and non-specific antibodies are adsorbed onto glutaraldehyde polymers of human serum and normal tissues; the specificity of the post-adsorption serum may then be assessed by immuno-electrophoresis (Volume I, Chapter 6) and haemagglutination (Volume I, Chapter 7). Affinity purification (Volume I, Chapter 5) may be omitted as it can cause loss of the highest-affinity antibodies, as discussed above (Section 2.1.2).

A specific antibody—antigen reaction may be demonstrated on tissue sections using, for example, the peroxidase—antiperoxidase technique (Chapter 7). Titre and affinity are tested by radioimmunoassay (Chapter 3) and protein concentration measured by optical density. The resultant purified specific antibody must then be radiolabelled and rendered sterile and pyrogen-free for use in human subjects. Factors of importance in radiolabelling are:

(i)   prevention of damage to the IgG molecule, particularly the antigen binding sites;
(ii)   protection of the worker from radiation exposure;
(iii)   ensuring a rapid, reliable and sterile procedure.

4.1 Purity of preparation

4.1.1 *Sterility*

(i) *Antibody preparation.* To ensure that bacterial contamination is minimal:

(1)   sodium azide (0.5%, w/v) should be added as soon as possible after collection of blood from immunized animals; this is toxic but will be separated from the antiserum by chromatography in the process of purification;
(2)   all containers should be cleaned, baked to destroy pyrogens, and sterilized according to established methods (27);
(3)   buffers should be made from analytical grade reagents, using either pyrogen-free or triple-distilled water;
(4)   dialysis tubing should be boiled before use;
(5)   column chromatography materials should be autoclaved and flushed with pyrogen-free buffer or sterilized by γ-irradiation.

Standard laboratory distilled water may be mildly pyrogenic and dialysis alone is insufficient to remove these pyrogens; ion-exchange chromatography is necessary in addition and must be carried out carefully using a low ionic strength starting buffer and collecting only the peak IgG fraction.

(ii) *Radiolabelling.* Labelling of antibodies is carried out in a downward laminar-flow cabinet which must be clinically clean. An adjacent clean area of the laboratory should be reserved for patients' materials. Sterile disposable gloves must be worn, and preferably a surgical gown, cap and face mask to reduce transmission to solutions for injection of infectious agents carried from other areas, or in the nose and throat. Radiation protection is considered in Section 4.1.4.

4.1.2 *Pyrogen testing*

Each batch of antibody must be tested in animals for the presence of pyrogens and this is usually carried out by independent laboratories according to a standard protocol (27). The antibody is diluted in saline (0.85%, w/v BP) to give five times the dose given

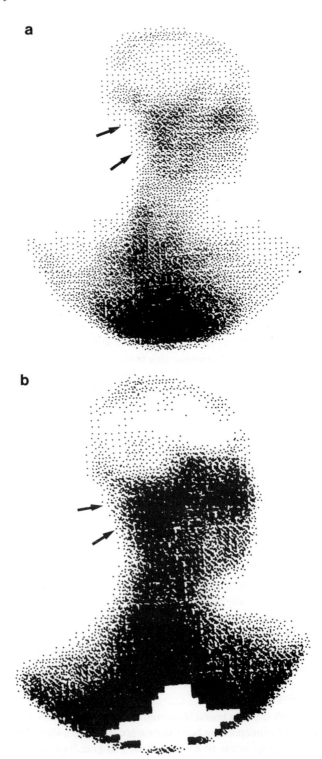

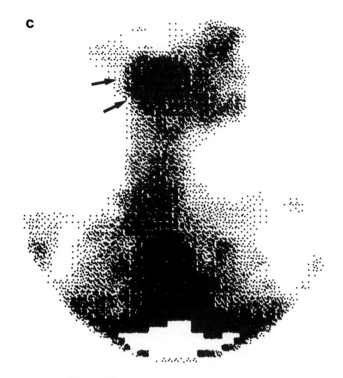

Figure 2. Comparison of [131]I- and [111]I-labelled anti-CEA in the same patient. All scans are unsubtracted and the arrows indicate a deposit of CEA-producing squamous carcinoma near the right temporomandibular joint. (**a**) [131]I scan at 24 h; (**b**) [111]In scan at 24 h; (**c**) [111]In scan at 5 days. The greater count rates from ^{111}In are seen together with its gradual accumulation in the tumour. (Reproduced from ref. 43 with permission.)

to humans to each of three rabbits. The antibody passes the test if the summed response of the three rabbits does not exceed 1.15°C, conversely the material fails if the summed response exceeds 1.15°C. Material for humans may only be administered if it passes this test. Equivocal responses are not acceptable.

4.1.3 *Storage*

Each batch of antibody should be clearly labelled in case adverse reactions should occur despite the above precautions. Storage should be in sterile tubes at −70°C in small aliquots (e.g. 0.5 ml).

4.1.4 *Radiation dosimetry*

Before working with any source of radiation it is essential to be familiar with the *Ionising Radiations Regulations* (28) and the local rules available in each authorized establishment. By adhering to standard precautions the dose received from handling the small amounts of radioactive substances involved in antibody labelling is minimized and should be negligible. For ^{131}I it has been measured at 0.27 pSv/Bq using finger dosemeters. This compares with the official permissable yearly dose limits of 500 mSv for the hands or 50 mSv for the whole body of non-pregnant workers over the age of 18. It is, however, advisable for the worker to take thyroid-blocking drugs (e.g. KI, 120 mg) before each iodination procedure to protect the thyroid in case of accidental ingestion of radioiodine.

4.2 Radiolabelling of antibodies by iodination

Many procedures have been described for the radioiodination of proteins (29). All involve methods of converting the relatively unreactive iodide into a more reactive species such as free iodine or the positively charged iodonium ion. Experience is required to perform any one method satisfactorily, which may explain why reliable methods continue to be preferred despite claims of superiority for others.

The number of iodine atoms substituted per protein molecule must be carefully controlled if the antibody is not to be damaged. Ideally, one iodine atom should be substituted onto each antibody molecule, since this will result in minimal damage. For Chloramine-T, an oxidizing agent to antibody ratio of 20:1 gives optimal and reliable radioiodination reactions. This has also been found to cause minimal damage to the antibody, while giving labelling efficiencies of up to 90%, and specific activities of up to 5 mCi/mg protein.

For radioimmunodetection $200-400$ μg of antibody is radiolabelled, taking aseptic precautions, with ^{131}I (Amersham International) using one of the methods given below. The radiolabelled antibody is separated from free iodine by gel chromatography (Sephadex G25) and then centrifuged overnight at 20 000 g to remove large protein complexes. Repeat 0.2 μm filtration is then performed and the antibody is dispensed into a sterile vial. The final activity is measured and the radiolabelled antibody can be administered to the patient intravenously as soon as is convenient. The dose is $1-1.5$ mCi for an investigational procedure.

4.2.1 *The Chloramine-T method*

This has been used extensively to iodinate various proteins (30). Chloramine-T is a potent oxidizing agent which converts iodine to a more reactive form. The reaction is classically terminated by the addition of a reducing agent, sodium metabisulphite, but this may be omitted and the reaction terminated instead by gel filtration on Sephadex G25 (*Table 2*). This avoids exposing antibody to harsh reducing conditions which may cause denaturation.

4.2.2 *The solid phase lactoperoxidase method*

Peroxidase-catalysed iodination takes longer than other methods but is easily controlled and requires almost negligible quantities of the oxidizing catalyst. It is a very gentle technique yielding labelled products with high immunoreactivity and minimal damage. Linked to an insoluble matrix or Sepharose beads and used as a suspension, the enzyme is easily removed by centrifugation: unlike soluble lactoperoxidase, the Sepharose-bound enzyme remains active after several iodinations (31) (*Table 3*).

4.2.3 *The Iodogen method*

Iodogen is an oxidant and virtually insoluble in water and so acts as a solid phase oxidizing system under aqueous conditions. It is removed from the reaction when the aqueous phase of the solution is decanted, and so reducing agents are not required.

Table 2. The Chloramine-T method.

1.   Drain the preservative from a 10 ml Sephadex G25 disposable column (PD10, Pharmacia) and wash through with 30 ml of sterile saline. Apply 1 ml of human serum albumin (HSA; 10% w/v, BTS, Blood Products Laboratory) followed by 10 ml of sterile saline.
2.   Place $200-400$ μg of IgG in a sterile reaction vial with 10 μl (or 10% of the total volume) of 0.3 M sodium phosphate buffer pH 7.0, $37-148$ MBq $(1-4$ mCi) of Na^{131}I (Amersham International, IBS 30) and 50 μl (20 μg) of Chloramine-T (Sigma; from a solution of 10 mg in 25 ml of sterile normal saline, made up immediately before use). Time reaction from addition of Chloramine-T.
3.   Mix for 1 min with a Finn pipette and then transfer into the gel filtration column.
4.   Add 1 ml of saline to the column followed by a further 4 ml.
5.   Collect the column eluate into a sterile centrifuge tube containing 1 ml of HSA.

Table 3. The solid phase lactoperoxidase method.

A. *Preparation of solid phase – lactoperoxidase suspension*

1.   Wash 15 ml of Sepharose 4B[a] with distilled water and inspect microscopically for bacterial contamination or bead breakage.
2.   Suspend in 15 ml of H_2O in an ice bath, maintaining a suspension with a magnetic stirrer throughout.
3.   Adjust to pH 11.0 with 10% NaOH.
4.   Add excess cyanogen bromide (CNBr) (4 g/30 ml of suspension).
5.   Monitor the pH, adding NaOH (10%) to keep it between $10.8-11.2$.
6.   On completion of the reaction wash rapidly on a coarse sintered glass funnel under gentle vacuum using ~ 5 vols of cold coupling buffer[b].
7.   Transfer the desired quantity of activated beads to a flask containing lactoperoxidase (Sigma) in $15-25$ ml of cold coupling buffer and agitate overnight at 4°C.
8.   Wash thoroughly with cold coupling buffer.
9.   Suspend in 0.2 M glycine containing 0.1 M NaPO$_4$ (pH 7.5) for at least 5 h in the cold.
10.   Wash thoroughly and store at 4°C in phosphate-buffered saline (PBS) (pH 7) containing 10^{-5} M merthiolate (wash off with PBS before use).

B. *Coupling of antibody to solid phase*

1.   Place $200-400$ μg of the antibody in 10 μl of 0.05 M sodium phosphate buffer pH 7.4, in a sterile vial with 20 μl of 0.5 M sodium phosphate buffer pH 7.4, $37-148$ MBq $(1-4$ mCi) Na^{131}I, $10-20$ μl of the solid phase – lactoperoxidase suspension and 10 μl of H_2O_2 solution (BDH Ltd; 100 vols diluted 1:100 000 with distilled water).
2.   Vortex-mix these reagents and leave for 10 min, then add 10 μl of H_2O_2 solution.
3.   Vortex-mix the iodination vial every 5 min throughout the reaction.
4.   After 30 min stop the reaction by adding 100 μl of 0.05 M sodium phosphate buffer pH 7.4, containing 0.1% sodium azide (to inhibit the enzyme) and 100 μl of 0.05 M phosphate buffer pH 7.4, containing 1% HSA (to act as a carrier for chromatography).
5.   Precipitate the solid phase lactoperoxidase by centrifugation (7000 g for 5 min) and apply the supernatant to the chromatography column as in *Table 2*.

[a]The solid phase can consist of either Sepharose 4B (Pharmacia) as above or a copolymer of maleic anhydride and butanediol divinyl ether (Merck).
[b]1 vol. 0.1 M NaCl, 1 vol. 0.01 M NaPO$_4$ pH 7.4.

However, a greater loss of immunoreactivity and more damage to proteins have been associated with this method (*Table 4*).

An alternative method is to use Iodogen as a thin film on the bottom of a glass vial using either methylene chloride or chloroform as the volatile solvent. With the aqueous suspension and above method, plastic ware can be used throughout.

Table 4. The Iodogen method.

1. Thoroughly disperse and suspend Iodogen (1,3,4,6-tetrachloro-3*a*,6*a*-diphenylglycoluril; Pierce Warriner) in 0.5 M sodium phosphate buffer pH 7.4, to a concentration of 1.0 mg/ml using a magnetic stirrer.
2. Place $200-400$ μg of IgG in a reaction vial with 10 μl of 0.5 M phosphate buffer pH 7.4, $37-148$ MBq $(1-4$ mCi) of Na[131]I and 30 μl of Iodogen suspension.
3. Vortex-mix and leave for 20 min.
4. Add 100 μl of 0.5 M phosphate buffer pH 7.4, and transfer into the chromatography column as in *Table 2*.

Table 5. The Bolton–Hunter method.

A. *Iodination of reagent*

To prevent inactivation of labelled SHPP by hydrolysis under the conditions of iodination, steps $2-7$ should be carried out as quickly as possible (~ 30 sec).

1. Place $0.2-0.25$ μg of crystalline SHPP (Sigma) in a sterile glass reaction vial at room temperature.
2. Add 50 μg of Chloramine-T in $10-20$ μl of 0.25 M sodium phosphate buffer pH 7.5 (made up immediately before use).
3. Add $37-148$ MBq $(1-4$ mCi) of Na[131]I.
4. Immediately add 120 μg sodium metabisulphite (120 μg per 10 μl of 0.05 M phosphate buffer pH 7.5) to stop the reaction.
5. Add 200 μg of KI as a carrier (200 μg per 10 μl of 0.05 M phosphate buffer pH 7.5).
6. Add 5 μl dimethyl formamide (DMF).
7. Extract into 2 vols of benzene (reagent grade), each 0.25 ml.

B. *Labelling of antibody*

1. Evaporate the benzene–DMF (containing 0.2 μg of ^{131}I-labelled SHPP) to dryness under a stream of dry nitrogen, taking precautions to trap any volatile radioactive material.
2. Cool the vial to 0°C.
3. Add $200-400$ μg of IgG in 10 μl of 0.1 M borate buffer pH 8.5.
4. Agitate the vial gently and allow the reaction to proceed for 15 min.
5. Add glycine (0.5 ml of a 0.2 M solution in 0.1 M borate buffer pH 8.5) to destroy any unreacted ester and agitate the mixture for 5 min.
6. Collect the labelled antibody by gel filtration on a Sephadex G50 (fine) column (Pharmacia) eluted with 0.05 M phosphate buffer pH 7.5, containing 0.25% (w/v) gelatin.

4.2.4 *The Bolton–Hunter method*

This is a technique in which a highly reactive compound, the 'Bolton–Hunter reagent' [succinimidyl 3-(*p*-hydroxyphenyl)propionate (SHPP)] is labelled with radioiodine by one of the above methods and separated from the iodination mixture before being allowed to react with the antibody (32). The second stage takes place under relatively mild conditions so that contact with potentially damaging oxidizing and reducing agents or high concentrations of radioactive iodine is avoided. The reagent may be purchased from Amersham International labelled with ^{125}I ready for reaction with antibody. For ^{131}I-labelling it is necessary to describe both stages (*Table 5*): SHPP may be iodinated with ^{131}I using the Chloramine-T method and the reaction terminated by adding a reducing agent to the reaction vial since no antibody is present at this stage.

4.3 **Radiolabelling of antibodies using indium**

4.3.1 *Conjugation methods with diethylene-triamine-pentaacetic acid (DTPA) for radiolabelling with metal ions*

A two-stage procedure is necessary to link metal ions to protein; first the covalent linkage (conjugation) of a chelating agent (DTPA) to the protein and then the addition of the metal ions. Alternatives to DTPA have been used but none has shown a particular advantage.

(i) *The mixed anhydride method.* In 1977 DTPA was linked to albumin and it was shown that, after labelling with ^{113m}In, it had a similar blood clearance to that of ^{125}I-labelled albumin (33). A mixed anhydride derivative of DTPA was then synthesized and reacted with the lysine amine groups on the protein molecule.

(ii) *The activated ester method.* This was devised in 1984 (34). The reactive derivative of DTPA is a mixed ester with *N*-hydroxysuccinimide, formed by heating with dicyclohexylcarbodiimide.

This method had several advantages over the mixed anhydride method. There were no long laboratory syntheses required, the labelling procedure being achieved in a matter of days rather than weeks. Drawbacks were that the requirement of carbodiimide and high concentrations of organic solvents in the protein-labelling mixture could result in precipitation of the antibody, and the mixed ester is extremely sensitive to hydrolysis, labelling efficiencies being low in comparison with the cyclic anhydride method.

(iii) *The cyclic anhydride method.* This method was first described for labelling albumin. The cyclic anhydride is synthesized from DTPA by refluxing with acetic anhydride (35). Its conjugation to antibody is described in *Table 7*. The advantages of labelling antibodies with this derivative are shown in *Table 7*.

4.3.2 *Indium-111 radiolabelling of DPTA-conjugated antibody*

(i) *Method.*

1. Add 2.5 M acetate buffer, pH 6.0, metal-free, (10% final volume) and $37-148$ MBq $(1-4$ mCi) of ^{111}In to a sterile reaction vial and mix well.
2. Add $200-400$ μg of DTPA-conjugated antibody (*Table 6*).
3. Mix the vial contents and incubate for at least 30 min.
4. Prepare a PD10 gel filtration column (*Table 2*, step 1).
5. Apply 1 ml of HSA (10%, w/v) to the column followed by a further 10 ml of sterile saline.
6. Apply the reaction mixture to the column.
7. Add 1 ml of sterile saline followed by a further 4 ml.
8. Collect the 5 ml eluate into a sterile centrifuge tube containing 1 ml of HSA.
9. Calculate the labelling efficiency (Section 4.4).
10. Centrifuge the radiolabelled antibody for 16 h at 20 000 *g* to sediment immune complexes.
11. Filter the antibody through a 0.2 micron filter into a sterile ampoule.

Table 6. Conjugation of antibody to the cyclic anhydride of DTPA.

A. Preparation of buffers

Metal ion contamination is reduced to a minimum by metal ion extraction with diphenylthiocarbazine (dithizone; Sigma) as follows. Concentrated buffers should be extracted then diluted.

1. Dissolve 40 mg of dithizone in 20 ml of chloroform (Fisons AR).
2. Place 100−200 ml of the buffer to be extracted, made up in pyrogen-free water (Section 4.1.1), in a 500 ml separating funnel.
3. Add 2 ml dithizone−chloroform.
4. Shake the funnel vigorously for 1 min.
5. Allow the dithizone−chloroform layer to separate. Its colour changes from green/blue to orange/red in the presence of metal ions but this may be masked by excess dithizone.
6. Remove the lower layer.
7. Repeat steps 3−6 until no colour change occurs.
8. Repeat steps 3−6 using 2 ml of chloroform only to extract dithizone.
9. Boil the buffer for 5 min to evaporate any remaining chloroform.
10. Store buffers in sterile 20 ml Universal containers at −20°C.

This method works poorly at low pH and so should precede correction of sodium acetate buffer to pH 6 (with metal-free HCl) for its use in the assessment of conjugation ratio as in C.

B. Antibody conjugation to DTPA

1. Dialyse 1 ml of antibody solution (10 mg/ml) extensively against 0.05 M sodium bicarbonate buffer, pH 8.5 before dithizone extraction.
2. Transfer the solution to a sterile reaction vial.
3. Add DTPA anhydride (mol. wt 357; D6148, Sigma) in dry dimethyl sulphoxide[a] (DMSO) (at a concentration of 10 mg/ml) to antibody in a 5:1 molar ratio and mix immediately.
4. Incubate the mixture for at least 15 min at room temperature.
5. Assess the conjugation ratio (see C).
6. Separate the antibody−DTPA conjugate from free DTPA by gel chromatography (see D).

C. Assessment of conjugation ratio

After incubation of antigen and DTPA (see step B4), 20 μl of the reaction mixture is trace-labelled with ^{65}Zn as follows.

1. Add 2 μl of ^{65}Zn to 2 μl of 2.5 M sodium acetate buffer pH 6.
2. Add a 20 μl aliquot of the reaction mixture to the vial.
3. Mix the vial contents and incubate for at least 15 min at room temperature.
4. Equilibrate a sterile disposable 10 ml Sephadex G25 column (PD10, Pharmacia) with 30 ml of 0.25 M sodium acetate buffer pH 6, and 1 ml HSA.
5. Apply the trace-labelled aliquot to the column and elute with the 0.25 M acetate buffer.
6. Collect ~20 fractions, each of 0.5 ml. Antibody-conjugated DTPA elutes in the void volume while free DTPA is retarded and elutes with a peak at fraction 12.
7. Count the radioactivity in each fraction and calculate the percentage of the total counts in the first peak.
8. The molar conjugation ratio can now be calculated.

D. Preparative gel chromatography of DTPA−antibody conjugation mixture

1. Prepare three PD10 columns as in C.
2. Divide the reaction mixture into three aliquots (333 μl each).
3. Apply each aliquot to a PD10 column and elute with 0.25 M acetate buffer pH 6.
4. Collect 10 fractions, each of 0.5 ml. Antibody elutes in fractions 6−8.
5. Pool fractions 6−8 from each column (three identical pools).
6. Trace-label an aliquot from each pool as in C to demonstrate freedom from free DTPA.

[a]Dry DMSO is produced by placing a dry molecular sieve (3A, BDH) in DMSO for 48 h.

Table 7. Advantages of the cyclic anhydride method for ^{111}In-labelling of antibodies.

1.	The cyclic anhydride is quite stable towards hydrolysis and may be stored for several months if kept anhydrous below 0°C, whereas the mixed anhydride deteriorates rapidly.
2.	The cyclic anhydride gives a much better labelling efficiency than the mixed anhydride (up to 70% compared with 0.3−4%). As a result of this, estimation of the number of DTPAs linked to an antibody becomes much more accurate.
3.	There is no complex organic chemistry required to synthesize the compound, which is marketed cheaply by Sigma and is ready for use.
4.	It is possible to conjugate the protein, remove free DTPA and label with metal ions in a matter of hours (compared with the weeks required by the mixed anhydride method).
5.	The absence of organic solvents in the protein/anhydride reaction mixture results in less damage to the antibody.
6.	Only minute quantities of the cyclic anhydride are needed to label quite large batches of protein. This allows the removal of non-conjugated DTPA from the antibody preparation on small columns, reducing contamination with metal ions.

4.4 Labelling ratios

After a labelling procedure ideally every antibody molecule should be radiolabelled but damage increases with the number of atoms added, both at the time of labelling and subsequently during storage. It has been shown that for iodine labelling more than one atom per protein molecule causes progressive damage (36). Since ^{131}I has, at best, an abundance of less than 20% when supplied, only one in five molecules will be labelled with an active atom. There is no need to label to higher specific activities unless the amount of target antigen is limited.

There has been considerable discussion about labelling carbohydrate side chains which would limit damage to the antibody binding site. This is particularly relevant when conjugating with chelates prior to metal labelling. However, since little damage to the antibody molecule is demonstrable with the cyclic anhydride technique, novel methods could at best have a small advantage.

4.4.1 *Calculation of radiolabelling efficiency*

Counts per minute are measured using an aliquot of the labelled antibody solution and a known amount of the radioisotope used for labelling and these values are used to calculate the labelling efficiency as follows.

Measure the background (bg) radioactivity, that of an aliquot of the total volume V_{ab} of the labelled antibody (Eluate) and that of an aliquot of a diluted sample of the isotope used for labelling (Standard), letting V_{is} equal the total volume added to antibody originally. The percentage labelling efficiency can then be calculated as

$$\frac{(\text{Eluate} - \text{bg}) \times (V_{ab}/\text{volume of aliquot})}{(\text{Standard} - \text{bg}) \times (\text{dilution factor}) \times (V_{is}/\text{volume of sample})} \times 100$$

Values of 80−90% can be achieved using standard methods.

4.5 Assessment of radiolabelled antibody *in vitro*

The immunoreactivity of the labelled antibody with a preparation of pure antigen can be assessed by an immunoradiometric assay (Chapter 3). Wells on a microtitre plate are sensitized with either antigen or control buffer. Serial dilutions of radiolabelled antibody are added to all wells and specific interaction of antibody with antigen assessed by the difference between the number of counts bound by the antigen-coated wells and those bound by the control wells.

5. SCANNING PROCEDURES FOR TUMOUR IMMUNODETECTION

5.1 **Patient preparation**

Uptake of radioactive antibody by the thyroid and stomach is blocked by giving 420 mg of KI and 400 mg of potassium perchlorate ($KClO_3$) 30 min before the ^{131}I-labelled antibody (37); followed by 120 mg of KI and 200 mg of $KClO_3$ every 6 h for 2 days. After the second scan only the KI is continued at 120 mg every 8 h (14).

Prior to injecting the labelled antibody a small amount is given i.v. to test for hypersensitivity and, provided there is no reaction, the remainder is given slowly. The documented side effects are remarkably few. An antibody-mediated response to injected antibody is possible. Pre-existing host antibodies specific for the heterologous injected immunoglobulin are unlikely except when repeat scans are performed (38). The quantity of injected antibody is small, less than 500 μg in most RAID studies if given i.v., and there have been no reports of severe immediate or delayed reactions after RAID. Much larger doses of antibody, up to 500 mg (39), have been administered repeatedly for passive serotherapy of cancer and reported toxicity has been minimal with low doses or with slow infusion of higher doses. Infusion rates faster than 500 μg per minute have induced dyspnoea. Fever, rigors and arthralgia have been observed occasionally in therapeutic studies and have frequently corresponded to rapid infusion rates, high doses, or the presence of large quantities of circulating antigen. These are likely to relate to immune complex formation and complement activation.

5.2 **Radiation protection**

As for preparation of radiopharmaceuticals, local rules dictate procedures also for their administration. Disposable gloves are worn throughout. The antibody is drawn up in a syringe and air bubbles expelled with care into cotton wool to contain the radioactive aerosol. The syringe is kept under a lead shield apart from during the actual injection after which all materials and gloves used are disposed of as radioactive waste, and workers's hands are monitored. No particular instructions need be issued to the patient for such small doses and there is no need for hospital admission on account of the scan. During the first 24 h post-injection, however, it is wiser for lactating mothers not to breast-feed, and patients with small children should avoid kissing and cuddling them as the effects of radiation are greater in children. For in-patients who may be incontinent, urinary catheterization is recommended to avoid contamination of linen, and nurses should be prepared for this possibility.

5.3 **Timing of scans**

Uptake ratios measured 1−2 weeks after injection may then be at a maximum due to the slower antibody clearance from the tumour compared with normal tissue. This apparent improvement is, however, illusory as count rates are then too low for useful imaging. In practice two scans are usual, at 24 and 48 h after injection. For subtracted

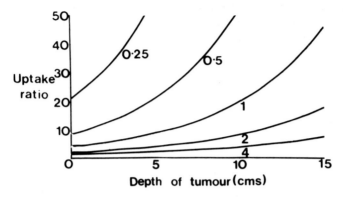

Tumour detection model.

Figure 3. Variation of minimum uptake ratio required for tumour detection with depth of tumour within patient. Contours on tumour area as seen by the γ camera. (Reproduced from ref. 24 with permission.)

scans (see Section 3.2.2) the patient receives 1 mCi ^{99m}Tc-pertechnetate 30 min before, and 1 mCi 5 min before imaging.

6. LIMITATIONS AND PROBLEMS

Overall, antibody uptake by tumours remains poor in spite of considerable research effort. Improvement is essential if RAID is to prove useful. It can be shown by calculations based on count rates, camera properties and tumour depth that substantially higher uptake ratios are required for really useful tumour detection (see *Figure 3* and *Table 1*). The main consideration is whether tumour imaging helps in patient management. There is limited value in locating tumours that cannot be removed or do not respond to therapy. Furthermore, RAID has to compete with other techniques in terms of sensitivity and cost. In the lungs, where density contrast is high, it is unlikely ever to compare favourably in sensitivity with computerized axial tomography (CAT) scanning or conventional radiology. In the abdomen the opposite is true however, and many workers have detected lesions missed by other methods.

One potential advantage of RAID over all other techniques is that highly specific antibodies should determine the tissue type of a known mass.

If the sensitivity of RAID improves sufficiently to detect lesions 0.5 cm in diameter then a variety of tumours could be usefully located. In particular, relatively benign endocrine tumors, such as those of the parathyroid glands, could be located prior to surgical excision. This level of sensitivity would then allow accurate staging of a wide range of tumours prior to surgery or chemotherapy. However, apart from the constraints of isotope and antibody properties on uptake ratios discussed earlier, there are a number of host factors which limit scan sensitivity and these are considered here.

6.1 Antibody access to tumour

Vascular access is essential for delivery of the injected radiolabelled antibody to a tumour. Areas of tumour which are underperfused are therefore less likely to be reliably imaged. A small tumour inevitably receives only a small fraction of the cardiac output and antibody diffuses slowly from the circulation into the extravascular space due to its large molecular size. Maximum uptake of intact IgG occurs 24−48 h after injection. If the tumour vascularity is greater than that of the surrounding tissue then circulating antibody may make a small positive contribution to the scan, similar to the tumour 'blush' effect seen in angiographic studies.

6.2 Circulating antigen

Unbound target antigen within the blood would be expected to be a barrier to successful RAID. Serum taken from a patient with circulating tumour antigen can inhibit antibody binding *in vitro* to tumour cells expressing this antigen (40); thus the presence of circulating antigen may decrease the ability of antibody to achieve tumour penetration *in vivo*. Tumours may, however, be detected even in the presence of high circulating levels of antigen (41). Circulating antigen may provide only a temporary barrier, or tumour localization may be due to the trapping of immune complexes within tumour interstices by tumour macrophages.

6.3 Antigen expression by tumour and normal tissue

Antibodies with absolute specificity for particular tumours have remained elusive and all target antigens used in RAID have been tumour-associated rather than tumour-specific. Thus expression of the target antigen by normal tissue will result in competition for labelled antibody and possible false positive localization. A quantitative difference in antigenic density between target (tumour) tissue and other tissues is a fundamental prerequisite for a favourable uptake ratio, and sufficient readily available tumour target antigen is required to avoid tumour saturation and antibody excess. Antigen saturation would be more likely to occur with monoclonal than polyclonal antibodies as the former recognize only a single epitope per tumour antigen molecule.

Tumour expresson of antigen is often heterogeneous and the expression of antigen by metastases may differ from that of the primary tumour. This also may prevent successful imaging.

6.4 Future prospects

As long as tumour uptake of antibody remains in the region of 0.005% of the injected dose per gram of tissue, radioimmunotherapy cannot be useful. To achieve predictable therapeutic benefit a substantial improvement in uptake ratios is essential, and to obtain tumour killing at least ten times the current values must be achieved. Higher values have been obtained in animals and reputedly in occasional patients but until such improvements are widely reproducible therapeutic studies seem inappropriate.

Improvements in the affinity and retention of the carrying antibody remain the primary aim of any future developments. Although antibodies remain the major subject of these studies other substances of metabolic importance to the cancer cell may later prove to be more successful. Solution of the problem is not necessarily immunological.

Animal and cell culture studies will continue to be helpful in selecting suitable antibodies whilst human scanning and tissue studies are essential for proper evaluation. Data collected by these methods will give clear indications of the value of potential reagents and whether therapeutic studies should follow. Overall, it is hoped that improved antibody localization will change a promising technique into one that is undeniably useful.

7. ACKNOWLEDGEMENTS

We are grateful to Dr D.B.Ramsden, for information and helpful comments and to Dr A.A.Keeling, Dr C.Chapman and Dr D.S.Fairweather whose PhD theses have contributed to this chapter.

8. REFERENCES

1. Hericourt,J. and Richet,C. (1895) *C.R. Acad. Sci.*, **120**, 948.
2. Hericourt,J. and Richet,C. (1895) *C.R. Acad. Sci.*, **121**, 567.
3. Pressman,D. (1949) *Cancer*, **2**, 697.
4. Pressman,D. and Korngold,L. (1953) *Cancer*, **6**, 619.
5. Pressman,D., Day,E.D. and Blau,M. (1957) *Cancer Res.*, **17**, 845.
6. Pressman,D. (1980) *Cancer Res.*, **40**, 2960.
7. Spar,I.L., Bale,W.F., Marrack,D., Dewey,W.C., McCardle,R.J. and Harper,P.V. (1967) *Cancer*, **20**, 865.
8. Goldenberg,D.M., DeLand,F.H., Kim,E., Bennett,S., Primus,F.J., van Nagell,J.R., Estes,N., DeSimone,P. and Rayburn,P. (1978) *N. Engl. J. Med.*, **298**, 1384.
9. Dykes,P.W., Hine,K.R., Bradwell,A.R., Blackburn,J.C., Reeder,T.A., Drolc,Z. and Booth,S.N. (1980) *Br. Med. J.*, **280**, 220.
10. Mach,J.-P., Carrel,S., Forni,M., Ritschard,J., Donath,A. and Alberto,P. (1980) *N. Engl. J. Med.*, **303**, 5.
11. Goldenberg,D.M., Kim,E.E., Deland,F.H., Van Nagell,J.R. and Javadpour,N. (1980) *Science*, **208**, 1284.
12. Halsall,A.K., Fairweather,D.S., Bradwell,A.R., Blackburn,J.C., Dykes,P.W., Howell,A., Reeder,A. and Hine,K.R. (1981) *Br. Med. J.*, **283**, 942.
13. Johnstone,A. and Thorpe,R. (1982) In *Immunochemistry in Practice*. Blackwell Scientific Publications, Oxford, p. 210.
14. Fairweather,D.S., Bradwell,A.R., Watson-James,S.F., Dykes,P.W., Chandler,S. and Hoffenberg,R. (1983) *Clin. Endocrinol.*, **18**, 563.
15. Larson,S.M. (1985) *J. Nucl. Med.*, **26**, 538.
16. Ballou,B., Reilznd,J.M., Levine,G., Taylor,R.J., Shen,W.-C., Ryser,H., Solter,D. and Hakala,T.R. (1986) *J. Surg. Oncol.*, **31**, 1.
17. Keeling,A.A., Bradwell,A.R., Fairweather,D.S., Dykes,P.W. and Vaughan,A. (1984) *Prot. Biol. Fluids*, **32**, 455.
18. Buraggi,G.L., Callegaro,L., Mariani,G., Turrin,A., Cascinelli,N., Attili,A., Bombardieri,E., Terno,G., Plassio,G., Dovis,M., Mazzuca,N., Natali,P.G., Scasselati,G.A., Rosa,U. and Ferrone,S. (1985) *Cancer Res.*, **45**, 3378.
19. Buchegger,F., Haskell,C.M., Shreyer,M., Scazziga,B.R., Randin,S., Carrel,S. and Mach,J.-P. (1983) *J. Exp. Med.*, **158**, 413.
20. Mach,J.-P., Chatal,J.-F., Lumbroso,J.-D., Buchegger,F., Ritschard,J., Berche,C., Douillard,J.-Y., Carrel,S., Herlyn,M., Steplewski,Z. and Korpowski,H. (1983) *Cancer Res.*, **43**, 5593.
21. Deland,F.H. and Goldenberg,D.M. (1985) *Semin. Nucl. Med.*, **15**, No. 1, p. 2.
22. Goodwin,D., Meares,C., Diamanti,C., McCall,M., Lai,C., Torti,F., McTigue,M. and Martin,B. (1984) *Eur. J. Nucl. Med.*, **9**(5), 209.
23. Bradwell,A.R., Fairweather,D.S., Keeling,A., Watson-James,S., Vaughan,A. and Dykes,P.W. (1983) *Clin. Sci.*, **65**, 31p.
24. Bradwell,A.R., Fairweather,D.S., Dykes,P.W., Keeling,A.A., Vaughan,A. and Taylor,J. (1985) *Immunol. Today*, **6**, 163.
25. Epenetos,A.A., Mather,S., Granowska,M., Nimmon,C.C., Hawkins,L.R., Britton,K.E., Shepherd,J., Taylor-Papadimitriou,J., Durbin,H., Malpas,J.S. and Bodmer,W.T. (1982) *Lancet*, **2**, 999.
26. Fairweather,D.S., Irwin,M., Bradwell,A.R., Dykes,P.W. and Flinn,R.M. (1983) *Prot. Biol. Fluids*, **31**, 285.
27. European pharmacopoeia (1971) **3**, 58.
28. *The Ionising Radiations Regulations* (1985) HMSO.
29. Edwards,R., Lalloz,M. and Pull,P.I. (1983) In *Immunoassays for Clinical Chemistry*. Hunter,W.M. and Corrie,J.E.T. (eds) Churchill Livingstone, 2nd edn, p. 277.
30. McConahey,P.J. and Dixon,F.J. (1980) In *Methods in Enzymology*, Volume 70. Colowick,S.P. and Kaplan,N.O. (eds), Academic Press, New York, p. 210.
31. David,G.S. and Reisfeld,R.A. (1974) *Biochemistry*, **13**, 1014.
32. Bolton,A.E. and Hunter,W.M. (1973) *Biochem. J.*, **133**, 529.

33. Krejcarek,G.E. and Tucker,K.L. (1977) *Biochem. Biophys. Res. Commun.*, **77**, 581.
34. Buckley,R.G. and Searle,F. (1984) *FEBS Lett.*, **166**, 202.
35. Hnatowich,D.J., Layne,W.W., Childs,R.L., Lanteigne,D., Davis,M.A., Griffin,T.W. and Doherty, P.W. (1983) *Science*, **220**, 613.
36. Greenwood,F.C., Hunter,W.M. and Glover,J.S. (1963) *Biochem. J.*, **89**, 114.
37. Bradwell,A.R., Dykes,P.W. and Fairweather,D.S. (1983) *J. Nucl. Med.*, **24**, 1081.
38. Goodman,G.E., Beaumier,P., Hellstrom,I., Fernyhough,B. and Hellstrom,K.E. (1985) *J. Clin. Oncol.*, **3**, No. 3, 340.
39. Houghton,A.N. and Scheinberg,D.A. (1986) *Semin. Oncol.*, **13**, 165.
40. Nadler,L.M., Stashenko,P., Hardy,R., Kaplan,W.D., Button,L.N., Kufe,D.W., Antman,K.H. and Schlossman,S.F. (1980) *Cancer Res.*, **40**, 3147.
41. Goldenberg,D.M., Kim,E., Deland,F.H., Spremulli,E., Nelson,M.O., Cockerman,J.P., Primus,F.J., Corgan,R.L. and Alpert,E. (1980) *Cancer*, **45**, 2500.
42. Dykes,P.W., Bradwell,A.R., Chapman,C.E. and Vaughan,A.T.M. (1987) *Cancer Treatment Rev.*, **14**, 87.
43. Fairweather,D.S., Bradwell,A.R., Dykes,P.W., Vaughan,A.T.M., Watson-James,S.F. and Chandler,S. (1983) *Br. Med. J.*, **287**, 167.

9. APPENDIX: REFERENCES FOR TABLE 1.

1. Goldenberg,D.M., DeLand,F.H., Kim,E., Bennett,S., Primus,F.J., van Nagell,J.R., Estes,N., DeSimone,P. and Rayburn,P. (1978) *N. Engl. J. Med.*, **298**, 1384.
2. Goldenberg,D.M., Kim,E.E., DeLand,F.H., van Nagell,J.R. and Javadpour,N. (1980) *Science*, **208**, 1284.
3. Ghose,T., Norvell,S.T., Alquino,J., Belitsky,P., Tai,J., Guclu,A. and Blair,A.H. (1980) *Cancer Res.*, **40**, 3018.
4. Dykes,P.W., Hine,K.R., Bradwell,A.R., Blackburn,J.C., Reeder,T.A., Drolc,Z. and Booth,S.N. (1980) *Br. Med. J.*, **280**, 220.
5. Mach,J.-P., Cartrel,S., Forni,M., Ritschard,J., Donath,A. and Alberto,P. (1980) *N. Engl. J. Med.*, **303**, 5.
6. Mach,J.-P., Buchegger,F., Forni,M., Ritschard,J., Berche,C., Lumbroso,J.-D., Schreyer,M.,Giardet,C., Accolla,R.S. and Carrel,S. (1981) *Immunol. Today*, **2**, 239.
7. Farrands,P.A., Perkins,A.C., Pimm,M.V., Hardy,J.D., Embleton,M.J., Baldwin,R.W. and Hardcastle,J.D. (1982) *Lancet*, **2**, 397.
8. Ishii,N., Nakata,K., Munehisa,T., Koji,T., Nishi,S. and Hirai,H. (1984) *Proc. Biol. Fluids*, **31**, 305.
9. Mach,J.-P., Chatal,J.F., Lumbroso,J.D., Buchegger,F., Forni,M., Ritschard,J., Berche,C., Douillard,J.-Y., Carrel,S., Herlyn,M., Steplewski,Z. and Koprowski,H. (1983) *Cancer Res.*, **43**, 5593.
10. Larson,S.M., Brown,J.P., Wright,P.W., Carrasquillo,J.A., Hellstrom,I. and Hellstrom,K.E. (1983) *J. Nucl. Med.*, **24**, 123.
11. Rainsbury,R.M., Ott,R.J., Westwood,J.H., Kalirai,T.S., Coombes,R.C., McCready,V.R., Neville,A.M. and Gazet,J.-C. (1983) *Lancet*, **2**, 934.
12. Armitage,N.C., Perkins,A.C., Pimm,M.V., Farrands,P.A., Baldwin,R.W. and Hardcastle,J.D. (1984) *Br. J. Surg.*, **71**, 407.
13. Chatal,J.F., Saccavini,J.C., Fumoleau,P., Douillard,J.-Y., Curtet,C., Kremer,M., LeMevel,B.Q. and Koprowski,H. (1984) *J. Nucl. Med.*, **25**, 307.
14. Thompson,C.H., Lichtenstein,M., Stacker,S.A., Leyden,M.J., Salehi,N., Andrews,J.T. and McKenzie,I.F.C. (1984) *Lancet*, **2**, 1245.
15. Buraggi,G.L., Callegaro,L., Marianai,G., Turrin,A., Cascinelli,N., Attili,A., Bombardieri,E., Terno,G., Plassio,G., Dovis,M., Mazzuca,N., Natali,P.G., Scassallati,G.A., Rosa,U. and Ferroni,S. (1985) *Cancer Res.*, **45**, 3378.
16. Epenetos,A.A., Snook,D., Durban,H., Johnson,P.M. and Taylor-Papadimitriou,J. (1986) *Cancer Res.*, **46**, 3183.
17. Epenetos,A.A., Carr,D., Johnson,P.M., Bodmer,W.F. and Lavender,J.P. (1986) *Br. J. Radiol.*, **59**, 117.
18. Armitage,N.C., Perkins,A.C., Pimm,M.V., Wastie,M., Hopkins,J.J., Dowling,F., Baldwin,R.W. and Hardcastle,J.D. (1986) *Cancer*, **58**, 37.

APPENDIX

Suppliers of specialist items

SUPPLIERS OF EQUIPMENT

The NIH microcytotoxicity test

Microwell (Terasaki) trays
BD Diagnostics (Falcon): *Between Towns Road, Cowley, Oxford OX4 3LY, UK*
Dynatech Laboratories Ltd (Greiner): *Daux Road, Billingshurst, West Sussex RH14 GSJ, UK*
Gibco Ltd (Nunc): *Trident House, Renfrew Road, Paisley PA3 4EF, UK*
Nycomed (UK) Ltd (Robbins): *211 Coventry Road, Sheldon, Birmingham B26 3EA, UK*
Sterilin Ltd (Sterilin): *Clockhouse Lane, Feltham, Middlesex TW14 8QS, UK*

Syringes and repeating dispensers
VA Howe Ltd (Hamilton): *12 – 14 St Annes Crescent, London SW18 2LS, UK*
Nycomed (UK) Ltd (Robbins)

Reagent stream splitters
Saxon Micro Ltd (One lambda): *PO Box 28, Newmarket, Suffolk CB8 8N7, UK*
Nycomed (UK) Ltd (Robbins)

Microcentrifuges
Scientific Instruments (Microcentaur MSE): *Sussex Manor Park, Gatwick Road, Crawley, Sussex RH10 2QQ*
Beckman-R116 (Microfuge): *Progress Road, Sands Industrial Estate, High Wycombe, Bucks HP12 4JL, UK*

Microwell tray oilers
Dynatech Laboratories Ltd (Greiner)
Nycomed (UK) Ltd (Robbins)

Microwell automatic serum dispensers
Biotest (UK) Ltd (Bio Tec): *Unit 21A, Monks Path Business Park, Stratford Road, Solihull, West Midlands B90 4NY, UK*
Dynatech Laboratories Ltd (Greiner)
Saxon Micro Ltd (Lambda Dot)

Microwell tray cell dispensers
Saxon Micro Ltd (Lambda Jet)

Spark generator
Saxon Micro Ltd (Lambda Zapper)

Automatic fluorescence readers
Astromed Ltd (Astroscan): *Innovation Centre, Science Park, Milton Road, Cambridge CB4 4GS, UK*
E.Leitz (Instruments) Ltd (Leitz MPV-MT): *48 Park Street, Luton LU1 3HP, UK*
Saxon Micro Ltd (Orac)
Carl Zeiss (Oberkochen) Ltd (Zeiss IM 35): *PO Box 78, Woodfield Road, Welwyn Garden City, Herts AL7 1LU, UK*

Programmable cell freezers
Cryoson (Ireland) Ltd (Cryoson): *PO Box 20, Bantry, Co. Cork, Ireland*
Planar Products (Planar): *110 Windmill Road, Sunbury-on-Thames, Middlesex TW16 7HD, UK*

HLA typing

Cell Washers
G.S.Ross Ltd, *Macclesfield, Cheshire, UK*
Ortho Diagnostic Systems Ltd, *High Wycombe, Bucks, UK*

Rabiolabelled assays

Hand gamma counters
Mini-instruments Ltd (Type 5.40. Serial No. 11798): *8 Station Industrial Estate, Burnham-on-Crouch, Essex CMO 8RN, UK*

Automated gamma counters
Nuclear Enterprises Ltd, *Bath Road, Beenham, Reading RG7 5PR, UK*
Pharmacia LKB Ltd, *Pharmacia House, Midsummer Boulevard, Milton Keynes MK9 3YY, UK*

Automated beta counters
Nuclear Enterprises Ltd
Pharmacia LKB Ltd

Refrigerated centrifuges (up to 10 000 r.p.m.)
Scientific Instruments (MSE)/Beckman/S.A.Jouan, *130 Western Road, Tring, Herts HP2 4BU, UK*

ELISA

Cuvettes
Corning Medical and Scientific Ltd, *Halstead, Essex CO9 2DX, UK*
(i) *Manual equipment*
  Gilford EIA manual reader for cuvettes 1414 × 13
(ii) *Automated equipment*
  Automatic pipettes/diluter/EIA printer with manual reader forms a manual system 1430 × 13
  PR-50 Processor/reader—automates coating, washing etc. with printout functions—1414 × 4

Nitrocellulose membrane—Hybond C

Amersham International plc, *Lincoln Place, Green End, Aylesbury, Bucks HP29 2TP, UK*

Plates

Dynatech Laboratories Ltd (Microelisa plates)

Dynatech Laboratories Inc. (Microelisa plates): *900 Slaters Lane, Alexandria, VA 22314, USA*

Flow Laboratories Ltd (PVC immunoassay microplates): *Woodcock Hill, Harefield Road, Rickmansworth, Herts WD3 1PQ, UK*

Gibco Europe Ltd (Nunc-Elisa plates): *Unit 4, Cowley Mill Trading Estate, Longbridge Way, Uxbridge UB8 27G, UK*

Readers—Plates

Available from Dynatech Laboratories Ltd

(i) *Manual equipment*

Accudrop ELISA reagent dispenser (AM58)

Microwash or Miniwash plate washers (AM50 or AM52)

Microelisa mini reader (MR590) or Mini-Elisa reader (AM114)

Shaker—Incubator for ELISA microplates (AM89)

(ii) *Automated equipment*

Dynadrop ELISA reagent dispenser (AM83)

Dynawasher (AM71)

Automatic ELISA reader AM120 or Microelisa auto reader (MR580)

Available from Flow Laboratories Ltd

(i) *Automated equipment*

Titertek autodrop 78-510-00

Titertek Multistopper 25/50 automated dispenser 77-940-00

Titertek microplate washer 78-430-00

Titertek Multiscan MC reader 78-530-00

(also automatic diluter, multi-diluter and multi-wash accessories)

(ii) *Automated equipment for strips*

Titertek miniscan reader 78-550-00 (about one-third the price of automated plate readers).

Pipettes

Alpha Laboratories/Eppendorf GmbH (Eppendorf micropipettes and tips): *169 Old Field Lane, Greenford, Essex UB6 8PW, UK*

V.A.Howe and Co. Ltd/Hamilton Bonaduz Ag (Microlitre syringes): *88 Peterborough Road, London SW6, UK*

Oxford Laboratories/Boehringer Corporation (Micropipettes and tips): *Bell Lane, Lewes, East Sussex BN7 1LG, UK*

Available from Flow Laboratories Ltd

Multichannel pipettes (4, 8 or 12 channel, $5-200$ μl or $5-50$ μl or $50-200$ μl variable volume)

Fixed volume and variable micropipettes and disposable tips
Plate sealers 77-400-05

Immunoperoxidase methods

Cryostats
E.Leitz (Instruments) Ltd, *48 Park Street, Luton, Beds LU1 3HP, UK*

Glass slides
Chance Propper Ltd, *PO Box 53, Spon Lane South, Smethwick, West Midlands B66 1NZ, UK*

Rockers
Denley Instruments Ltd, *Natts Lane, Billingshurst, Sussex RH14 9EY, UK*

Analytical pipettes
Anachem Ltd, *Anachem House, 20 Charles Street, Luton, Beds LU2 0EB, UK*

Disposable tips
Boehringer Corp. (London) Ltd, *BCL, Bell Lane, Lewes, East Sussex BN7 1LG, UK*

Disposable tubes
Starstedt Ltd, *68 Boston Road, Beaumont Leys, Leicester LE4 1AW, UK*

Immunofluorescence

Multispot slides
C.A.Hendley Ltd, *Oakwood Hill Industrial Estate, Elstree, UK*

Tissue freezers
South London Electrical Equipment Co. Ltd, *Lanier Works, Hither Green Lane, London, UK*

Cryostats
Bright Equipment Co. Ltd, *Clifton Road, Huntingdon, Cambridgeshire, UK*

Fluorescent microscopes
Zeiss, *PO Box 78, Woodfield Road, Welwyn Garden City, Herts AL7 1LU, UK*
E.Leitz, *48 Park Street, Luton, Beds LU1 3HP, UK*

Cytocentrifuges
Shandon Southern Products, *Chadwick Road, Astmoor, Runcorn, Cheshire, UK*

SUPPLIERS OF REAGENTS

HLA typing

The NIH microcytotoxicity test

Ready-made density centrifugation media
Flow Laboratories Ltd (Lymphocyte separation medium): *Woodcock Hill, Rickmansworth, Herts WD3 1PQ, UK*
Nycomed (UK) Ltd (Lymphoprep®): *211 Coventry Road, Sheldon, Birmingham B26 3EA, UK*

Pharmacia Diagnostics Ltd (Ficoll-Paque®): *Pharmacia House, Midsummer Boulevard, Milton Keynes, Bucks MK9 3HP, UK*
Sigma−Aldrich (Histopaque®): *The Old Brick Yard, New Road, Gillingham, Dorset SP8 4JL, UK*

Density media components
Nycomed (UK) Ltd (Isopaque®)
Pharmacia Diagnostics Ltd (Ficoll 400 and Percoll®)

Cell separation reagents
Biotest (UK) Ltd (Sepracell®): *Unit 21A, Monks Park Business Park, Stratford Road, Solihull, West Midlands, B90 4NY, UK*
Dynal (UK) Ltd (Dynabeads®): *26 Grove Street, New Ferry, Wirral L62 5AZ, UK*
Fenwal Travenol Ltd (Nylon wool): *Telford, Norfolk, UK*
Saxon Micro Ltd (Lymphoqwik®): *PO Box 28, Newmarket, Suffolk CB8 8N7, UK*

Typing reagents
The serum catalogues list individual sera and ready-made comprehensive typing trays
Behring Hoescht (UK) Ltd, *50 Salisbury Road, Hounslow, Middlesex TW4 6JH, UK*
Biotest (UK) Ltd
Merieux, Institut Merieux, *17 rue Bourgelat, 69002 Lyon, France*
Pel Freeze, *9099 N.Deerbrook Trail, Brown Deer, WI 53223, USA*
Saxon Micro Ltd (One Lambda)

Rabbit complement
Biotest (UK) Ltd
Behring Hoescht (UK) Ltd
Buxted Rabbit Co. Ltd, *Great Totease Farm, Buxted, Sussex TW22 4LR, UK*
North East Biomedical Laboratory: *PO Box 45, Uxbridge, Middlesex UB9 5QD, UK*
Saxon Micro Ltd
Sera Laboratory Ltd, *Crawley Down, Sussex RH10 4FF, UK*

Blood grouping reagents
Alpha Laboratories Ltd
Blood Products Laboratory (Diagnostics), *Oxford, UK*
Biotest (UK) Ltd
Lorne Laboratories Ltd, *Twyford, Berks, UK*

Radiolabelled assays

Hormones
New England Nuclear, DuPont (UK) Ltd, *Biotechnology Systems Division, NEN Research Products, Wedgewood Way, Stevenage, Herts SG1 4QN, UK*
Weddel Pharmaceuticals Ltd, *Union International Research Centre, Old London Street, St Albans, Herts, UK*
Steraloids Ltd, *31 Radcliffe Road, Croydon CRO 5QJ, UK*

Appendix

Immunoperoxidase methods

Antisera

Bio-Nuclear Services Ltd, *24 Westleigh Drive, Sonning Common, Reading RG4 9LB, UK*

Biotest (UK) Ltd, *Unit 21A, Monkspath Business Park, Highlands Road, Shirley, Solihull, West Midlands B90 4NZ, UK*

DAKO Ltd, *22 The Arcade, The Octagon, High Wycombe, Bucks HP11 2HT, UK*

Cryo-M-Bed

Bright Instrument Co. Ltd, *St Margaret's Way, Stukeley Meadows Industrial Estate, Huntingdon, Cambridgeshire PE18 6EB, UK*

FACS

CD4 monoclonal antibody

Becton Dickinson, *Between Towns Road, Cowley, Oxford OX4 3LY, UK*

CD45R (2H4) monoclonal antibody

Coulter Electronics Ltd, *Northwell Drive, Luton, Beds LU3 3RH, UK*

Chicken red blood cells (fixed)

Sigma Chemical Co. Ltd, *Fancy Road, Poole, Dorset, UK*

Fluorescent beads

Flow Cytometry Standards Corp., *PO Box 12621, Research Triangle Park, NC 27709, USA*

Lymphocyte separation medium

Flow Laboratories Ltd, *Woodcock Hill, Rickmansworth, Herts WD3 1PQ, UK*

Immunofluorescence

Teflon spray

Marshall Howlett, *PO Box 39, Betsham Road, Gravesend Kent, UK*

Diazabicyclooctane (DABCO) (Fluorescence fading retardant)

Aldrich Chemicals Co. Ltd, *The Old Brickyard, New Road, Gillingham, Dorset SP8 4JL, UK*

OCT compound

Miles Laboratories Inc., *Naperville, IL 60566, USA*

Antibody radiolabelling

^{131}I, ^{111}In, ^{65}Zn

Amersham International plc, *UK Sales office, Lincoln Place, Green End, Aylesbury, Bucks HP20 2TP, UK*

Column media

Pharmcia LKB Ltd

Molecular sieves

BDH Ltd

250

Iodogen
Pierce & Warriner, *44 Upper Northgate Street, Chester, Cheshire CH1 4EF, UK*

General chemicals
Aldrich Chemical Co. Ltd, *Gillingham, Dorset, UK*
BDH, *Broom Road, Poole, Dorset BH12 4NN, UK*
David Bull Laboratories, *Warwick, UK*
Fisions Scientific Apparatus, *Loughborough, Leicestershire, UK*
Hughes and Hughes Ltd, *Harold Wood, Essex, UK*
Oxoid Ltd, *Wade Road, Basingstoke, Hants RG24 OPW, UK*
Sigma Chemical Co. Ltd

Culture media and animal reagents
Flow Laboratories
Gibco Ltd
Imperial Labs Ltd, *West Portway, Andover, Hampshire SP10 3LF, UK*
Organon-Teknika Ltd, *Science Park, Milton Road, Cambridge CB4 4BH, UK*

Antisera
Miles Laboratory, *PO Box 37, Stoke Poges, Slough SL2 4L7, UK*

SEROLOGICAL RED CELL REFERENCE LABORATORIES IN THE UK

Blood Group Reference Laboratory, *Oxford, UK*
Regional Transfusion Centres

INDEX